Opportunistic Intracellular Bacteria and Immunity

INFECTIOUS AGENTS AND PATHOGENESIS

Series Editors: Mauro Bendinelli, *University of Pisa*
Herman Friedman, *University of South Florida*
College of Medicine

Recent volumes in the series:

DNA TUMOR VIRUSES
Oncogenic Mechanisms
Edited by Giuseppe Barbanti-Brodano, Mauro Bendinelli, and
Herman Friedman

ENTERIC INFECTIONS AND IMMUNITY
Edited by Lois J. Paradise, Mauro Bendinelli, and Herman Friedman

FUNGAL INFECTIONS AND IMMUNE RESPONSES
Edited by Juneann W. Murphy, Herman Friedman, and
Mauro Bendinelli

HERPESVIRUSES AND IMMUNITY
Edited by Peter G. Medveczky, Herman Friedman, and
Mauro Bendinelli

MICROORGANISMS AND AUTOIMMUNE DISEASES
Edited by Herman Friedman, Noel R. Rose, and Mauro Bendinelli

NEUROPATHOGENIC VIRUSES AND IMMUNITY
Edited by Steven Specter, Mauro Bendinelli, and Herman Friedman

OPPORTUNISTIC INTRACELLULAR BACTERIA AND IMMUNITY
Edited by Lois J. Paradise, Herman Friedman, and Mauro Bendinelli

PSEUDOMONAS AERUGINOSA AS AN OPPORTUNISTIC
PATHOGEN
Edited by Mario Campa, Mauro Bendinelli, and Herman Friedman

PULMONARY INFECTIONS AND IMMUNITY
Edited by Herman Chmel, Mauro Bendinelli, and Herman Friedman

RAPID DETECTION OF INFECTIOUS AGENTS
Edited by Steven Specter, Mauro Bendinelli, and Herman Friedman

RICKETTSIAL INFECTION AND IMMUNITY
Edited by Burt Anderson, Herman Friedman, and Mauro Bendinelli

A Continuation Order Plan is available for this series. A continuation order will bring
delivery of each new volume immediately upon publication. Volumes are billed only
upon actual shipment. For further information please contact the publisher.

Opportunistic Intracellular Bacteria and Immunity

Edited by

Lois J. Paradise and
Herman Friedman
University of South Florida College of Medicine
Tampa, Florida

and

Mauro Bendinelli
University of Pisa
Pisa, Italy

Plenum Press • New York and London

Library of Congress Cataloging-in-Publication Data

Opportunistic intracellular bacteria and immunity / edited by Lois J.
Paradise and Herman Friedman and Mauro Bendinelli.
    p.   cm. -- (Infectious agents and pathogenesis)
  Includes bibliographical references and index.
  ISBN 0-306-45894-2
  1. Bacterial diseases. 2. Opportunistic infections.
3. Immunodeficiency. 4. Immunosuppression.   I. Paradise, Lois J.
II. Friedman, Herman, 1931-   . III. Bendinelli, Mauro.
IV. Series.
  [DNLM: 1. Bacterial Infections--immunology. 2. Opportunistic
Infections--immunology. 3. Immunity, Cellular.   WC 200 O619 1998]
QR201.B34O67 1998
616.9'2--dc21
DNLM/DLC
for Library of Congress   98-42016
                                                              CIP

ISBN 0-306-45894-2

© 1999 Plenum Press, New York
A Division of Plenum Publishing Corporation
233 Spring Street, New York, N.Y. 10013

http://www.plenum.com

10 9 8 7 6 5 4 3 2 1

Printed in the United States of America

Contributors

LINDA B. ADAMS • G. W. Long Hansen's Research Center, Laboratory Research Branch, Louisiana State University, Baton Rouge, Louisiana 70803

BURT E. ANDERSON • Department of Medical Microbiology and Immunology, University of South Florida, College of Medicine, Tampa, Florida 33612

CYNTHIA L. BALDWIN • Department of Veterinary and Animal Sciences, Paige Laboratory, University of Massachusetts, Amherst, Massachusetts 01003

ANDREW W. O. BURGESS • Department of Medical Microbiology and Immunology, University of South Florida, College of Medicine, Tampa, Florida 33612

GERALD I. BYRNE • Department of Medical Microbiology and Immunology, University of Wisconsin Medical School, Madison, Wisconsin 53706

FRANK M. COLLINS • Laboratory of Mycobacteria, CBER, FDA, Bethesda, Maryland 20852

PATRICIA A. DARRAH • Department of Microbiology and Immunology, Temple University School of Medicine, Philadelphia, Pennsylvania 19140

ROLIEN DE JONG • Department of Immunohematology and Blood Bank, Leiden University Medical Center, 2333 ZA Leiden, The Netherlands

RENÉ R. P. DE VRIES • Department of Immunohematology and Blood Bank, Leiden University Medical Center, 2333 ZA Leiden, The Netherlands

JON S. FRIEDLAND • Department of Infectious Diseases, Imperial College, Hammersmith Hospital, London, W12 ONN, England

HERMAN FRIEDMAN • Department of Medical Microbiology and Immunology, University of South Florida, College of Medicine, Tampa, Florida 33612

RAFAEL GARDUNO • Department of Microbiology and Immunology, Dalhousie University, Halifax, Nova Scotia B3H 3H7, Canada

DAVID L. HAHN • Arcand Park Clinic, Dean Medical Center, Madison, Wisconsin 53705

ROGELIO HERNANDEZ-PANDO • Department of Pathology, Instituto Nacional de la Nutricion, Salvador Zubrian, Delegacion Tlalpan, 1400 Mexico DF

M. B. HEVIN • Unité d'Immunophysiologie Cellulaire, Institut Pasteur, 75724 Paris-Cedex 15, France

HERBERT HOF • Institute of Medical Microbiology and Hygiene, Faculty of Clinical Medicine Mannheim, University of Heidelberg, Manheim D-68165, Germany

PAUL S. HOFFMAN • Departments of Microbiology, Immunology, and Medicine, Division of Infectious Diseases, Dalhousie University, Halifax, Nova Scotia B3H 3H7, Canada

MARY K. HONDALUS • Howard Hughes Medical Research Institute, Albert Einstein College of Medicine, Bronx, New York 10461

DAVID JOHNSON • Infectious Diseases Section, Department of Veterinary Affairs Medical Center, Bay Pines, Florida 33744

MURAT V. KALAYOGLU • Department of Medical Microbiology and Immunology, University of Wisconsin Medical School, Madison, Wisconsin 53706

THOMAS W. KLEIN • Department of Medical Microbiology and Immunology, University of South Florida, College of Medicine, Tampa, Florida 33612

JAMES L. KRAHENBUHL • G. W. Long Hansen's Research Center, Laboratory Research Branch, Louisiana State University, Baton Rouge, Louisiana 70803

M. LEBASTARD • Unité d'Immunophysiologie Cellulaire, Institut Pasteur, 75724 Paris-Cedex 15, France

DANIELLE MALO • Departments of Medicine and Human Genetics, McGill University, and Centre for the Study of Host Resistance, Montreal General Hospital, Montreal, Quebec H3G 1A4, Canada

G. MILON • Unité d'Immunophysiologie Cellulaire, Institut Pasteur, 75724 Paris-Cedex 15, France

DAVID M. MOSSER • Department of Microbiology and Immunology, Temple University School of Medicine, Philadelphia, Pennsylvania 19140

CHARLES NAUCIEL • Faculté de Médecine de Paris-Ouest, Université Paris 5, 92380 Garches, France

CATHERINE NEWTON • Department of Medical Microbiology and Immunology, University of South Florida, College of Medicine, Tampa, Florida 33612

PETER H. NIBBERING • Department of Infectious Diseases, Leiden University Medical Center, 2333 ZA Leiden, The Netherlands

TOM H. M. OTTENHOFF • Department of Immunohematology and Blood Bank, Leiden University Medical Center, 2333 ZA Leiden, The Netherlands

LOIS J. PARADISE • Department of Medical Microbiology and Immunology, University of South Florida, College of Medicine, Tampa, Florida 33612

SALMAN T. QURESHI • Departments of Medicine and Human Genetics, McGill University, and Centre for the Study of Host Resistance, Montreal General Hospital, Montreal, Quebec H3G 1A4, Canada

GRAHAM A. W. ROOK • Department of Bacteriology, University College London Medical School, London, W1P 6DB, England

R. MARTIN ROOP II • Department of Microbiology and Immunology, Louisiana State University Medical Center, Shreveport, Louisiana 71130-3939

JULIUS SCHACHTER • Department of Laboratory Medicine, University of California, San Francisco, San Francisco, California 94110

EMIL SKAMENE • Departments of Medicine and Human Genetics, McGill University, and Centre for the Study of Host Resistance, Montreal General Hospital, Montreal, Quebec H3G 1A4, Canada

ERIC SPIERINGS • Department of Immunohematology and Blood Bank, Leiden University Medical Center, 2333 ZA Leiden, The Netherlands

YOSHIMASA YAMAMOTO • Department of Medical Microbiology and Immunology, University of South Florida, College of Medicine, Tampa, Florida 33612

Preface to the Series

The mechanisms of disease production by infectious agents are presently the focus of an unprecedented flowering of studies. The field has undoubtedly received impetus from the considerable advances recently made in the understanding of the structure, biochemistry, and biology of viruses, bacteria, fungi, and other parasites. Another contributing factor is our improved knowledge of immune responses and other adaptive or constitutive mechanisms by which hosts react to infection. Furthermore, recombinant DNA technology, monoclonal antibodies, and other newer methodologies have provided the technical tools for examining questions previously considered too complex to be successfully tackled. The most important incentive of all is probably the regenerated idea that infection might be the initiating event in many clinical entities presently classified as idiopathic or of uncertain origin.

Infectious pathogenesis research holds great promise. As more information is uncovered, it is becoming increasingly apparent that our present knowledge of the pathogenic potential of infectious agents is often limited to the most noticeable effects, which sometimes represent only the tip of the iceberg. For example, it is now well appreciated that pathologic processes caused by infectious agents may emerge clinically after an incubation of decades and may result from genetic, immunologic, and other indirect routes more than from the infecting agent in itself. Thus, there is a general expectation that continued investigation will lead to the isolation of new agents of infection, the identification of hitherto unsuspected etiologic correlations, and, eventually, more effective approaches to prevention and therapy.

Studies on the mechanisms of disease caused by infectious agents demand a breadth of understanding across many specialized areas, as well as much cooperation between clinicians and experimentalists. The series *Infectious Agents and Patho-genesis* is intended not only to document the state of the art in this fascinating and challenging field but also to help lay bridges among diverse areas and people.

M. Bendinelli
H. Friedman

Preface

Opportunistic, intracellular bacterial infections are in the forefront today because of the challenges they present for the treatment of the patient who is immuno-compromised due to underlying, chronic disease and/or to radiation or chemo-therapy for that disease, which have caused the weakened host defenses of innate or specific immunity, for treatment of the opportunistic infection, and for identi-fication of new species that appear in this role. Many of the bacteria that are associated with these infections are acquired from environmental niches, not transmitted from other infected persons. On the other hand, some of the infec-tions are already present in body orifices and are able to cause disease because they can invade due to compromised defense mechanisms of the patient. In this volume, pathogenesis and immune reactions of some these intracellular infections are featured and problems related to antimicrobial chemotherapy and how they are being solved are discussed as well.

The editors wish to express their gratitude to Ilona M. Friedman for her organizing abilities and for her patience, persistence, and fortitude in dealing with problems that arose during the editorial process.

Lois J. Paradise
Herman Friedman
Mauro Bendinelli

Contents

2. **Genetic Regulation of Host Responses to** *Salmonella*
   typhimurium

SALMAN T. QURESHI, EMIL SKAMENE,
AND DANIELLE MALO

3. **Host Resistance and** *Mycobacterium tuberculosis* **Infection**

JON S. FRIEDLAND

4. The Influence of Adrenal Steroids on Macrophage and T-Cell Function in Tuberculosis

GRAHAM A. W. ROOK
AND ROGELIO HERNANDEZ-PANDO

7. *Mycobacterium avium*-**Complex Infections**
and Immunodeficiency

FRANK M. COLLINS

8. **Pathogenesis of** *Legionella pneumophila* **Infection**

PAUL S. HOFFMAN AND RAFAEL GARDUNO

11. *Rhodococcus equi:* Pathogenesis and Replication in Macrophages

PATRICIA A. DARRAH, MARY K. HONDALUS,
AND DAVID M. MOSSER

12. *Bartonella* Infections in the Immunocompromised Host

ANDREW W. O. BURGESS, DAVID JOHNSON,
AND BURT E. ANDERSON

13. *Chlamydia trachomatis* Infections

JULIUS SCHACHTER

14. *Chlamydia* Infection and Pneumonia

MURAT V. KALAYOGLU, DAVID L. HAHN,
AND GERALD I. BYRNE

15. *Brucella* **Infections and Immunity**

CYNTHIA L. BALDWIN AND R. MARTIN ROOP II

16. Antibiotic Treatment of Infections with Intracellular Bacteria

HERBERT HOF

Introduction and Perspectives

LOIS J. PARADISE

OPPORTUNISM AND BACTERIAL INFECTIONS

In recent years, attention has been increasingly focused on those bacteria that are relatively or completely innocuous to immunocompetent individuals, but produce disease once they can invade those who have lowered nonspecific/innate or specific/immune defenses against infection. In describing the difference between opportunists and pathogens, Relman and Falkow[1] refer to "'principal' pathogens, which *regularly* cause disease in some proportion of susceptible individuals with apparently *intact* specific and nonspecific defense systems" as opposed to opportunists which have the ability to proliferate and cause disease in humans, but require a diminution of normal host defenses to establish the infection at a site in the host that allows them to do so.

The enhanced susceptibility to skin infection by *Staphylococcus aureus* in patients having predisposing factors such as subcutaneous gut sutures and by *Pseudomonas aeruginosa* in burned patients has long been called opportunism. In the industrialized world today, opportunistic infections confronting us are increasingly those in organ transplant patients, cancer patients, and others receiving immunosuppressive chemotherapeutic measures; those harboring immunosuppressive microorganisms such as human immunodeficiency virus, and in the very elderly whose immune functions are modulating[2] or decreasing in certain respects. In addition to these, worldwide there is malnutrition, a condition with marked adverse effects on both innate and immune defenses.[3] Some bacteria now

LOIS J. PARADISE • Department of Medical Microbiology, University of South Florida, College of Medicine, Tampa, Florida 33612.

Opportunistic Intracellular Bacteria and Immunity, edited by Lois J. Paradise *et al.* Plenum Press, New York, 1999.

known to be opportunists previously were not suspected of being able to cause human infections, for example, *Legionella* spp. and *Rhodococcus equi*. Their habitats are in the external human environment, although some may also infect animals, and their association with human disease was unknown until they were identified in immunocompromised humans. Other bacteria, such as *Mycobacterium tuberculosis* and *Mycobacterium leprae*, are associated with diseases that have been known for centuries and now have recognized roles as opportunists. Primary tuberculosis is an acute inflammatory disease that is controlled adequately in immunocompetent persons. In some patients, however, lowered resistance allows post-primary tuberculosis to occur and chronic disease results. This is largely an immunopathological condition with tissue damage resulting from cellular activities, production of cytokines, and other mediators rather than microbial factors.

SURVIVAL OF BACTERIA WITHIN MACROPHAGES

When bacteria invade and are in the extracellular microenvironment, they are exposed to phagocytic cells [polymorphonuclear leukocytes, (PMNs), and macrophages] as well as molecules such as complement system components and perhaps immunoglobulins that opsonize the bacteria and enhance phagocytosis. Bactericidal factors of these cells kill most bacterial species readily. However, some bacteria have properties that protect them from this. When PMNs do not kill them, they are taken up by the longer lived macrophages. Within macrophages then, they survive, multiply, and cause disease directly (damaging tissue cells by their own action) or indirectly (e.g., by stimulation of immune responses that damage tissues) while they are protected from the extracellular nonspecific and specific defense mechanisms. Because activities surrounding phagocytosis by macrophages which may include activation, phagolysosome formation, signaling, and cytokine production comprise a complex system of interactions, there are many sites at which bacterial virulence factors may inhibit completion of killing mechanisms. In the chapters that follow, the current status of knowledge of such activities of bacterial opportunists, bacteria that act as opportunists under certain conditions (e.g., *Chlamydia trachomatis*), and primary pathogens, such as *Brucellae* and *Chlamydia pneumoniae*, that also interrupt macrophage killing are detailed. Although the primary focus of this volume is on opportunists, it was felt that the greater breadth of coverage that was presented concerning intracellular survival of a wide range of bacteria should be valuable in providing greater insight regarding possible mechanisms for those opportunists for which they have not been elucidated. The entire story is not known for any facultative intracellular bacterial species as far as its interactions with macrophages and the stimulation of immune reactions are concerned.

PHAGOCYTOSIS AND KILLING IN NORMAL MACROPHAGES

A brief outline of endocytosis and killing of bacteria (see ref. 4 for a review) cannot detail all the complexities of the system, but, it is hoped, will serve as a framework for the discussions that follow. Once bacteria have invaded tissues and are contacted by macrophages, they may bind to the macrophage cell membrane by some nonspecific molecule, by complement component C3b, or, in a host previously exposed to one or more of the bacterial antigens, by specific immunoglobulins. Adherence of bacteria to the macrophages stimulates pseudopod engulfment of the particles and endocytosis with the bacteria now residing within the cell-membrane-bound vacuole, the phagosome. Formation of the phagosome stimulates the movement of lysosomal granules toward it; membranes of the two organelles fuse; and antibacterial enzymes, cationic proteins, and other molecules are released within the phagolysosome. Acidification of the internal environment, stimulation of the hexose monophosphate shunt with formation of NADP and ultimate production of oxidative bactericidal molecules and ions (hydrogen peroxide, superoxide anions, singlet oxygen, hydroxyl radicals) mark the initiation of attempts to kill the invaders. Acidification promotes bacterial cell damage by the cationic proteins and lactoferrin and enzymes aid in completion of the killing process. Once the microbes are destroyed, enzymes break down their remains. When this is complete, the phagosome moves toward and fuses with the macrophage cell membrane and discharges the debris into the external environment.

Destruction of the intracellular bacteria is more rapid if they have induced activation of the macrophages or if production of interferon-γ by T lymphocytes or NK (natural killer) cells has been stimulated by the infection. Activated macrophages produce interleukins (IL-1, IL-6, IL-8, IL-10, IL-12) and other cytokines (e.g., tumor necrosis factor-α and transforming growth factor-β). Some of these promote the inflammatory response, but IL-10 and transforming growth factor-β appear to regulate their actions by antagonizing them. Bacteria that do not induce macrophage activation enhance their own intracellular survival obviously.

In the chapters that follow, the mechanisms by which various bacteria affect host defense mechanisms are described. Initially immune and genetic factors of resistance to infectious agents are considered. Several aspects of infection and resistance by mycobacterial species are presented. Tuberculosis is the model for a discussion of the effects of adrenal steroids on macrophage and T-cell functions, which points out the importance of neuroendocrine involvement in these activities. Experimental studies of *Listeria monocytogenes* infection in mice are detailed. Other intracellular species discussed have been mentioned earlier. The final chapter covers an important aspect of problems presented by intracellular bacterial infections. These microorganisms are protected from chemotherapeutic agents by their intracellular location. In addition, those opportunists that are acquired from the external environment, that are not transmitted from person to person, but invade the host due to lowered resistance, tend to be resistant to many chemotherapeutic agents. Presentation of the problem and progress being made in development of chemotherapy for these infections is presented.

REFERENCES

1. Relman, D. A., and Falkow, S., 1990, A molecular perspective of microbial pathogenicity, in: *Principles and Practice of Infectious Diseases*, 3rd Ed. (G. L. Mandell, R. G. Douglas, and J. E. Bennett, eds.), Churchill Livingstone, New York, pp. 25–32.
2. Franceschi, C., Monti, D., Sansoni, P., and Cossarizza, A., 1995, The immunology of exceptional individuals: The lesson of centenarians, *Immunol. Today* **16:**12–16.
3. Morris, J. G., Jr., and Potter, M., 1997, Emergence of new pathogens as a function of changes in host susceptibility, *Emerg. Infect. Dis.* **3:**435–441.
4. van Furth, R., 1996, Intracellular antimicrobial mechanisms in macrophages, in: *Intracellular Bacterial Infections* (J-C. Pechere, ed.), Cambridge Medical Publications, Worthing, England, pp. 1–6.

Immune Defenses against Intracellular Bacterial Infections

CHARLES NAUCIEL

Intracellular bacteria have the capacity to persist and multiply within resident macrophages. This intracellular location protects them from humoral defense mechanisms and probably from more aggressive phagocytic cells such as neutrophils. As macrophages are long-lived cells, they can constitute a microbial niche allowing the development of subacute or chronic infections, associated with a granulomatous reaction.

Acquired resistance to intracellular bacteria is essentially T-cell-mediated and the main effector cells of the immune response are activated macrophages. Macrophages therefore can be both the targets of intracellular bacterial infections and the effectors of defense mechanisms. The use of monoclonal antibodies and mice with targeted gene disruption[1] has yielded a better understanding of the role of various components of the nonspecific and specific responses to infection by intracellular bacteria.

1. HOST INVASION BY INTRACELLULAR BACTERIA

Although some facultative intracellular bacteria may penetrate through the skin (e.g., *Francisella tularensis*), most enter through the mucosa. *Mycobacterium tuberculosis* and *Legionella pneumophila* enter the body via the respiratory tract. *Salmonella,*

CHARLES NAUCIEL • Faculté de Médecine de Paris-Ouest, Université Paris 5, 92380 Garches, France.

Opportunistic Intracellular Bacteria and Immunity, edited by Lois J. Paradise *et al.* Plenum Press, New York, 1999.

Listeria monocytogenes, and *Brucella* usually enter via the intestine, and *Chlamydia trachomatis* gains access via the genital or conjunctival mucosa.

Intracellular bacteria have the capacity to adhere to host cells and to induce their own ingestion, even by nonprofessional phagocytes. These processes are induced by proteins expressed at the bacterial surface (adhesins and invasins) that interact with host cell receptors.[2] The triggering of host cell receptors activates intracellular signaling pathways and results in cytoskeletal rearrangements and endocytosis (as in professional phagocytes).

The interaction between bacteria and host cells also induces the synthesis of new proteins by the bacteria. This probably reflects an adaptive response to a new environment and illustrates the crosstalk between bacteria and host cells.

The main target of bacteria penetrating via the intestine are M cells. These cells are specialized in transepithelial transport from the lumen to organized lymphoid tissues within the mucosa, such as Peyer's patches.

After the bacteria have passed through the epithelial layer they are ingested by phagocytic cells, especially macrophages. Ingestion is mediated by binding to various cell receptors, including complement receptors (CR1 or CR3), the mannose receptor, the fibronectin receptor, and scavenger receptors. The role of CR3 in the ingestion of several intracellular bacteria (e.g., *M. tuberculosis, M. leprae, L. pneumophila*) has been demonstrated. Following ingestion bacteria are located in a membrane-bound vacuole, the phagosome. The phagosome fuses with lysosomes to generate a phagolysosome, where acidification and bacteriolytic processes may occur.

A major property of facultative intracellular bacteria is their ability to survive and replicate within macrophages. Intracellular bacteria have developed various strategies to escape killing by phagocytic cells. Some bacteria such as *M. tuberculosis* are able to inhibit fusion between the phagosome and lysosomes, as well as phagolysosome acidification. *L. monocytogenes* escapes from the phagosome after lysing the phagosome membrane by listeriolysin O. The bacterium is then able to move into the cytosol by inducing actin polymerization and to invade the neighboring cell.

Following infection macrophages may be killed, in some cases by apoptosis. Alternatively, quiescent bacteria may persist for a long time within macrophages.

The infection may spread locally near its portal of entry (lungs or intestine), reaching regional lymph nodes. When systemic infection occurs, bacteria diffuse through the bloodstream and may localize in various organs, where they are trapped by resident macrophages, mainly in the liver, spleen, and bone marrow. In the liver, intracellular bacteria such as *L. monocytogenes* and *Salmonella* may spread from Küpffer cells to hepatocytes. Facultative intracellular bacteria can be found in the extracellular milieu, especially at advanced stages of the disease. Obligate intracellular bacteria (e.g., *Rickettsiae,* and *Chlamydiae*) replicate mainly in nonprofessional phagocytes such as endothelial or epithelial cells.

When mice are infected with a sublethal dose of *L. monocytogenes*, bacteria are eradicated from the organs within 8 to 10 days. In contrast, other intracellular bacteria induce long-lasting infections.

2. NONSPECIFIC RESPONSE TO INTRACELLULAR BACTERIAL INFECTIONS

When bacteria have passed through the epithelial barrier that protects the host, resistance is based initially on nonspecific (or innate) mechanisms. This innate resistance is very important for host survival prior to the development of the specific immune response several days later, particularly for rapidly growing organisms. Animals with defective specific immune responses such as *nude* and *scid* mice are good models to analyze the respective roles of specific and nonspecific mechanisms of resistance to infection. In fact nonspecific and specific mechanisms are tightly interconnected.

2.1. Inflammatory Response

Nonspecific resistance is based mainly on an inflammatory response that attracts and activates phagocytic cells at the site of infection. The inflammatory response can be triggered by various pathways. Bacteria can activate complement by the alternative pathway. The production of C5a and C3a contribute to the inflammatory response. Moreover, coating of bacteria with complement will induce their binding to the complement receptors of phagocytic cells and, hence, their ingestion. Following the ingestion of bacteria or the interaction with some bacterial components, such as lipopolysaccharide (through CD14) or peptidogylcan, macrophages secrete a variety of proinflammatory cytokines and chemokines. It appears that the pattern of macrophage responses may differ according to the receptor used for bacterial internalization.[3] Cells other than macrophages (e.g., intestinal[4] and endothelial cells) can also produce cytokines when invaded by bacteria. Messenger RNAs for inflammatory cytokines are produced within the first few hours of infection.

The critical role of cytokines in innate resistance is demonstrated by the effect of administering neutralizing antibodies against interferon-γ[5] (IFN-γ), tumor necrosis factor-α (TNF-α), or interleukin-12 (IL-12). These treatments strongly depress resistance to infection by intracellular bacteria during the first few days[6] (Fig. 1). Resistance to *L. monocytogenes* is also depressed by blocking IL-1 and IL-6 activities[7].

Proinflammatory cytokines may also diffuse through the bloodstream and reach the central nervous system, where IL-1 and TNF-α can induce fever, and the liver, where IL-6 induces the synthesis of acute-phase reactants. Antiinflam-

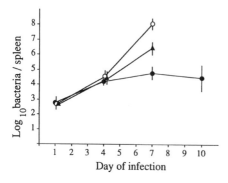

FIGURE 1. Time course of infection in mice inoculated with 10^3 CFUs of *S. typhimurium* C5 and treated at day 0 with anti-IFN-γ(○), anti-TNF-α (▲), or control antibodies (●). Data are the geometric mean numbers ± standard deviations of bacteria recovered from the spleens. (From ref. 6, with permission.)

matory cytokines (IL-4, IL-10, IL-13, TGF-β) can be produced to regulate the host response and inhibit macrophage activation. Administration of neutralizing antibodies against IL-4 or IL-10 may increase resistance against some intracellular bacteria.

In most instances cytokines act locally. IL-1 α, IL-1 β, and TNF-α induce the production of inflammatory mediators (prostaglandin E_2) and increase the expression of E-seletins and intercellular adhesion molecules of the immunoglobulin superfamily (intercellular adhesion molecule-1 [ICAM-1], vascular cell adhesion molecule-1 [VCAM-1]) on endothelial cells. The local production of inflammatory molecules results in capillary dilation and plasma leakage, but the main event in resistance to infection is the influx of phagocytic cells.

This phenomenon is a multistep process regulated by the interaction of a set of soluble mediators and cell receptors.[8] Leukocytes expressing L-selectins first attach to endothelial cells expressing E- and P-selectins in a rolling interaction. Selectins mediate a labile adhesion through the binding of carbohydrate ligands. Then various chemoattractants direct the migration of leukocytes and increase the adhesiveness of integrins. Classic chemoattractants include *N*-formyl peptides (produced by bacteria), C5a, leukotriene B4, and platelet-activating factor.

More recently, chemoattractive cytokines, termed chemokines, have been characterized. Chemokines contain two cysteine residues near the NH_2 terminus. These two residues are either adjacent (CC-chemokines) or separated by an additional amino acid (CXC-chemokines). The CC-chemokines, which include MCP-1, MIP-1α, MIP-1β, and RANTES, act mainly on monocytes, whereas CXC-chemokines, such as IL-8, act on neutrophils. Leukocyte chemoattractants interact with G-protein-coupled receptors possessing seven transmembrane domains. Their specificity is regulated by the cellular distribution of their receptors.

Chemoattractants increase integrin adhesiveness on leukocytes. β2 integrins such as MAC-1 and lymphocyte function antigen-1 (LFA-1) allow firm adhesion to endothelial cells by their binding to members of the immunoglobulin super-

TABLE I
Interaction between Integrins and Immunoglobulin Superfamily Molecules

Integrins[a]	Expressed by	Ig superfamily molecules[b]	Expressed by
αLβ2 (LFA-1)	Lymphocytes, monocytes, neutrophils	ICAM-1 ICAM-2	Inflamed endothelium Endothelium
αMβ2 (MAC-1)	Monocytes, neutrophils	ICAM-1	Inflamed endothelium
α4β1	T lymphocytes, monocytes	VCAM-1	Inflamed endothelium
α4β7	Lymphocytes	MAdCAM-1	Mucosal endothelium

[a]Integrin adhesiveness is increased by chemoattractants (e.g., chemokines).
[b]Expression of Ig superfamily molecules is increased by IL-1 and TNF-α on inflamed endothelial cells.

family (Table I). Leukocytes can then migrate through the capillary endothelium and reach the tissue where bacteria have triggered an inflammatory response. Neutrophils appear rapidly at the site of infection but are shortlived. They are followed by mononuclear phagocytes (monocytes / macrophages) endowed with a longer life span.

2.2. Neutrophils

The role of neutrophils in resistance against intracellular bacteria has recently been demonstrated. The administration of monoclonal antibodies that deplete granulocytes or inhibit their influx decreases resistance against *L. monocytogenes, Salmonella typhimurium, and Francisella tularensis* infection. Neutrophils are necessary for the initial destruction of bacteria, during the first hours following intravenous challenge. They are also involved in the lysis of hepatocytes that are invaded by bacteria during the first few days of infection.[9]

2.3. Mononuclear Phagocytes

The influx of mononuclear phagocytes, derived from blood monocytes, is necessary for the development of resistance to intracellular bacteria.[10] Mononuclear phagocytes need to be activated to express their antibacterial activities. The most potent macrophage activator is INF-γ. A T-independent pathway of macrophage activation has been demonstrated in *scid* mice.[11] It involves the production of IL-12 by macrophages; this cytokine, in synergy with TNF-α, stimulates the production of INF-γ by natural killer cells that in turn activate macrophages. Several reports indicate that activation of macrophage microbicidal activity by IFN-γ does not occur in the presence of anti-TNF-α antibodies, suggesting the participation of TNF-α in macrophage activation through an autocrine pathway.[12]

Microbicidal activity is related mainly to the production of NADPH-oxidase, which initiates the production of reactive oxygen intermediates and, at least in mice, to the induction of NO synthetase, which produces reactive nitrogen intermediates. Macrophages also synthesize a variety of other compounds with antimicrobial activities (Fig. 2).

2.4. Genetic Control of Nonspecific Resistance

Susceptibility to infection varies widely among individuals. Comparative studies in various mouse strains have characterized some of the genes controlling the level of innate resistance. Susceptibility to listeriosis was found to be linked to a deficiency of the C5 component of complement. The gene that has been most extensively studied was designated *Lsh, Ity,* or *Bcg* and is now termed *Nramp*[13] (natural resistance-associated macrophage protein). This gene is located on mouse chromosome 1, and controls natural resistance against *Leishmania donovani, S. typhimurium,* and several mycobacterial species (*M. bovis* BCG, *M. lepraemurium, M. avium*). There are two alleles in mice, susceptible and resistant, the latter being dominant. The replication rate of the aforementioned pathogens is slower in

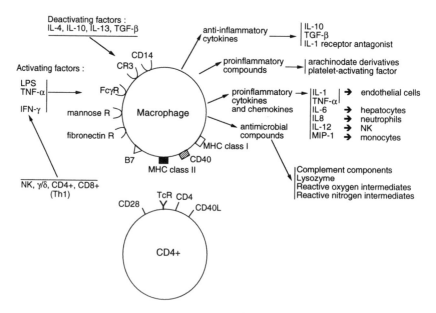

FIGURE 2. The pivotal role of macrophages in resistance to intracellular bacteria.

resistant than in susceptible mice. Susceptibility is associated with a glycine-to-aspartic acid substitution at position 169 of the gene product. The protein encoded by *Nramp* is expressed in macrophages and is not detected in mice homozygous for the susceptibility allele. Its precise function is not known. A homologous gene has been found in various species, including humans. There is great polymorphism in the human gene but no clear correlation between suscep-tibility to mycobacterial infection and a given allele has yet been found.

3. SPECIFIC IMMUNE RESPONSE TO INTRACELLULAR BACTERIAL INFECTIONS

3.1. Role of T Cells in the Immune Response to Intracellular Bacteria

Acquired resistance to intracellular bacteria is expressed by the capacity to control bacterial growth, to gradually clear the bacteria from the organs, and to resist reinfection. Resistance to reinfection is nonspecific as long as the host harbors bacteria from the primary infection.[14] For instance, mice infected with *Brucella abortus* are resistant to *L. monocytogenes*. However, when the primary inoc-ulum is cleared, animals display increased resistance only against the homologous bacterium.

Protective immunity is generally induced by live bacteria only. The immune response to infection is associated with delayed-type hypersensitivity (DTH) to antigens of the causative organism. Like DTH, acquired resistance to infection by intracellular bacteria cannot be passively transferred with the serum of immune animals. In contrast, a strong level of resistance to *L. monocytogenes* can be passively transferred with T lymphocytes[15] (Fig. 3). In infections with other intracellular bacteria, the level of resistance that can be transferred by T cells is generally lower.

The role of T cells in immunity against intracellular bacteria is also sup-ported by the outcome of experimental infections in mice devoid of T cells (e.g., *nude* and *scid* mice). Although these mice are more resistant than controls during the first few days (by nonspecific mechanisms), they are unable to control the growth of bacteria in their organs. Patients with T-cell deficiencies [acquired immunodeficiency syndrome (AIDS), immunosuppressive therapy, etc.] are prone to infection by intracellular bacteria.

3.2. T-Cell Traffic

After maturation in the thymus, where selection of the T-cell repertoire occurs, T cells bearing clonally distributed receptors continuously recirculate from blood to secondary lymphoid tissues.[8] This process increases the likelihood

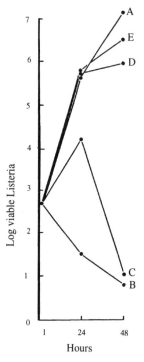

FIGURE 3. Growth curves showing the protective effect of varying numbers of *Listeria*-immune lymphoid cells from the spleens of 7-day immune donors. Recipients were injected with 2×10^8 normal cells (A) or immune cells in doses of 2×10^8 (B), 4×10^7 (C), 8×10^6 (D), and 2×10^6 (E) and challenged with 3.7×10^4 *Listeria monocytogenes*. (From ref. 15, with permission.)

that T cells will encounter their cognate antigens (in particular invading pathogens). Naive T cells emigrate through high endothelium venules, either into peripheral lymph nodes or mucosal lymphoid tissues. Emigration of lymphocytes from blood involves mechanisms similar to those previously described for phagocytic cells. L-selectin expressed by lymphocytes interacts in the lymph nodes with a peripheral lymph node adressin. Interaction between the integrin $\alpha 4\beta 7$ and the mucosal adressin MAdCAM-1 allows homing to mucosal lymphoid tissues (Table I). After 10 to 20 h, naive T cells leave secondary lymphoid tissues through efferent lymphatic vessels and reach the blood through the thoracic duct. When T cells interact with antigen they are retained and expand clonally. The resulting activated T cells exhibit an increased capacity to migrate through inflamed endothelium, even in nonlymphoid tissues. This is how activated T lymphocytes accumulate at sites of inflammation. T cells expressing CLA preferentially accumulate in inflamed skin (they participate in particular in DTH reactions). Several CC-chemokines participate in this influx of T lymphocytes (macrophage inflammatory protein-1β [MIP-1β], monocyte chemoattractant protein-1 [MCP-1], and RANTES). They are produced by macrophages, endothelial cells, and activated T cells themselves. Persistence of intracellular bacteria contributes to maintaining an inflammatory process. Local accumulation of mononuclear phagocytes and T lymphocytes leads to the formation of granulomas. Local production of TNF-α is necessary to their development.[16]

Memory T cells generated during the immune response retain the migratory characteristics of activated T cells. They are able to respond to antigen in non-lymphoid tissues and they are more likely to return to the tissue where they first encountered the antigen. They are a key element in resistance to reinfection.

3.3. T-Cell Subsets

T cells do not recognize free antigens, but only peptides presented on the cell surface by molecules of the major histocompatibility complex (MHC). When cells are infected by intracellular pathogens, peptides derived from the pathogen are expressed on the cell surface in association with MHC molecules and can trigger a T-cell response. It is noteworthy that MHC molecules expression is increased by IFN-γ and TNF-α, both of which are produced at an early stage of infection.

T cells comprise several subsets which may play various roles in resistance to infection. The respective roles of T-cell subsets in resistance to experimental infections has been determined by selective depletions with monoclonal antibodies or targeted gene disruption (knockout mice). The bulk of T cells express a T receptor made of α and β chains. This population is divided into CD4+ and CD8+ subpopulations, both of which can participate in resistance to intracellular bacteria. A minor population of T cells bears a receptor made of γ and δ chains.

3.3.1. CD4+ T Cells

This subpopulation recognizes epitopes presented by the polymorphic MHC class II molecules. Only a limited number of cell types constitutively express MHC class II molecules and behave as antigen-presenting cells (mainly macrophages, B cells, dendritic cells, and Langerhans cells).

Bacteria or bacterial components can be ingested by antigen-presenting cells. In the endosomal compartment, proteins are fragmented by proteases into peptides that bind into a groove of MHC class II molecules. The peptide-loaded class II molecules are then expressed on the cell surface, where they can interact with the receptor of CD4+ T cells.

T-cell activation requires a costimulatory signal, the best characterized of which results from the interaction between CD28 on T cells and B7−1 or B7−2 molecules on antigen-presenting cells. Expression of costimulatory molecules on antigen-presenting cells can be modulated by bacteria. For instance, lipopolysacharide and *L. monocytogenes* have been shown to increase their level of expression, whereas *M. tuberculosis* has the opposite effect.[17]

T cells seem to be devoid of direct antibacterial activity. Their role is to recruit and activate mononuclear phagocytes. Activated CD4$^+$ T lymphocytes, expressing CD40 ligand, can interact with CD40 on macrophages and stimulate various macrophage functions (e.g., proinflammatory cytokine production) (Fig. 2). Mice with targeted gene disruption of CD40 ligand display increased susceptibility to the intracellular parasite *Leishmania major*.[18] CD4$^+$ T cells act mainly by the production of cytokines. According to their pattern of cytokine production, CD4$^+$ T cells have been subdivided into Th1 cells (producing IL-2, IFN-γ, and TNF-β) and Th2 cells (producing IL-4, IL-5, IL-6, and IL-10) (Table II).

Th1 cells play a critical role in resistance to intracellular bacteria by their ability to produce IFN-γ, the main activator of macrophages. They also mediate DTH. In contrast, Th2 cells, which favor the differentiation of B cells and antibody production, have a detrimental effect on infections due to intracellular pathogens.[19] Indeed, Th2 cells produce IL-4 and IL-10, which inhibit macrophage activation.

As IFN-γ inhibits the development of Th2 cells and IL-4 inhibits the development of Th1 cells, theoretically the immune response is dominated either by Th1 or by Th2 cells. The differentiation of CD4$^+$ T cells into Th1 or Th2 cells appears to be determined by the cytokines produced during the early phase of the infection (Fig. 4). IL-12, produced primarily by macrophages, promotes the differentiation and growth of Th1 cells. IL-12 production by macrophages is induced by the ingestion of various intracellular bacteria. Thus, in most cases, the immune response against intracellular bacteria is of the Th1 type and depletion of CD4$^+$ T cells or neutralization of IFN-γ by monoclonal antibodies exacerbates many experimental infections induced by intracellular bacteria, for example, *M. tuberculosis*, and *S. typhimurium*.[20] During pregnancy Th1 response appears to be suppressed[19] and this may increase susceptibility to intracellular bacterial infections.

IL-4 favors the development of a Th2 response. A potential source of early IL-4 in mice seems to be a subpopulation of CD4$^+$ cells expressing the NK1.1 antigen. The detrimental effect of the type 2 response on resistance to intracellu-

TABLE II
Cytokine Production Patterns of CD4$^+$ T Cells

Th1	Th2^a	Both subsets
IL-2	IL-4	IL-3
IFN-γ	IL-5	GM-CSF
TNF-β	IL-6	TNF-α
	IL-9	chemokines
	IL-10	
	IL-13	

^{a} Th0 cells can produce both type 1 and type 2 cytokines.

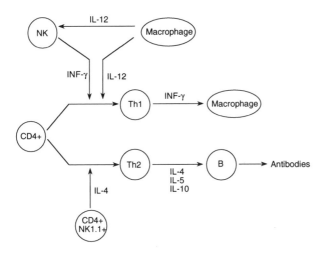

FIGURE 4. Differentiation of CD4+ T cells.

lar pathogens was initially demonstrated in *Leishmania major* infection in mice, and later in human leprosy. In the most severe form of the latter disease, lepromatous leprosy, mRNAs coding for IL-4, IL-5, and IL-10 are found in the lesions, whereas mRNAs for IL-2 and IFN-γ are present in tuberculoid lesions.[21]

Yet the polarization of CD4+ T cells toward the secretion of type 1 or type 2 cytokines is not always absolute. Th1 and Th2 cytokines can be produced simultaneously; in particular, IL-12 can induce the production of both IFN-γ and IL-10,[22] and simultaneous production of these cytokines can be found during infections.

3.3.2. CD8+ T Cells

CD8+ T cells recognize peptides presented by MHC class I molecules. Class I molecules are expressed by the majority of cells. Proteins in the cytosol are hydrolyzed by a proteolytic particle, the proteasome, and the resulting peptides are transported into the rough endoplasmic reticulum by a transporter associated with antigen processing (termed TAP). Peptides are then loaded on newly synthesized class I molecules and brought to the cell surface. It was initially believed that peptides derived from cytosolic proteins were exclusively synthesized endogenously and, therefore, that a CD8 response could be induced only by pathogens replicating in the cytosol, such as viruses and bacteria able to escape from the phagolysosome (e.g., *L. monocytogenes*). Indeed, CD8+ T cells play a major role in resistance to *L. monocytogenes* infection.[7] Yet CD8+ T cells also play a role in resistance to *M. tuberculosis,* as shown by the susceptibility of mice lacking class I

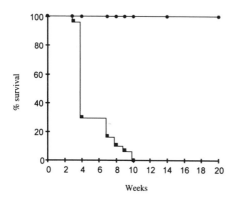

FIGURE 5. Survival curves of β2m$^{-/-}$ (devoid of CD8$^+$ T cells) (■) and C57BL/6 (●) mice infected with *M. tuberculosis.* (From ref. 23, with permission.)

molecules and, consequently, CD8$^+$ T cells[23] (Fig. 5). *M. tuberculosis* remains in the endosomal compartment, and other bacteria located in the same compartment (e.g., *S. typhimurium*) can elicit a CD8$^+$ T cell response. Two possible pathways have been described to explain how peptides from the endosomal compartment can bind class I MHC molecules.[24] The first involves transfer by an unknown mechanism from the phagosome to the cytosol. The second involves regurgitation of peptides, which can then bind to class I molecules on the cell surface.

CD8$^+$ T cells may participate in resistance to intracellular bacteria either by the production of cytokines, such as IFN-γ, or by their cytolytic activity. Evidence for the second mechanism has been obtained with perforin-deficient mice. In such mice the number of CD8$^+$ T cells is normal, but their cytolytic activity is impaired. Perforin-deficient mice are more susceptible to *L. monocytogenes* infection than controls, especially against a secondary infection.[7] Moreover, CD8$^+$ T immune cells from IFN-γ knockout mice can protect naive recipients. It is generally believed that the lysis of infected cells (permissive cells) induces the release of bacteria that can then be ingested by activated phagocytic cells.[25]

It must also be remembered that CD8$^+$ T cells can produce type 2 cytokines that may exert a detrimental effect on infections due to intracellular bacteria. This has been shown, for instance, in the lepromatous form of leprosy.

3.3.3. γδ T Cells

These cells form a minority of circulating T cells.[26] They are preferentially located near epithelia in contact with the external environment. γδ T cells differ markedly from αβ T cells in their recognition properties. Antigens appear to be recognized directly without prior processing. Antigens are generally not presented by classic MHC molecules, and γδ T cells can recognize nonpeptide antigens.

A large proportion of γδ T cells from mice and humans respond to heat-killed mycobacteria. In humans the major stimulatory components are small nonpeptidic phosphorylated molecules. They are recognized by Vγ9/Vδ2 bearing cells. The role of γδ T cells in infection was initially suspected because these cells accumulate rapidly at the site of bacterial replication. Depletion of γδ T cells by monoclonal antibodies or targeted gene disruption confirmed their role in resistance (especially in the early phase) to several infections due to intracellular bacteria (e.g., *L. monocytogenes*, *M. bovis* BCG, *M. tuberculosis*, and *S. typhimurium*). Depletion of γδ T cells has less of an effect than depletion of αβ T cells. In addition compensatory mechanisms between the two T-cell populations appear to exist.[1]

The mechanisms allowing γδ T cells to participate in resistance to infection are not precisely known. γδ T cells may act as αβ T cells, as they can produce cytokines (particularly IFN-γ), and express cytolytic activity.

3.4. Target Antigens of the T-Cell Response

A great variety of bacterial antigens can induce, *in vitro*, the proliferation of T cells from immune hosts and the production of cytokines. As discussed previously, the T-cell receptor usually interacts with peptide fragments presented by MHC class I or class II molecules. Moreover, αβ T cells can also recognize glycopeptides. It has also been found that some bacterial components (formylpeptides) can be presented by nonclassic MHC molecules (H-2M3). Nonpeptide antigens such as bacterial lipids (e.g., mycolic acids from *Mycobacteria*) and glycolipids (e.g., lipoarabinomannan from *M. leprae*) can be presented by molecules of the CD1 family.[27] These molecules have a structure similar to that of MHC class I or class II molecules, but are not polymorphic and are encoded by genes that are unlinked to the MHC. The range of molecules that can be recognized by T cells therefore appears to be very broad. The characterization of antigens eliciting protective immunity would be of great interest to improve vaccination against intracellular bacteria. Some data suggest that proteins secreted by bacteria may play an important role. In *L. monocytogenes* infection, secreted listeriolysin O and p60 are the targets of CD8+ T cells conferring significant protection. Immunization with secreted proteins from *M. tuberculosis* can induce protective immunity in mice.[28]

3.5. Role of the MHC in the Genetic Control of Resistance to Intracellular Bacteria

In mice the late phase of infection by *S. typhimurium*[29] (Fig. 6), *M. tuberculosis*, and *M. lepraemurium* is controlled by the MHC. In humans, progression toward the lepromatous or tuberculoid form of leprosy is controlled by MHC class II molecules.

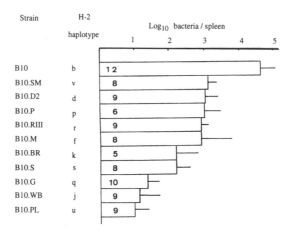

FIGURE 6. Bacterial counts in the spleens of various H-2 congenic mice 21 days after infection with an attenuated strain of *S. typhimurium*. The number of animals used is indicated in each bar. (From ref. 29, with permission.)

As discussed previously the function of polymorphic MCH class I and class II molecules is to present antigen fragments to T cells, a given allele being able to present a given set of peptides. The role of the MHC in the genetic control of the immune response was initially demonstrated by using synthetic antigens bearing a small number of epitopes. The fact that the course of infection can be influenced by the host MHC suggests that a limited number of epitopes are the target of the protective T cell response. Yet the MHC also encodes class III molecules such as TNF-α, which can also play a role in resistance to infection.

3.6. Role of Antibodies

Antibodies do not seem to play a role in resistance to some intracellular bacterial infections (e.g., *L. monocytogenes*, *M. tuberculosis*). The role of antibodies in *S. typhimurium* infection has been a subject of controversy. Antibodies can protect mice when the challenge is given by the intraperitoneal route or when mice are naturally resistant. Synergistic interaction between immune serum and immune T cells has been reported in an adoptive transfer of immunity model.[30] These results in mice may explain some of the protective effects of killed vaccines against human typhoid.

A role for antibodies has also been found in *Francisella tularensis* and *Brucella*[31] infections. The mechanism of action of antibodies against intracellular bacteria remains unclear. It is noteworthy that opsonization by antibodies, which allows internalization by phagocytic cells via the Fc receptor, induces the production of reactive oxygen intermediates, whereas this is not the case when internalization occurs via the complement receptor type 3 (CR3).

4. CONCLUSIONS

Resistance to intracellular bacterial infections involves almost all the components of the immune system and mainly T cells. The immune response tends to contain the invading pathogens in localized foci of inflammation, where complex interactions among phagocytic cells, endothelial cells, and T cells take place. These interactions are mediated by soluble molecules (cytokines and chemokines) and adhesion molecules and result in the accumulation of activated phagocytic cells. The inflammatory response is triggered initially by nonspecific mechanisms, and then by the interaction between T-cell receptors and bacterial antigens. Characterization of bacterial antigens able to induce protective immunity would be of great value to improve vaccination strategies.

REFERENCES

1. Kaufmann, S. H. E., 1994, Bacterial and protozoal infections in genetically disrupted mice. *Curr. Opin. Immunol.* **6:**518–525.
2. Galan, J. E., 1994, Interactions of bacteria with non-phagocytic cells, *Curr. Opin. Immunol.* **6:** 590–595.
3. Yamamoto, Y., Klein, T. W., and Friedman, H., 1996, Induction of cytokine granulocyte-macrophage colony-stimulating factor and chemokine macrophage inflammatory protein 2 mRNAs in macrophages by *Legionella pneumophila* or *Salmonella typhimurium* attachment requires different ligand-receptor systems, *Infect. Immun.* **64:**3062–3068.
4. Eckmann, L., Kagnoff, M. F., and Fierer, J., 1993, Epithelial cells secrete the chemokine interleukin-8 in response to bacterial entry, *Infect. Immun.* **61:**4569–4574.
5. Buchmeier, N. A., and Schreiber, R. D., 1985, Requirement of endogenous interferon-γ production for resolution of *Listeria monocytogenes* infection, *Proc. Natl. Acad. Sci. USA* **82:**7404–7408.
6. Nauciel, C., and Espinasse-Maes, F., 1992, Role of gamma interferon and tumor necrosis factor alpha in resistance to *Salmonella typhimurium* infection, *Infect. Immun.* **60:**450–454.
7. Harty, J. T., Lenz, L. L., and Bevan, M. J., 1996, Primary and secondary immune responses to *Listeria monocytogenes*, *Curr. Opin. Immunol.* **8:**526–530.
8. Springer, T. A., 1994, Traffic signals for lymphocyte recirculation and leukocyte emigration: The multistep paradigm, *Cell* **76:**301–314.
9. Conlan, J. W., 1997, Critical roles of neutrophils in host defense against experimental systemic infections of mice by *Listeria monocytogenes*, *Salmonella typhimurium*, and *Yersinia enterolitica*, *Infect. Immun.* **65:**630–635.
10. North, R. J., 1970, The relative importance of blood monocytes and fixed macrophages to the expression of cell-mediated immunity to infection, *J. Exp. Med.* **132:**521–534.
11. Bancroft, G., 1993, The role of natural killer cells in innate resistance to infection, *Curr. Opin. Immunol.* **5:**503–510.
12. Langermans, J. A. M., Van Der Hulst, M. E. B., Nibbering, P. H., and Van Furth, R., 1992,

Endogenous tumor necrosis factor alpha is required for enhanced antimicrobial activity against *Toxoplama gondii* and *Listeria monocytogenes* in recombinant gamma interferon-treated mice, *Infect. Immun.* **60:**5107–5112.

13. Vidal, S. M., Mallo, D., Vogan, K., Skamene, E., Gros, P., 1993, Natural resistance to infection with intracellular parasites: Isolatin of a candidate for *Bcg*, *Cell* **73:**469–485.

14. Mackaness, G. B., 1964, The immunological basis of acquired cellular resistance, *J. Exp. Med.* **120:**105–120.

15. Mackaness, G. B., 1969, The influence of immunologically committed lymphoid cells on macrophage activity *in vivo*, *J. Exp. Med.* **129:**973–992.

16. Kindler, V., Sappino, A. P., Grau, G. E., Piguet, P. F., and Vassalli, P., 1989, The inducing role of tumor necrosis factor in the development of bactericidal granulomas during BCG infection, *Cell* **56:**731–740.

17. Kaye, P. M., 1995, Costimulation and the regulation of antimicrobial immunity, *Immunol. Today,* **16:**423–427.

18. Campbell, K. A., Ovendale, P. J., Kennedy, M. Y., Fanslow, W. C., Reed, S. G., and Maliszewski, C. R., 1996, CD40 ligand is required for protective cell-mediated immunity to *Leishmania major, Immunity* **4:**283–289.

19. Mosmann, T. R., and Sad, S., 1996, The expanding universe of T-cell subsets: Th1, Th2 and more, *Immunol. Today,* **17:**138–146.

20. Nauciel, C., 1990, Role of CD4+ T cells and T-independent mechanisms in acquired resistance to *Salmonella typhimurium* infection. *J. Immunol.* **145:**1265–1269.

21. Yamamura, M., Uyemura, K., Deans, R. J., Weinberg, K., Rea, T. H., Bloom, B. R., and Modlin, R. L., 1991, Defining protective responses to pathogens: Cytokine profiles in leprosy lesions, *Science* **254:**277–279.

22. Gerosa, F., Paganin, C., Peritt, D., Paiola, F., Scupoli, M. T., Aste-Amezaga, M., Frank, I., and Trinchieri, G, 1996, Interleukin-12 primes human CD4 and CD8 T cell clones for high production of both interferon-γ and interleukin-10, *J. Exp. Med.* **183:**2559–2569.

23. Flynn, J. L., Goldstein, M. M., Triebold, K. L., Koller, B., and Bloom, B. R., 1992, Major histocompatibility complex class I-restricted T cells are required for resistance to *Mycobacterium tuberculosis* infection, *Proc. Natl. Acad. Sci. USA* **89:**12013–12017.

24. Rock, K. L., 1996, A new foreign policy: MHC class I molecules monitor the outside world, *Immunol. Today* **17:**131–137.

25. Kaufmann, S. H. E., 1995, Immunity to intracellular microbial pathogens, *Immunol. Today* **16:**338–342.

26. Chien, Y. H., Jores, R., and Crowley, M. P., 1996, Recognition by γ/δ T cells, *Annu. Rev. Immunol.* **145:**511–532.

27. Porcelli, S. A., Morita, C. T., and Modlin, R. L., 1996, T-cell recognition of nonpeptide antigens, *Curr. Opin. Immunol.* **8:**510–516.

28. Andersen, P., 1994, Effective vaccination of mice against *Mycobacterium tuberculosis* infection with a soluble mixture of secreted mycobacterial proteins, *Infect. Immunol.* **62:**2536–2544.

29. Nauciel, C., Ronco, E., Guenet, J. L., and Pla, M., 1998, Role of H-2 and non-H-2 genes in control of bacterial clearance from the spleen in *Salmonella typhimurium*-infected mice, *Infect. Immunol.* **56:**2407–2411.

30. Mastroeni, P., Villarreal-Ramos, B., and Hormaeche, C. E., 1993, Adoptive transfer of immunity to oral challenge with virulent salmonellae in innately susceptible BALB/c mice requires both immune serum and T cells, *Infect. Immun.* **61:**3981–3984.

31. Araya, L. N., Elzer, P. H., Rowe, G. E., Enright, F. M., and Winter, A. J., 1989, Temporal development of protective cell-mediated and humoral immunity in BALB/c mice infected with *Brucella abortus, J. Immunol.* **143:**3330–3337.

2

Genetic Regulation of Host Responses to *Salmonella typhimurium*

SALMAN T. QURESHI, EMIL SKAMENE, and DANIELLE MALO

1. INTRODUCTION

From birth, mammals live in a close yet generally imperceptible relationship with bacteria. Microorganisms that form the normal host flora serve a number of useful roles in maintaining a state of health by priming the immune system, participating in the breakdown and synthesis of nutrients, and preventing colonization by pathogens. Yet despite the seemingly beneficial or symbiotic nature of this relationship, organisms forming the indigenous flora as well as their pathogenic counterparts residing in the environment also pose a continuous challenge to the host. Even a brief period of uncontrolled growth within the host or spread of these organisms beyond normal anatomic boundaries may create a serious and imminent threat to its survival.

Of necessity, therefore, mammals have developed a sophisticated network of host defenses to provide constant surveillance against even the smallest threat of infection. This system is organized into two functional compartments: a series of rapidly acting antimicrobial mechanisms that form the "innate" or natural im-

DANIELLE MALO, SALMAN T. QURESHI, and EMIL SKAMENE • Departments of Medicine and Human Genetics, McGill University, and Centre for the Study of Host Resistance, Montreal General Hospital, Montreal, Quebec H3G 1A4 Canada.

Opportunistic Intracellular Bacteria and Immunity, edited by Lois J. Paradise *et al.* Plenum Press, New York, 1999.

mune response and an elaborate, diverse repertoire of effector lymphocytes that generate an adaptive immune response through clonal expansion.[1] These components serve distinct and highly complementary roles in protection of the host. Innate immune mechanisms are functional prior to the first encounter with an invader and protect the host in the earliest stages of infection through sensitive, nonspecific pathogen recognition mechanisms. This allows time for the generation of a slower, yet highly specific adaptive immune response that confers effective and long-lasting protection against reinfection through the production of antibodies and/or cytotoxic lymphocytes.

Progress toward understanding the basis of innate immunity has been facilitated through the study of mouse models of human infectious diseases, which have clearly demonstrated that such protection is under genetic control.[2] Naturally occurring variation in susceptibility to bacterial, viral, and parasitic infection among inbred strains of laboratory mice has been extensively studied during the past half century, leading to the description of numerous loci important to effective host defense.[3] One of the most well-characterized systems used for identification of such host resistance loci is murine infection with *Salmonella typhimurium*, a classic model of human typhoid fever. To date, five distinct loci *(Ity, Lps, xid, nu, H2)* have been described that influence the outcome of early (<10 days) or late-phase (>10 days) infection among inbred mouse strains. Until recently, limitations in the technology and resources for genomic analysis precluded the systematic identification of the genes encoded by these loci. Rapid advances in genetic and physical mapping techniques, large-capacity cloning vectors, and novel transcript identification techniques over the past several years have facilitated the definitive identification of three of these genes *(Nramp1* for *Ity, Btk* for *xid, Hfh11* for *nu)* and progress toward the characterization of *Lps* and members of the *H2* complex is well underway. Furthermore, studies of *Salmonella* infection in mice with specifically induced mutations have uncovered other genes such as nuclear protein interleukin (IL)-6 (IL-6)(Nfil6) that are critical to the complex network of robust host defense. In this chapter we review selected aspects of the genus *Salmonella*, describe the course of experimental murine infection with this agent, and give a detailed description of the host resistance loci that have been identified to date, including where applicable, information about the relevant gene. Finally, we discuss future prospects and directions for identification of other novel genes that participate in the host defense against *Salmonella* spp. and other opportunistic bacterial pathogens. Readers interested in the methodology and techniques of genetic analysis are referred to a recently published text[4] and reviews.[3,5]

2. DESCRIPTION OF THE PATHOGEN

Gram-negative bacilli of the genus *Salmonella* are ubiquitous in nature, inhabiting the gastrointestinal tracts of domesticated and wild mammals, reptiles, birds, and even insects.[6] They are effective pathogens, capable of producing a spectrum of clinical illness in both animals and man ranging from asymptomatic carriage to life-threatening sepsis. More than 2000 serotypes have been described through analysis of the cell wall and flagellar antigens; in the past each has been assigned a separate species designation. Current taxonomy based on DNA analysis recognizes all isolates as a single species, *Salmonella enterica*, with seven subgroup designations.[7] In the following discussion, we retain the traditional nomenclature as used by investigators in this research field.

Individual *Salmonella* serotypes exhibit different patterns of host specificity, some restricted to humans *(S. typhi, S. paratyphi)*, whereas others are more broadly adapted to both animals and humans *(S. typhimurium)*. Human infection occurs in two major patterns, a systemic disease known as enteric fever or a gastrointestinal illness termed salmonellosis. Other classic syndromes include bacteremia and vascular infection, a variety of focal extraintestinal infections, and a chronic carrier state. On a global scale, typhoid fever continues to be a major cause of morbidity and mortality; surveys by the World Health Organization Diarrheal Disease Control Program have estimated that approximately 12.5 million cases of typhoid fever occur annually.[8] Most of the disease burden is in areas of the world with inadequate human waste disposal facilities and lack of a clean water supply. In North America the incidence of typhoid fever has declined dramatically since 1920; fewer than 500 cases were reported in the United States during 1991 and most of these were related to foreign travel. Conversely, the incidence of reported nontyphoidal salmonellosis has increased dramatically since 1980. At present, up to 3.7 million cases of salmonellosis are estimated to occur annually in the United States.[9] Surveillance data from the United States Centers for Disease Control for 1993–94 indicates that *S. enteritidis* had become the most common serotype isolated, surpassing *S. typhimurium*.[10] Increasingly efficient multistate distribution of inadvertently contaminated food products such as ice cream has resulted in well-documented epidemics involving several hundred thousand people.[11]

3. RECOGNIZED HOST SUSCEPTIBILITY FACTORS

Host susceptibility factors have been observed mainly at the organ system level through studies of *Salmonella* infection in specific patient populations. Immaturity of immune function may explain why neonates are at high risk of infection and development of severe manifestations of disease including meningitis and septicemia.[12] Disruption of the normal gastrointestinal barrier at any of several sites, including reduction of gastric acidity, alteration of the normal intestinal flora, and chronic inflammatory or malignant bowel disease may predispose individuals to clinically significant disease from a smaller infectious dose.[13] Chronic asymptomatic carriage and fecal shedding is more frequent among those with anatomical or functional abnormalities of the biliary tract. *Salmonella* was the second most common cause of bacterial infection in a series of patients with chronic granulomatous disease[14] and is the most common cause of osteomyelitis among patients with sickle cell hemoglobinopathy.[15] Abnormalities of phagocytic function are characteristic of both of these inherited diseases. Deficient cell-mediated immunity associated with chronic lymphoproliferative disease, organ transplantation, and the acquired immune deficiency syndrome (AIDS) increases the risk of severe disease. North Americans with AIDS are at risk for severe, recurrent nontyphoidal *Salmonella* bacteremia[16] that may progress despite therapy; a similar increase in typhoid fever among HIV-infected persons from endemic areas has also been observed.[17] Finally, clustering of reactive *Salmonella*-triggered arthritis within families suggests that genetic factors may also play a role in the development of postinfectious sequelae.[18]

4. OVERVIEW OF EXPERIMENTAL INFECTION

Experimental primary infection of inbred strains of laboratory mice with *S. typhimurium* has been used extensively as a model of human typhoid fever. In contrast to natural infection where *Salmonella* must first overcome the antibacterial mechanisms of the gastrointestinal tract (low pH, competing bacterial flora, epithelial barriers, and lymphatic channels) to successfully establish systemic infection, in the experimental setting the route of acquisition is parenteral (intravenous, intraperitoneal, subcutaneous). Following bloodstream dissemination, however, the courses of natural and experimental infection are equivalent. Study of sublethal inocula of *S. typhi* in mice has led to the identification of four distinct phases of infection.[19] The first involves rapid (<2 after inoculation) clearance of the organism from the intravascular compartment mediated by complement and resident macrophages. The rate of organism clearance is dependent upon bacterial virulence factors and the presence or absence of preexisting antibody. A small fraction (10%) of the initial inoculum will survive and be localized to the liver and spleen within macrophages and polymorphonuclear leukocytes.[20] The bacteria that survive within this "safe site" of the reticuloendothelial system then divide exponentially for the first week after infection. The macrophage appears to exert an important regulatory function during this phase; administration of silica, a macrophage poison, greatly enhances bacterial growth.[21] At the completion of this phase, bacterial growth is halted by the macrophage, resulting in a plateau. Production of tumor necrosis factor (TNF) and interferon-γ (IFN-γ) are also required to establish and maintain the plateau phase; administration of neutralizing antibodies against either of these mediators enhances bacterial proliferation in the spleen, thereby converting a sublethal infection into a lethal one.[22] Finally, in the late phase, T lymphocytes mediate clearance of bacteria from the reticuloendothelial system.

Genetic variation in susceptibility of mice to lethal *Salmonella* infection has been recognized for more than 50 years. Through selective breeding, Webster was able to develop two outbred lines that differed in their resistance to experimental challenge with *Salmonella*.[2] Using a virulent clinical isolate of *S. typhimurium*, Robson and Vas[23] classified common inbred strains into three categories. Susceptible strains (C57BL/6J, BALB/cJ, and C3H/HeJ) uniformly succumbed in the first week after infection regardless of the inoculum size. One strain (DBA/2J) had intermediate susceptibility when challenged with lower inocula, surviving from 1 to 4 weeks, while another strain (A/J) could survive for at least 28 days with a challenge of $<10^4$ colony-forming units (CFUs) and was considered resistant. These differences were recognized to be under genetic control however, no specific loci were proposed as susceptibility candidates. Subsequent studies by several groups have revealed at least six distinct loci that exert an important influence on the course of experimental infection and are responsible for the observed differences among inbred strains. *Ity* (for immunity to *S. typhimurium*), *Lps* (lipopolysaccharide responsiveness), and *Nfil6* (nuclear protein Il-6) control the rate of exponential bacterial growth in the reticuloendothelial organs during phase 2 of experimental infection. Three other loci, *nu* (nude), *xid* (X-linked immunodeficiency), and certain *H2* (major histocompatibility complex) haplotypes act during the late phase of infection through their effects on the acquired immune response. In the following sections each of these genetic loci is described in greater detail along with a review of the evidence supporting their involvement in the host defense against *S. typhimurium*.

5. DESCRIPTION OF INDIVIDUAL HOST RESISTANCE LOCI

5.1. *Ity*

The mouse *Ity* locus is involved in the differential resistance/susceptibility of inbred strains of mice to infection with several *Salmonella* species including *S. typhimurium*, *S. enteritidis*, and *S. abortusovis*. the major effect of the *Ity* gene is to modulate the growth rate of *Salmonellae* in cells of the reticuloendothelial system (RES) during the early phase of infection. *Ity* is present in two allelic forms in inbred strains of mice: the resistance *(Ity^r)* and the susceptibility *(Ity^s)* alleles. Resistant and susceptible strains are distinguished by the kinetics of infection and by survival rate. The *Ity^s* allele causes a higher net growth rate of *Salmonellae* in the RES during the early nonimmune phase of infection (exponential growth) and decreases the LD_{50} after lethal challenge with a high dosage of *S. typhimurium*. Crosses between resistant and susceptible strains demonstrated that resistance segregates as a dominant single gene trait.[24] *Ity* (also named *Bcg* and *Lsh*) appears to control resistance to infection with other taxonomically and antigenically unrelated intracellular pathogens including *Mycobacterium bovis* (BCG), *M. lepraemurium*, *M. intracellulare (Bcg)*, and *Leishmania donovani (Lsh)*. Linkage studies in recombinant inbred strains of mice and segregation analysis in backcross progeny indicated that *Ity*, *Bcg*, and *Lsh* were either identical or very closely linked genes on mouse chromosome 1.[25]

In vivo and *in vitro* studies using bone marrow radiation chimeras and explanted cell populations have suggested that the mature tissue macrophage is the cell type expressing *Ity*, *Bcg*, and *Lsh*.[26-30] *Ity/Bcg/Lsh* has many pleiotropic effects on the macrophage including enhanced production of reactive oxygen and nitrogen intermediates, increased expression of surface activation markers (Ia and AcM.1) upon *in vitro* and *in vivo* stimulation with IFN-γ and BCG, upregulation of TNF production and increased IL-1β expression.[31] The exact mechanism responsible for enhanced cytocidal and/or cytostatic activity of the *Ity[r]* allele against *S. typhimurium* and other unrelated intracellular pathogens remains unknown but it is clear that *Ity/Bcg/Lsh* plays an important role in regulating macrophage functions that affect innate resistance to infection.

Nramp1 (for natural resistance-associated macrophage protein 1) was identified by positional cloning as a candidate for *Bcg*.[32] *Nramp1* is expressed exclusively in reticuloendothelial organs and in explanted macrophages derived from them and its expression can be modulated by treatment with lipopolysaccharide (LPS) and IFN-γ.[33] *Nramp1* encodes a novel integral membrane phosphoglycoprotein of apparent MW 90 to 100 kDa composed of 12 highly hydrophobic, putative transmembrane (TM) domains, a predicted extracellular glycosylated loop, several consensus sites for phosphorylation by protein kinase C, and a consensus transport motif known as the "binding-dependent inner membrane component transport signature" in the predicted intracytoplasmic loop linking TM8 and TM9.[32,34] This motif is present in a large number of prokaryotic periplasmic transport proteins and in a few eukaryotic membrane proteins, including CrnA (a nitrate concentrator of *Aspergillus*).[32] In addition, this region shares several conserved residues with a highly conserved region corresponding to the permeation pathway of animal voltage-gated potassium channels.[35]

Susceptibility to infection in inbred mice is caused by a single nonconservative glycine to aspartic acid substitution at position 169 within TM4 of Nramp1 protein.[32,36] Analysis of a total 27 *Bcg[r]* and *Bcg[s]* mouse strains for nucleotide sequence variations within the coding region of *Nramp1* has shown that Gly[169] was always associated with *Bcg[r]* and Asp[169] with *Bcg[s]* strains. Haplotype analysis of *Nramp1* and the region surrounding it indicated that the Gly[169] to Asp mutation occurred only once on a particular ancestral chromosome and that Gly[169] is the wild-type allele of *Nramp1*.[36] Gene knockout experiments were used to test directly whether *Nramp1* deficiency results in a Bacillus Calmette Guérin (BCG)-susceptible phenotype and to determine if *Bcg*, *Ity*, and *Lsh* are indeed the same gene.[37] Targeting of *Nramp1[Gly169]* abrogated resistance to infection with BCG, *S.*

typhimurium, and *L. donovani*, and therefore proved that *Nramp1*, *Bcg*, *Ity*, and *Lsh* are the same gene.[37] Mice homozygous for *Nramp1^Asp169* are equally susceptible to infection with *S. typhimurium* as *Nramp1^-/-*.[37] In fact, Nramp1 protein polypeptide is completely absent in macrophages from inbred mice homozygous for *Nramp1^Asp169*, which implies that the mutation causes a structural alteration that somehow prevents accumulation of the mature Nramp1 protein in macrophages.[34]

Nramp1 belongs to a small gene family with at least two other members in the mouse, *Nramp1-rs*,[38] which has been mapped to mouse chromosome 17, and *Nramp2*, on mouse chromosome 15.[39] *Nramp2* is expressed in all tissues, and encodes an integral membrane protein that shares 78% homology with *Nramp1*. In humans two *NRAMP* genes have been identified, *NRAMP1* on chromosome 2q[40] and *NRAMP2* on chromosome 12.[41] The highest level of human NRAMP1 expression is the peripheral blood leukocytes followed by the lungs and spleen.[40] Within the peripheral blood leukocyte population, *NRAMP1* is expressed in both polymorphonuclear leukocytes (PMNs) and monocytes however, the level of expression is higher in PMNs when compared to monocytes.[42] Sequence comparisons of the mouse and human Nramp1/NRAMP1 proteins revealed a very high degree of conservation between the two species (88% identity and 93% similarity), with the most conserved regions being the predicted TM domains and the intracellular loop containing the consensus sequence motif.

The pattern of *Nramp1/NRAMP1* gene expression and sequence analyses are indicative that Nramp1/NRAMP1 proteins may represent a new class of ubiquitous transporters or channels of professional phagocytes.[35] Recent studies have shown that Nramp1 protein is located within the plasma membrane of late endocytic vesicles of resting macrophages.[43] Upon phagocytosis, Nramp1 protein is recruited to the phagosome membrane and remains associated with this structure through it maturation into phagolysosome.[43] This observation supports a potential function for Nramp1 protein in controlling the replication of intracellular parasites by altering the intravacuolar environment of the phagosome containing microorganisms.

Homologues of *Nramp* have been identified in several phylogenically distant organisms including other mammalian species (cow, pig, rat, rabbit, sheep, etc.), birds, insects, plants, yeast, and bacteria.[35,43] Phylogenic analysis of these distantly related Nramp proteins has identified a common hydrophobic topology consisting of 10 TM domains with a very high degree of sequence homology including the predicted intracytoplasmic loop following TM8 (which might correspond to a functional transport motif).[35] Mutant phenotypes have been associated with some of these distantly related members of the *Nramp* family. In the chicken, *NRAMP1* is also expressed in reticuloendothelial organs (spleen and liver) and shows a high degree of amino acid sequence identity (68%) with mouse and human sequences. In addition, several promoter consensus elements such as the myeloid specific PU.1/Spi-1, IFN-γ-responsive elements, and binding sites for

NF-IL6 and NF-κB are present in chicken, mouse, and human promoters.[44] Taken together these data were suggestive that the NRAMP1 protein exerts similar roles *in vivo* both in mice and birds. In fact, allelic variation at *NRAMP1* has been associated with differential resistance/susceptibility of inbred chicken lines to infection with *S. typhimurium*.

In the fly *Drosophila melanogaster* and in the yeast *Saccharomyces cerevisiae*, null mutations have been created for homologues of *Nramp*. Mutations within *Drosophila Nramp* homolog named *malvolio (mlv)*, which is expressed in neurons and phagocytes and shares 70% amino acid identity with NRAMP1 or NRAMP2 proteins, are associated with a behavioral defect in taste discrimination.[45] In the yeast, *Nramp* homologs, *SMF1* and *SMF2*, show significant sequence homology (40% to 45% identity) with mammalian *NRAMP*. The yeast *SMF1* and *SMF2* genes were originally isolated in a genetic suppression assay devised to identify components of the import pathway of mitochondrial proteins. More recently, *SMF1* was identified in an assay for survival to lethal concentration of the metal chelating agent EGTA.[46] *SMF1* encodes for a plasma membrane protein and deletion of *SMF1* results in decreased cellular uptake of Mn^{2+} whereas overexpression of the gene leads to an increase in Mn^{2+} uptake by cells, suggesting a role of *SMF1* as a Mn^{2+} transporter. Finally, an *NRAMP* homologue that shares 37% identity with its mammalian counterpart was identified in *Mycobacterium leprae*.[35] Gros and colleagues proposed that the mammalian *NRAMP1* could antagonize the transport of a substrate (Mn^{2+} or other divalent cations) essential for intracellular survival of the bacterium into the phagosomes.[35,43] Mn^{2+} is an essential cofactor of superoxide dismutase (SOD), an enzyme that neutralizes reactive oxygen and nitrogen and that is present in the three pathogens *(S. typhimurium, M. bovis,* and *L. donovani)* known to be under the control of *Nramp1*.

5.2. Lps

The *Lps* locus was originally identified during studies of the sensitivity of five inbred mouse strains to the lethal effect of *in vivo* challenge with purified LPS.[47,48] The C3H/HeJ inbred strain was found to be naturally resistant to challenge with pure LPS derived from the outer membrane of several different Gram-negative bacteria, withstanding up to 40 times the lethal dose (LD_{50}) for other inbred strains. This phenotype was not observed in its progenitor strain, C3H/He, from which C3H/HeJ had been derived in 1947, nor was it present in closely related substrains such as C3H/HeN. Further *in vivo* and *in vitro* studies revealed that C3H/HeJ mice were hyporesponsive to many, if not all, of the immunostimulatory properties of LPS or its biologically active moiety, lipid A. A number of different cell types from these mice exhibit phenotypic hyporesponsiveness to LPS stimulation. C3H/HeJ splenocytes fail to mount an immune response or undergo polyclonal activation in response to *in vitro* stimulation with LPS and are unresponsive to its mitogenic and adjuvant properties.[49] C3H/HeJ fibroblasts show altered baseline glucose consumption and do not exhibit normal LPS-induced metabolic activation.[50] Most importantly, macrophages derived from C3H/HeJ mice have a defective activation phenotype and fail to differentiate to a fully competent state; as a result they are incapable of mediating the immunostimulatory properties of LPS. These defects include negligible LPS-stimulated secretion of several proinflammatory mediators including IL-1, IL-6, IL-12, TNF, IFN-γ, granulocyte-colony-stimulating factor (CSFG) and prostaglandin E_2, reduced *in vitro* tumoricidal capacity, impaired phagocytosis of IgG or C3 opsonized sheep erythrocytes and resistance to the lethal effect of high *in vitro* LPS concentrations. Through a formal backcross analysis and subsequent analysis of BXH recombinant inbred strains, control of B-cell LPS-responsiveness and other pleiotropic cellular phenotypes has been attributed to a single autosomal codominant gene that maps to mid-chromosome 4.[51] Two alleles have been assigned to the *Lps* gene, *Lps^n* (responsive) and *Lps^d* (hyporesponsive). It is believed that the recessive hyporesponsive allele of *Lps* arose through spontaneous mutation in the C3H/HeJ strain between 1960 and 1965. Two other mouse strains, C57B10/ScCR and its progenitor C57B10/ScN, were also characterized as LPS-hyporesponders and are phenotypically indistinguishable from the C3H/HeJ strain. The defect in both of these has also been mapped to chromosome 4, and F1 progeny from C3H/HeJ × C57B10/ScCR fail to exhibit complementation, suggesting that these mutations are within the same genetic locus.

Despite their natural resistance to purified bacterial LPS, C3H/HeJ mice are highly susceptible to lethal infection with *S. typhimurium*. The LD_{50} for C3H/HeJ mice with *S. typhimurium* is <2 organisms, while the LD_{50} for genetically related LPS-responsive strains such as C3H/HeN is >2 × 10^3 CFUs.[52] The death of C3H/HeJ mice following infection appears to result from an inability to restrict multiplication of the infecting organism in the RES of the mice, as measured by CFUs/g spleen tissue.[52] C3H/HeJ mice show a geometric increase in net bacterial growth beginning 72 h after infection and all died within 2 weeks, whereas LPS-responsive control mice show lower net bacterial growth with a plateau phase beginning 10 days after infection and all survive. Genetic linkage between LPS hyporesponsiveness and susceptibility to lethal infection with *Salmonella typhimurium* was studied using a panel of 27 backcross progeny. Although the cosegregation of these two traits was not exact in the original study, concordant inheritance was established in recombinant progeny from a total of 325 (DBA/2J × C3H/HeJ)F1 × C3H/HeJ backcross animals by successive phenotyping of LPS responsiveness and bacterial growth in the spleen,[53] supporting the hypothesis that *Lps* is a *Salmonella* susceptibility locus.

A great deal of effort has been made to understand the exact nature of the *Lps* defect by studying the normal pathway of LPS-induced cellular activation.[54] In the current model, LPS from the outer membrane of Gram-negative bacteria is bound by lipopolysaccharide binding protein (LBP), a 60-kDa glycoprotein synthesized in the liver. LBP is an acute phase reactant that is a member of a family of proteins that bind amphipathic molecules and transport them in aqueous environments. LBP functions by facilitating LPS binding to membrane CD14 (mCD14), a glycosylphosphatidylinositol (GPI)-anchored glycoprotein that is a major cellular receptor for LPS. A soluble form of CD14 (sCD14) is also present in plasma that delivers LPS to cells lacking mCD14, such as endothelium and B cells. The mechanism by which CD14 triggers ligand-specific cellular activation remains unclear, especially because GPI-anchored proteins lack a transmembrane domain and cannot directly communicate with the interior of the cell. Despite this incomplete understanding, the importance of this signaling pathway has been verified through gene-targeting; mice deficient in CD14 are resistant to lethal challenge with purified LPS and exhibit marked reduction in bacterial dissemination after parenteral infection.[55] Analysis of intracellular signaling pathways triggered by LPS–CD14 interactions have demonstrated the activation by phosphorylation of multiple MAP kinase-related families,[56] yet the events preceding these enzymatic cascades remain obscure.

The complexity and interrelated nature of these signaling pathways and pleiotropy of other LPS responses has thus far made it difficult to pinpoint the specific defect caused by the *Lps^d* allele. Therefore, an effort to identify the *Lps* gene by positional cloning has been initiated.[53] Using two panels of backcross mice segregating the defective *Lps* allele, a high-resolutin genetic map of mid-chromosome 4 has been constructed. The *Lps* gene has been localized to a 1.1cM interval, flanked proximally by a gene cluster *(Ambp, Tnc, Cd301)* and distally by a pair of microsatellite markers *(D4Mit7, D4Mit178)*. This region is homologous to human chromosome 9; a syntenic breakpoint exists in the vicinity of *Lps*, indicating that the human homologue may be located near either 9p22-pter or 9q33–9q34. Current efforts are underway to further narrow this genetic interval and generate a physical map of the chromosomal region to precisely identify the *Lps* gene.

5.3. NF-IL-6

Nuclear protein (NF-IL-6) is a member of the CCAAT enhancer-binding protein (C/EBP) family of basic-leucine zipper transcription factors.[57] It was originally described as a nuclear factor that binds to the IL-1 response element of the human IL-6 gene, and subsequently identified as a transcriptional activator of a variety of genes. High expression levels of NF-IL-6 are observed during macrophage activation and NF-IL-6 binding motifs are found in the functional regulatory regions of genes specifically induced in activated macrophages including *Il6*, *Il1*, *Il8*, *Tnf*, *Csfg*, *Nos*, and lysozyme. It is therefore believed that this transcription factor is necessary for the coordinate expression of a group of genes that specifically participate in macrophage activation and differentiation.

Mice that have been rendered deficient in *NfιIl6* are highly susceptible to lethal infection with *S. typhimurium* compared to controls (LD$_{50}$: 1 × 10^4 CFUs vs. 3 × 10^5 CFUs, respectively).[57] Death following experimental infection all occurred within 6 days; a similar susceptibility pattern was observed after experimental infection with 5 × 10^2 CFUs of *Listeria monocytogenes*. Impaired macrophage bactericidal capacity secondary to defective transcriptional activation was proposed to account for the findings, although the exception of *Csfg*, expression levels of all other inflammatory cytokines measured, including IFN-γ and TNF, were unchanged. Further investigation including a search for other genes under the regulation of *NfιIl6* will be required to explain the mechanism of susceptibility in these knockout mice.

5.4. *xid*

The role of intact humoral immunity in resistance to the late stage of experimental *Salmonella* infection has been studied using the CBA/N inbred mouse strain. CBA/N mice carry an X-linked immunodeficiency mutation *(xid)* characterized by defects in peripheral B-cell activation and function.[58] The bone marrow of these mice has normal numbers of pro-B and pre-B cells while the peripheral B-cell pool is reduced. Those B cells that are present have an immature surface marker phenotype including a reduced number of complement receptors and high surface IgM to IgD ratio. B-cell proliferation triggered through the surface IgM receptor is impaired as is the response to LPS, IL-5, IL-10, CD38, and CD40 ligand. Consistent with these cellular abnormalities, CBA/N mice have low serum IgM and IgG$_3$ levels and are unable to mount an antibody response to polysaccharide antigens or hapten–polysaccharide conjugates. T-cell function as measured by skin graft rejection, proliferative response to Concanavalin A, or *in vitro* cellular cytotoxicity is preserved.

Infectious challenge of CBA/N mice with *S. typhimurium* demonstrated marked susceptibility relative to their immunologically normal progenitor strain, CBA/CaHN (LD$_{50}$ 20 CFUs vs. LD$_{50}$ 2 × 10^4 CFUs at 28 days, respectively).[59] Inheritance of the susceptibility trait is X-linked and recessive, affecting hemizygous males and female mice homozygous for the defective *xid* allele. B lymphocytes from heterozygous females exhibit preferential inactivation of the chromosome carrying the defective *xid* allele, thereby creating a normal phenotype. Linkage of *xid* with *Salmonella* susceptibility was suggested by experiments using backcross and F2 progeny derived from CBA/N and DBA/2N parental strains. The X-linked susceptibility phenotype was not observed early (<10 days) after infection, indicating that functional expression of *xid* occurs primarily during the late phase. Impaired generation of IgG anti-*Salmonella* antibodies by *xid* male mice appears to confer susceptibility; passive transfer of immune serum from heterozygous female mice increased their resistance, whereas serum that had been preabsorbed with the bacterium was ineffective. Other measures of impaired immune function among susceptible male mice including quantitation of early net bacterial growth in the spleen or the absence of a delayed-type hypersensitivity response to *Salmonella* were not observed.[60]

Positional cloning and a candidate gene approach disclosed the genetic basis of *xid* and its human counterpart, X-linked agammaglobulinemia (XLA).[61-63] The defective gene, named *Btk* (Bruton agammaglobulinemia tyrosine kinase), encodes a cytoplasmic tyrosine kinase with significant similarity to a subfamily of the *src* nonreceptor kinases including Tec II, Itk, Txk, and Bmx. In the C-terminus Btk contains a catalytic Src-homology 1 (SH1) domain; the N-terminus contains an SH2 and and SH3 domain that interact with motifs containing phosphotyrosine and proline, respectively as well as two domains of unknown function designated pleckstrin homology (PH) and tec homology (TH). Btk is expressed at all stages of B-cell development but is found at negligible levels in T cells and is specifically downregulated in plasma cells. Like other tyrosine kinases, Btk is presumed to mediate intracellular signal transduction but is precise role in B-cell development has not yet been defined.

In mouse, *Btk* and *xid* were mapped to the same genetic interval in two independent backcross panels.[64,65] Sequence analysis revealed a cytosine to thymidine transition at position 219 that resulted in an Arg^{28} to Cys^{28} substitution in the N-terminal region of Btk outside of the known functional domains. *Btk* expression levels in resting B cells or those stimulated with IL-4 or LPS are equivalent in CBA/N mice compared to CBA/CaHN; therefore, a functional alteration of the Btk unique region is hypothesized to disrupt the signaling pathway of normal B cell development in mutant mice. Targeted disruption of *Btk* has also been achieved by two groups;[66,67] complete absence of expression decreases the expansion of B-cell progenitors and reproduces the naturally occurring *xid* phenotype.

In human XLA, two sequential steps of normal B-cell growth and development within the marrow are interrupted, resulting in severely reduced B-cell numbers in the peripheral blood and lymphoid organs compared to *xid*. Pro-B cells, the earliest recognizable precursor committed to the B-cell lineage, generate reduced numbers of next stage pre-B cells. Development beyond the pre-B-cell stage is also blocked, resulting in virtually no mature B cells. The original mutation described in XLA was a missense mutation in the BTK kinase domain; since then more than 175 different mutations involving all parts of the gene have been recorded in a database (Btkbase).[61] Correlation of a specific mutation with a functional abnormality or clinical phenotype has not been possible, and is complicated by the variable disease severity observed within families with XLA. The spectrum of infections in patients with XLA is also more diverse than in mouse. Bacterial infections involving the respiratory tract are the most frequent and are usually due to encapsulated organisms that require opsonization for efficient clearance, such as *Streptococcus pneumoniae*, *Haemophilus influenzae*, *Staphylococcus aureus and Pseudomonas* spp. Intestinal infections with a variety of organisms including *Salmonella* sp. and refractory disease due to *Campylobacter jejuni* have also been described. Resistance to other classes of pathogens including viruses is generally intact in patients with XLA, with the exception of the enteroviruses (poliovirus, echovirus, coxsackie virus). These infect patients via the gastrointestinal tract and then may disseminate to secondary targets via the bloodstream. Because neutralization by antibody is important during intravascular transit, untreated XLA patients may develop chronic, disseminated infection with these agents. Based on knowledge of this genetic defect carrier detection and prenatal diagnosis of XLA are now possible. Prophylaxis of infection with intravenous immunoglobulin and appropriate treatment with antibiotics have markedly improved the long-term prognosis of these patients.[61]

5.5. *nu*

The role of T lymphocytes in the control of *Salmonella* infection during both the early and late phases of experimental infection in the mouse has been facilitated by use of the nude *(nu / nu)* mouse mutant.[68] Nude mice (and rats) have a pleiotropic phenotype characterized by congenital lack of hair and athymia, due to a spontaneous recessive mutation at a single locus on chromosome 11. Hair follicles are normal at birth yet undergo faulty keratinization, producing the hairlessness. The thymic defect results from a failure of normal ectodermal proliferation, resulting in a rudimentary organ with undifferentiated stroma that cannot attract T-lymphocyte precursors. As a result, these mice have a profoundly reduced lymphocyte population composed almost entirely of B cells. With a virtual absence of cell-mediated immunity they are incapable of allogeneic graft rejection and are profoundly susceptible to infection with a variety of pathogens.

Participation of T cells in the regulation of *Salmonella* growth during the early phase of experimental infection was studied by intravenous challenge of CD1, CD1 *nu / nu* mice and heterozygous CD1 *nu / +* littermate controls with *S. typhimurium*.[26] No significant difference in kinetics of *S. typhimurium* growth in the spleen or liver were observed among the three genotypes during the first 10 days, indicating that T cells are not required for early-stage host defense. Nevertheless by day 17, CD1 *nu / nu* mice began to die, and all succumbed by day 26. None of the CD1 *nu / +* died, suggesting that the nude phenotype is relevant to late-stage immunity against *Salmonella*. Confirmation that early suppression of *Salmonella* is independent of T cells was found using an acute depletion model.[69] In this system, irradiated mice were reconstituted with T-cell-depleted marrow and then treated with anti-CD4 and anti-CD8 monoclonal antibodies. Both controls and animals lacking functional T lymphocytes were able to suppress bacterial growth in the liver and spleen one week after sublethal challenge and go on to the plateau phase of infection.

More detailed investigation of the role of CD4[+] and CD8[+] T lymphocytes in defense against a temperature-sensitive mutant of *S. typhimurium* (C5TS) was carried out using depletion and adoptive transfer experiments.[70] Administration of monoclonal antibodies against CD4 resulted in a significant increase in the number of bacteria in the spleen of BALB/c mice on day 21 compared to controls, suggesting that these cells are involved in clearance of the organism during the late phase. Treatment with anti-CD8 also caused a smaller rise in the same parameter. Simultaneous adoptive transfer of immune spleen cells with *Salmonella* challenge reduced the splenic bacterial load beginning 6 days after infection in naive recipients; this effect was eliminated by pretreatment of donor cells with anti-CD4 or anti-CD8, suggesting that both subsets play a role in acquired resistance to *S. typhimurium.* Finally, athymic *(nu/nu)* mice challenged with the C5TS strain showed lower spleen counts relative to euthymic controls during the first week after infection; this reversed during the subsequent 2 weeks, again suggesting that T cells are involved in control of the late stage of infection.

The nude locus (*Hfh11* for hepatocyte nuclear factor-3/forkhead homolog 11) has been identified in mouse and rat using a positional cloning approach.[71] *Hfh11* was mapped to mouse chromosome 11 and the homologous region of the rat genome on chromosome ten.[68] The nude gene is a member of the winged-helix domain family of transcription factors, named for a structural motif of the DNA binding domain as determined by X-ray crystallographic analysis.[72] Members have been identified in yeast *Drosophila* and vertebrates including rat, mice, frogs, and humans. All of these proteins are characterized by a highly conserved region of 100 amino acids which appears to be necessary and sufficient for site-specific DNA binding; approximately half of the residues in this domain are conserved in all family members. *In situ* hybridization and antibody studies have suggested wide-ranging roles for various members of the family during development; the first member to be identified was a *Drosophila* nuclear protein termed forkhead, named because mutant embryos were defective in the formation of terminal structures that normally give rise to the anterior and posterior gut, resulting in two spiked head structures. In the adult this family of proteins has a limited tissue distribution and is involved in cell-specific regulation of gene expression.

Sequence analysis of the eight coding exons and flanking intron sequence from wild-type C57BL/6J mice and the congenic strain C57BL/6J/Han carrying the original nude allele showed a single base-pair (G) deletion in exon 3, causing a frameshift terminating in exon 6.[71] The resulting aberrant protein does not contain the DNA-binding domain essential for function. Reverse-transcription–polymerase chain reaction studies in normal mice show skin and thymus-specific expression patterns consistent with the observed phenotype. Embryonic expression is evident by day 9, the time when thymic stroma undergoes differentiation into cortical and medullary compartments. Analysis of the rat nude allele showed a nonsense mutation at bp 1429, also preventing production of functional protein containing the DNA binding domain. These mutations in the mouse and rat are analogous to mutations in the *Drosophila* forkhead gene that result in a complete loss of function phenotype.

5.6. *H2*

The major histocompatibility complex of mouse (MHC, also named *H2*) on chromosome 17 contains a series of closely linked genes that have a central role in tissue graft rejection and control of the cellular interactions responsible for immune responses. These loci play a critical role in restriction of immune responses to foreign antigen-presenting cells for recognition by the T cell receptor of CD4$^+$ or CD8$^+$ lymphocytes. Genes of the MHC are among the most highly polymorphic loci known and have codominant expression, attributes that allow efficient presentation of peptides from a broad range of different infectious agents that themselves exhibit polymorphism.studies have implicated *H2* in resistance to *Toxoplasma gondii*, *Mycobacterium lepraemurium*, and *L. donovani* in mouse, as well as severe *Plasmodium falciparum* infection in humans.[73]

Late susceptibility to infection with *S. typhimurium* of intermediate virulence and its association with *H2* was studied in C57BL/10 congenic lines carrying the *Nramp1^s* allele.[74] Inbred mouse strains carrying the *H2^b* and *H2^d* haplotypes were more susceptible (LD^{50}<10^3 CFU) than those carrying the *H2^a*, *H2^k*, and *H2^f* haplotypes (LD$_{50}$≥10^4 CFUs). Backcross studies to each parental strain of F1 progeny derived from *H2^b* and *H2^f* congenics showed codominant inheritance more closely resembling the resistant phenotype. Susceptibility of backcross mice with the *H2^{b/b}* haplotype was apparent 4 weeks after infection, with maximum differences at 7 to 8 weeks. Using several congenic strains with recombinant *H2* haplotypes, susceptibility was mapped to the I-Eα subregion. Study of the kinetics of infection among susceptible *(H2^b)* and resistant *(H2^k)* C57BL/10 congenic strains revealed 10- to 100-fold higher viable bacterial counts in the spleen and liver of susceptible animals 3 weeks after infection that persisted for the duration of observation (10 weeks). Spleen weight in susceptible mice was more than double that in resistant animals and weight increase persisted for twice as long before declining. The observed differences in mortality and bacterial load in the reticuloendothelial organs were attributed to differences in development of a cell-mediated immune response although no specific mechanism was proposed.

In another series of experiments using *S. typhimurium* C5TS, three phenotypic groups were observed by comparison of late bacterial clearance among *H2* congenic mice on a C57BL/10 genetic background.[75] The lowest rate of bacterial clearance was observed in *H2^b*; intermediate clearance in *H2^d*, *H2^f*, *H2^k*, *H2^p*, *H2^r*, *H2^s*, and *H2^v*; and high clearance in *H2^j*, *H2^q*, and *H2^u*. The influence of the *H2* haplotype on low *(H2^b)* and high *(H2^k)* clearance was apparent although influenced by different genetic backgrounds. The overall conclusion from these results was that although certain *H2* haplotypes such as *H2^b* confer late-phase susceptibility, several non-*H2*-linked genes must also participate in the clearance of *Salmonella*. Further analysis using *H2* recombinant congenic mice on a C57BL/10 genetic background suggested that at least two regions of the *H2* complex, D and K-Aα, are involved in determining the late clearance phenotype.[76] The mechanisms by which *H2*-linked genes influence host responses to infectious agents remain an area in need of further investigation. The inherent complexity and polymorphism of *H2* will continue to pose a formidable challenge to investigators attempting to define specific susceptibility candidates using conventional genetic approaches.

6. CONCLUSION

Knowledge of the host genes governing susceptibility or resistance to infection with a particular pathogen is as fundamental to the understanding of infectious disease pathogenesis as the study of microbial virulence factors. As a group, microbes may be regarded as having the most intimate understanding of host defense mechanisms.[77] Many successful pathogens, including *Salmonella*, have developed means to subvert or employ host defenses to create their own survival advantage. Our challenge is also to uncover the spectrum of molecular mechanisms that have evolved to maintain the integrity of the host and use the knowledge to ensure a healthy state. In the foreseeable future, advances in whole-genome genetic and physical maps as well as large-scale production of expressed sequence tags will put a wealth of genetic information at our disposal. This, coupled with accelerating production of single and multiple knockout mice, will help establish the relationships among various host resistance genes.[78] Defining the physiologic role of each of these factors is the next step, and will surely assume increasing importance in the future study of host resistance.

In this chapter, we have summarized the advances that have come about through the study of a single model of host–pathogen interaction. The knowledge derived from these studies will have applications that go beyond the model organism, *Salmonella typhimurium*. Genes such as *Nramp1* clearly demonstrate that each host defense factor participates in the control and elimination of many different pathogens undoubtedly many more than we currently appreciate. Ultimately, elucidating the function of these genes will give us a better insight and better means of prevailing in the molecular battle waged between host and pathogen.

REFERENCES

1. Nathan, C., 1995, Natural resistance and nitric oxide, *Cell* **82:**873–876.
2. Rosenstreich, D. L., Weinblatt, A. C., and O'Brien, A. D., 1982, Genetic control of resistance to infection in mice, in: *CRC Critical Reviews in Immunology*, **3:**263–330.

3. Malo, D., and Skamene, E., 1994, Genetic control of host resistance to infection, *Trends Genet.* **10:**365–371.
4. Silver, L. M., 1995, *Mouse Genetics*, Oxford University Press, New York.
5. Nadeau, J. H., Arbuckle, L. D., and Skamene, E., 1995, Genetic dissection of inflammatory responses, *J. Inflamm.* **45:**27–48.
6. Miller, S. I., Hohmann, E. L., and Pegues, D. A., 1995, *Salmonella* (including *Salmonella typhi*), in *Principles and Practice of Infectious Disease*, 4th Ed. (G. E. Mandell, J. E. Bennett, and R. Dolin, eds.), Churchill Livingston, New York, pp. 2013–2033.
7. Gray, L. D., 1995, *Escherichia, Salmonella, Shigella and Yersinia*, in: *Manual of Clinical Microbiology*, 6th Ed. (P. R. Murray, E. J. Baron, M. A. Pfaller, F. C. Tenover, and R. H. Yolken, eds.), ASM Press, Washington D.C., pp. 450–456.
8. Edelman, R., and Levine, M. M., 1986, Summary of an international workshop on typhoid fever, *Rev. Infect. Dis.* **8:**329–349.
9. Chalker, R. B., and Blaser, M. J., 1988, A review of human salmonellosis III: Magnitude of *Salmonella* infection in the United States, *Rev. Infect. Dis.* **10:**111–124.
10. Centers for Disease Control and Prevention, 1995, *Salmonella* surveillance: Annual tabulations summary, 1993–1994, Atlanta.
11. Hennessy, T. W., Hedberg, C. W., Slutsker, L., White, K. E., Besser-Wiek, J. M., Moen, M. E., Feldman, J., Coleman, W. W., Edmonson, L. E., MacDonald, K. L., and Osterholm, M. T., 1996, A national outbreak of *Salmonella enteritidis* infections from ice cream, *N. Engl. J. Med.* **334:**1281–1286.
12. Butler, T., Islam, A., Kabir, I., and Jones, P. K., 1991, Patterns of morbidity and mortality in typhoid fever dependent on age and gender: Review of 552 hospitalized patients with diarrhea, *Rev. Infect. Dis.* **13:**85–90.
13. Pavia, A. T., Shipman, L. D., Wells, J. G., Puhr, N. D., Smith, J. D., McKinley, T. W., and Tauxe, R. V., 1990, Epidemiologic evidence that prior antimicrobial resistance decreases resistance to infection by antimicrobial-sensitive *Salmonella*, *J. Infect. Dis.* **161:**255–260.
14. Mouy, R., Fischer, A., Vimer, E., Seger, R., and Griscelli, C., 1988, Incidence, severity, and prevention of infections in chronic granulomatous disease, *J. Pediatr.* **114:**555–560.
15. Diggs, L. W., 1967, Bone and joint lesions in sickle cell disease, *Clin. Orthop.* **52:**119–143.
16. Levine, W. C., Beuhler, J. W., Bean, N. H., and Tauxe, R. V., 1991, Epidemiology of nontyphoidal *Salmonella* bacteremia during the human immunodeficiency virus epidemic, *J. Infect. Dis.* **164:**81–87.
17. Gutozzo, E., Frisancho, O., Sanchez, J., Liendo, G., Carrillo, D., Black, R. E., and Morris, J. G., 1991, Association between the acquired immunodeficiency syndrome and infection with *Salmonella typhi* or *Salmonella paratyphi* in an endemic typhoid area, *Arch. Intern. Med.* **151:**381–382.
18. Aragon, A., and Perez-Navarro, A. D., 1996, Familial *Salmonella*-triggered reactive arthritis, *Br. J. Rheum.* **35:**908–912.
19. Mastroeni, P., Harrison, J. A, and Hormaeche, C. E., 1994, Natural resistance and acquired immunity to *Salmonella*, *Fund. Clin. Immunol.* **2:**83–95.
20. Dunlap, N. E., Benjamin, W. H., Berry, A. K., Eldridge, J. H., and Briles, D. E., 1992, A "safe site" for *Salmonella typhimurium* is within splenic polymorphonuclear cells, *Microb. Pathogen.* **13:**181–190.
21. O'Brien, A. D., Scher, I., and Formal, S. B., 1979, Effect of silica on the innate resistance of inbred mice to *Salmonella typhimurium* infection, *Infect. Immun.* **25:**513–520.
22. Nauciel, C., and Espinasse-Mase, F., 1992, Role of gamma interferon and tumor necrosis factor alpha in resistance to *Salmonella typhimurium* infection, *Infect. Immun.* **60:**450–454.
23. Robson, H. G., and Vas, S. I., 1972, Resistance of inbred mice to *Salmonella typhimurium*, *J. Infect. Dis.* **126:**378–386.

24. Plant, J. E., and Glynn, A., 1976, Genetics of resistance to infection with *Salmonella typhimurium* in mice, *J. Infect. Dis.* **133:**72–78.
25. Skamene, E., Gros, P., Forget, A., Kongshavn, P. A. L., St-Charles, C., and Taylor, B. A., 1982, Genetic regulation of resistance to intracellular pathogens, *Nature* **297:**506–509.
26. O'Brien, A. D. and Metcalf, E. S., 1982, Control of early *Salmonella typhimurium* growth in innately *Salmonella*-resistant mice does not require functional T lymphocytes, *J. Immunol.* **129:**1349–1351.
27. Gros, P., Skamene, E., and Forget, A., 1983, Cellular mechanisms of genetically controlled host resistance to *Mycobacterium bovis* (BCG), *J. Immunol.* **133:**1966–1972.
28. Lissner, C. R., Swanson, R. N., and O'Brien, A. D., 1983, Genetic control of the innate resistance of mice to *Salmonella typhimurium:* Expression of the *Ity* gene in peritoneal and splenic macrophages isolated *in vitro*, *J. Immunol.* **131:**3006–3013.
29. Stach, J. L., Gros, P., Forget, A., and Skamene, E., 1984, Phenotypic expression of genetically controlled natural resistance to *Mycobacterium bovis* (BCG), *J. Immunol.* **132:**888–892.
30. Olivier, M., and Fernes, C. E., 1987, Susceptibilities of macrophage populations to infection *in vitro* by *Leishmania donovani*, *Infect. Immun.* **55:**467–471.
31. Buschman, E., Taniyama, T., Nakamura, R., and Skamene, E., 1989, Functional expression of the *Bcg* gene in macrophages, *Res. Immunol.* **140:**793–797.
32. Vidal, S., Malo, D., Vogan, K., Skamene, E., and Gros, P., 1993, Natural resistance to infection with intracellular parasites: Isolation of a candidate gene for *Bcg*, *Cell* **73:**469-485.
33. Govoni, G., Vidal, S., Cellier, M., Lepage, P., Malo, D., and Gros, P., 1995, Structural organization and cell specific expression of the mouse *Nramp1* gene, *Genomics* **27:**9–19.
34. Vidal, S. M., Pinner, E., Lepage, P., Gauthier, S., and Gros, P., 1996, Natural resistance to intracellular infections—*Nramp1* encodes a membrane phosphoglycoprotein absent in macrophages from susceptible mouse strains, *J. Immunol.* **157:**3559–3568.
35. Cellier, M., Belouchi, A., and Gros, P., 1996, Resistance to intracellular infections: Comparative genomic analysis of *Nramp*, *Trends Genet.* **12:**201–204.
36. Malo, D., Vogan, K., Vidal, S., Hu, J., Cellier, M., Schurr, E., Fuks, A., Bumstead, N., Morgan, K., and Gros, P., 1994, Haplotype mapping and sequence analysis of the mouse *Nramp* gene predict susceptibility to infection with intracellular parasites, *Genomics* **23:**51–61.
37. Vidal, S., Tremblay, M. L., Govoni, G., Gauthier, S., Sebastiani, G., Malo, D., Skamene, E., Olivier, M., Jothy, S., and Gros, P., 1995, The *Ity/Lsh/Bcg* locus: Natural resistance to infection with intracellular parasites is abrogated by disruption of the *Nramp1* gene, *J. Exp. Med.* **182:**655–666.
38. Dosik, J. K., Barton, C. H., Holiday, D. L., Krall, M. M., Blackwell, J. M., and Mock, B. A., 1994, An *Nramp*-related sequence maps to mouse chromosome 17, *Mamm. Genome* **5:**458–460.
39. Gruenheid, S., Cellier, M. Vidal, S., and Gros, P., 1995, Identification and characterization of a second mouse *Nramp* gene, *Genomics* **25:**514–525.
40. Cellier, M., Govoni, G., Vidal, S., Kwan, T., Groulx, N., Liu, J., Sanchez, F., Skamene, E., Schurr, E., and Gros, P., 1994, Human natural resistance-associated macrophage protein: cDNA cloning, chromosomal mapping, genomic organization, and tissue-specific expression, *J. Exp. Med.* **180:**1741–1752.
41. Vidal, S., Belouchi, A. -M., Cellier, M., Beatty, B., and Gros, P., 1995, Cloning and characterization of a second human *NRAMP* gene on chromosome 12q13, *Mamm. Genome* **6:**224–230.
42. Cellier, M., Shustik, C., Dalton, W., Rich, E., Hu, J., Malo, D., Schurr, E., and Gros, P., 1996, The human *NRAMP1* gene as a marker of professional primary phagocytes: Studies in blood cells, and in HL-60 promyelocytic leukemia, *J. Leuk. Biol.* **61:**96–105.
43. Gruenheid, S., Pinner, E., Desjardins, M., and Gros, P., 1997, Natural resistance to infection with intracellular pathogens—the *Nramp1* protein is recruited to the membrane of the phagosome, *J. Exp. Med.* **185:**717–730.
44. Hu, J., Bumstead, N., Skamene, E., Gros, P., and Malo, D., 1996, Structural organization,

sequence and expression of the chicken *NRAMP1* gene encoding the natural resistance associated macrophage protein 1, *DNA Cell Biol.* **15:**113–123.

45. Rodrigues, V., Cheah, P. Y., Ray, K., and Chia, W., 1995, *Malvolio,* the *Drosophila* homologue of mouse *Nramp-1 (Bcg)* is expressed in macrophages and in the nervous system and is required for normal taste behavior, *EMBO J.* **14:**3007–3020.

46. Supek, F., Supekova, L., Nelson, H., and Nelson, N., 1996, A yeast manganese transporter related to the macrophage protein involved in conferring resistance to mycobacteria. *Proc. Natl. Acad. Sci. USA* **93:**5105–5110.

47. Rosenstreich, D. L., 1985, Genetic control of endotoxin response: C3H/HeJ mice, in: *Handbook of endotoxin,* Vol. 3: *Cellular Biology of Endotoxin* (L. J. Berry, ed.), Elsevier Science, Amsterdam, pp. 82–122.

48. Vogel, S. N., 1992, The *Lps* gene: Insights into the genetic and molecular basis of LPS responsiveness and macrophage differentiation, in: *Tumor Necrosis Factors: The Molecules and Their Emerging Role in Medicine* (B. Beutler, ed.), Raven Press, New York, pp. 485–513.

49. Skidmore, B. J., Chiller, J. M., Morrison, D. C., and Weigle, W. O., 1975, Immunologic properties of bacterial lipopolysaccharide (LPS): Correlation between the mitogenic, adjuvant, and immunogenic activities, *J. Immunol.* **114:**770–775.

50. Ryan, J. L., and McAdam, K. P. W. J., 1977, Genetic non-responsiveness of murine fibroblasts to bacterial endotoxin, *Nature* **269:**153–155.

51. Watson, J., Riblet, R., and Taylor, B., 1978, The genetic mapping of a defective LPS response gene in C3H/HeJ mice, *J. Immunol.* **120:**422–424.

52. O'Brien, A. D., Rosenstreich, D. L., Scher, I., Campbell, G. H., MacDermott, R. P., and Formal, S. B., 1980, Genetic control of susceptibility to *Salmonella typhimurium* in mice: Role of the *Lps* gene, *J. Immunol.* **124:**20–24.

53. Qureshi, S. T., Larivière, L., Sebastiani, G., Clermont, S., Skamene, E., Gros, P., and Malo, D., 1996, A high-resolution map in the chromosomal region surrounding the *Lps* locus, *Genomics* **31:**283–294.

54. Ulevitch, R. J., and Tobias, P. S., 1995, Receptor-dependent mechanisms of cell stimulation by bacterial endotoxin, *Annu. Rev. Immunol.* **13:**437–457.

55. Haziot, A., Ferrero, E., Köntgen, F., Hijiya, N., Yamamoto, S., Silver, J., Stewart, C. L., and Goyert, S., 1996, Resistance to endotoxin shock and reduced dissemination of gram-negative bacteria in CD14-deficient mice, *Immunity* **4:**407–414.

56. Sanghera, J. S., Weinstein, S. L., Aluwalia, M., Girn, J., and Pelech, S. L., 1996, Activation of multiple proline-directed kinases by bacterial lipopolysaccharide in murine macrophages, *J. Immunol.* **156:**4457–4465.

57. Tanaka, T., Akira, S., Yoshida, K., Umemoto, M., Yoneda, Y., Shirafuji, N., Fujiwara, H., Suematsu, S., Yoshida, N., and Kishimoto, T., 1995, Targeted disruption of the *NF-IL6* gene discloses its essential role in bacteria killing and tumor cytotoxicity by macrophages, *Cell* **80:**353–361.

58. Scher, I., 1982, The CBA/N mouse strain: An experimental model illustrating the influence of the X-chromosome on immunity, *Adv. Immunol.* **33:**1–71.

59. O'Brien, A. D., Scher, I., Campbell, G. H., MacDermott, G. H., and Formal, S. B., 1979, Susceptibility of CBA/N mice to infection with *Salmonella typhimurium:* Influence of the X-linked gene controlling B lymphocyte function, *J. Immunol.* **123:**720–724.

60. O'Brien, A. D., Scher, I., and Metcalf, E., 1981, Genetically-conferred defect in anti-*Salmonella* antibody formation renders CBA/N mice innately susceptible to *Salmonella typhimurium* infection, *J. Immunol.* **126:**1368–1372.

61. Ochs, H. D., and Edvard Smith, D. I., 1996, X-linked agammablobulinemia. A clinical and molecular analysis, *Medicine* **75:**287–299.

62. Vetrie, D., Vorechovsky, I., Sideras, P., Holland, J., Davies, A., Flinter, F., Hammarström, L.,

Kinnon, C., Levinsky, R., Bobrow, M., Edvard Smith, C. I., and Bentley, D. R., 1993, The gene involved in X-linked agammaglobulinemia is a member of the *src* family of protein-tyrosine kinases, *Nature* **361:**226–233.

63. Tsukada, S., Saffran, D. C., Rawlings, D. J., Parolini, O., Allan, R. C., Klisak, I., Sparkes, R. S., Kubagawa, H., Mohandas, T., Quan, S. Belmont, J. W., Cooper, M. D., Conley, M. E., and Witte, O. N., 1993, Deficient expression of a B cell cytoplasmic tyrosine kinase in human X-linked agammaglobulinemia, *Cell* **72:**279–290.

64. Thomas, J. D., Sideras, P., Edvard Smith, C. I., Vorechovsky, I., Chapman, V., and Paul, W. E., 1993, Colocalization of the XLA and X-linked immunodeficiency genes, *Science* **261:**355–358.

65. Rawlings, D. J., Saffran, D. C., Tsukada, S., Largespada, D. A., Grimaldi, J. C., Cohen, L., Mohr, R. N., Bazan, J. F., Howard, M., Copeland, N. G., Jenkins, N. A., and Witte, O., 1993, Mutation of unique region of Bruton's tyrosine kinase in immunodeficient XID mice, *Science* **261:**358–361.

66. Kamer, J. D., Appleby, M. W., Mohr, R. N., Chien, S., Rawlings, D. J., Maliszewski, C. R., Witte, O. N., and Perlmutter, R. N., 1995, Impaired expansion of mouse B cell progenitors lacking Btk, *Immunity* **3:**301–312.

67. Khan, W. N., Alt, F. W., Gerstein, R. M., Malynn, B. A., Carsson, I., Rathbun, G., Davidson, L., Müller, S., Kantor, A. B., Herzenberg, L. A., Rosen, F. S., and Sideras, P., 1995, Defective B cell development and function in Btk-deficient mice, *Immunity* **3:**283–299.

68. Segre, J. A., Nemhauser, J. L., Taylor, B. A., Nadeau, J. H., and Landers, E. S., 1995, Positional cloning of the *nude* locus: Genetic, physical and transcription maps of the region and mutations in the mouse and rat, *Genomics* **28:**549–559.

69. Hormaeche, E. E., Mastroeni, P., Arena, A., Uddin, J., and Joysey, H. S., 1990, T cells do not mediate the initial suppression of a *Salmonella* infection in the RES, *Immunology* **70:**247–250.

70. Nauciel, C., 1990, Role of CD4+ T cells and T-independent mechanisms in acquired resistance to *Salmonella typhimurium* infection, *J. Immunol.* **145:**1265–1269.

71. Nehls, M., Pfeifer, D., Schorpp, M., Hedrich, H., and Boehm, T., 1994, New member of the winged-helix protein family disrupted in mouse and rat nude mutations, *Nature* **372:**103–106.

72. Lai, E., Clark, K. L., Burley, S. K., and Darnell, J. E. Jr., 1993, Hepatocyte nuclear factor 3/fork head or "winged helix" proteins: A family of transcription factors of diverse biologic function, *Proc. Natl. Acad. Sci. USA* **90:**10421–10423.

73. McLeod, R., Buschman, E., Arbuckle, L. D., and Skamene, E., 1995, Immunogenetics in the analysis of resistance to intracellular pathogens, *Curr. Opin. Immunol.* **7:**539–552.

74. Hormaeche, C. E., Harrington, K. A., and Joysey, H. S., 1985, Natural resistance to Salmonellae in mice: Control by genes within the major histocompatibility complex, *J. Infect. Dis.* **152:**1050–1055.

75. Nauciel, C., Ronco, E., Guenet, J. L., and Pla, M., 1988, Role of *H-2* and non *H-2* genes in control of bacterial clearance from the spleen in *Salmonella typhimurium*-infected mice, *Infect. Immun.* **56:**2407–2411.

76. Nauciel, C., Ronco, E., and Pla, M., 1990, Influence of different regions of the *H-2* complex on the rate of clearance of *Salmonella typhimurium*, *Infect. Immun.* **58:**573–574.

77. Jones, B. D., and Falkow, S., 1996, Salmonellosis: Host immune responses and bacterial virulence determinants, *Annu. Rev. Immunol.* **14:**533–561.

78. Kaufmann, S. H. E., 1994, Bacterial and protozoal infections in genetically disrupted mice, *Curr. Opin. Immunol.* **6:**518–525.

3

Host Resistance and *Mycobacterium tuberculosis* Infection

JON S. FRIEDLAND

1. INTRODUCTION

Mycobacterium tuberculosis is a non-spore-forming, anaerobic bacillus that is acid-alcohol fast and usually less than 5 μm long. This small organism kills more people worldwide each year than any other single infectious agent. In richer areas of the world, including the United States and Europe, there has been a resurgence of the disease, particularly in poorer subgroups of the population and in immunosuppressed individuals, notably those with concomitant human immunodeficiency virus (HIV) infection. The emergence of multidrug-resistant bacteria has been an added source of concern, with the possibility that some strains may soon be untreatable even with second-line agents. This has led to renewed interest in the genetics and immunology of the host response to *M. tuberculosis*. Such study is the necessary prerequisite for the future development of novel immunotherapeutic agents.

A relevant question in the context of this book is whether *M. tuberculosis* is an opportunistic or endemic pathogen. The first part of the chapter examines the evidence, focusing on the difference between asymptomatically infected individu-

JON S. FRIEDLAND • Department of Infectious Diseases, Imperial College, Hammersmith Hospital, London W12 0NN, England.

Opportunistic Intracellular Bacteria and Immunity, edited by Lois J. Paradise *et al.* Plenum Press, New York, 1999.

als and patients who are affected by clinically significant disease. Tuberculosis in the immunosuppressed patient is specifically reviewed. The remainder of the chapter addresses the specific issues concerning host resistance to *M. tuberculosis*. The pathological response to *M. tuberculosis* is granuloma formation. Phagocytosis of the pathogen by fixed tissue macrophages is the initial stimulus to cellular recruitment to areas of infection. The principal cells involved in the granuloma are monocytes, monocyte-derived cells such as epithelioid cells and multinucleate giant cells, and T lymphocytes. Thus, this chapter concentrates on the role of these cell types in host resistance to tuberculosis. As yet, there are scanty data on the involvement of other accessory cell types in protective immune responses to tuberculosis. Knowledge concerning immune responses comes mainly from cellular systems or animal models of infection, although recently more information is being sought in clinically based research. This is critical, for although cellular models are extremely helpful in dissecting out specific immune responses, they lack the complexity found in human disease. Although animal models are more complex and allow some unique experiments, particularly those involving gene knockout animals, they do have limitations including the fact that acquisition of infection is carefully controlled and there are very significant differences between host immune responses of different species.

2. *MYCOBACTERIUM TUBERCULOSIS* AS AN OPPORTUNISTIC INFECTION

In this section, evidence is presented that supports the view that *M. tuberculosis* is an opportunistic pathogen that causes disease only in the presence of altered or inadequate host immune resistance. In normal circumstances, infection is contained and the organism either lies dormant or replicates at extremely low levels within the host.

2.1. Primary Infection

One third of the world's total population are infected by *M. tuberculosis*.[1] Of these 1.6 billion people, approximately 15 million have active disease and 3 million people die each year. Although the number of deaths is high, in terms of the total number of infected individuals only a relatively small proportion are involved. This suggests that the host immune response in patients who fail to contain the disease is in some way compromised. In other words, the development of disease could be considered to be consistent with the opportunistic behavior of a ubiquitous pathogen than is normally contained, although seldom completely eliminated, by the immune response. Exactly what compromises the immune response in these patients is unknown. However, the majority of cases of tuberculosis occur in poorer areas of the world and there is a clear relationship between income and incidence of tuberculosis. It is possible that poor nutrition may be an important factor in development of disease.

It is also increasingly apparent that there are certain groups of people who have a genetic predisposition to developing clinical tuberculosis. In animal models, sensitivity to *M. bovis* Bacillus Calmette Gúerin (BCG) strain is associated with expression of the *Nramp* gene, and segregation of this gene in man may relate to development of clinical tuberculosis. More graphically, people who are homozygous for mutations in the interferon-γ (IFN-γ) receptor have been shown to be susceptible to recurrent, often fatal mycobacterial infections.[2,3] However, there may be more subtle effects that allow *M. tuberculosis* infection to progress to disease. Clinical infection has been associated with a variety of HLA types including B15 and DR2. Other areas that are currently being investigated include the effects of specific polymorphisms in genes coding for tumor necrosis factor-α (TNF-α) and the vitamin D receptor. It is probable that there will turn out to be many genes that influence whether or not infection with *M. tuberculosis* is clinically significant but the independent effect of any single gene is likely to be low in population studies.

2.2. Reactivation of Infection

Many clinical cases of tuberculosis are due to reactivation of infection that was acquired years earlier and contained by the immune system. The stimulus to reactivation is often not identified but may be overt, significant immunosuppression. However, some obviously immunosuppressive therapies are not necessarily sufficient to reactivate *M. tuberculosis*. For example, high doses of steroids given to a patient for a variety of clinical indications may cause reactivation of tuberculosis. Presentation to the physician is often atypical or delayed because the symptoms of infection may mimic symptoms of the disease for which steroids were being prescribed. In contrast, tuberculosis does not appear more common in asthmatic individuals maintained on daily low doses of steroids, which is initially extremely surprising. It is possible that another factor is at work and that the disparate T helper cell responses in asthma and tuberculosis are involved.[4]

Many other clinical conditions are associated both with reactivation of tuberculosis and with relatively mild, often poorly characterized, immune deficiencies. These include end-stage renal disease, diabetes mellitus, lung malignancy, silicosis, extremes of age, and gastrectomy. Malignancy has two distinct effects on tuberculosis granulomas. The first is related to anatomical disruption of the granuloma that is secondary to invading tumor and the second is a more subtle immune dysfunction. The particular influences of immunosuppression due to HIV infection and organ transplantation are considered in the next section. In summary, in very many if not all patients, *M. tuberculosis* infection is generally contained by the human immune system, but if circumstances are opportune then the pathogen replicates and disease supervenes.

2.3. Infection in Immunosuppressed Individuals

Relatively trivial, nonspecific impairment of host immune responses may be associated with reactivation of tuberculosis. However, there are two particular features of 20th century medical practice that have important and generalized effects on infection due to *M. tuberculosis* and these merit more detailed consideration. The first is HIV infection and the second is organ transplantation.

2.3.1. HIV Infection

Coinfection with HIV and tuberculosis occurs in approximately 8 million people, the majority of whom live in the poorer countries of the world. However, the problem is widespread and in the United States tuberculosis patients are offered HIV screening tests. HIV-seropositive patients appear more susceptible to infection by *M. tuberculosis* and rates of reactivation of tuberculosis may be more than 20 times greater than in controls of similar ages.[5] Clinical tuberculosis, which is often atypical and disseminated, is also associated with shorter survival in acquired immunodeficiency syndrome (AIDS) patients. Not only does HIV infection increase the incidence of clinical tuberculosis, but infection with *M. tuberculosis* appears to increase viral replication and HIV disease progression.[6] A full discussion of this topic is beyond the scope of this chapter, but this interaction is in part due to tuberculosis activating NF-κB (nuclear factor-κB)-dependent transcription of the HIV genome.[7,8]

The reasons that underlie the susceptibility of HIV-seropositive individuals to tuberculosis are complex. At the simplest level HIV infection causes a progressive depletion of $CD4^+$ T lymphocytes, which are a critical part of the immune response to tuberculosis. In addition, in HIV, there appears to be a shift away from generation of the T helper 1 (Th1) responses that are critical in effective immunity to infection.[9] HIV infection of monocytes and macrophages has a multitude of generally downregulatory effects on the important proinflammatory activity of these cells, altering cytokine secretion and interactions with other cell types. Some of these changes are explored in more detail in Section 3. The net effect is to make such cells more susceptible to infection by *M. tuberculosis* and less able to eradicate the pathogen. Tuberculosis clearly acts as an overt opportunist pathogen in such immunocompromised hosts.

2.3.2. Transplantation

There is no doubt that in all parts of the world transplantation puts patients at risk of both primary infection with and reactivation of latent *M. tuberculosis*.[10,11]

The numbers of people receiving transplants is increasing and the length of post-surgery survival is steadily improving. Thus, tuberculosis can expect to be seen with increasing frequency in this context despite the widespread policy of offering prophylactic therapy to those with evidence of prior healed tuberculosis. Tuberculosis occurs at an increased frequency in all solid organ transplants including those of kidney, liver, and lung. In addition, there is a small group of unfortunate patients who have received active *M. tuberculosis* along with their graft. The reason for the increased risk of infection is that, for successful transplantation, it is necessary to prevent T-lymphocyte-mediated graft rejection. This is achieved by use of immunosuppressive agents including high-dose steroids, cyclosporin A, and therapies such as antilymphocyte globulin. The problem is that all such treatments have nonspecific effects on T-cell function and therefore also reduce the response to mycobacterial antigens. Thus, *M. tuberculosis* is presented with another context in which it may act as an overt opportunistic pathogen.

Because it is clear that *M. tuberculosis* appears to behave in an opportunistic manner in many if not all active infections, it is clearly important to understand the normal immune response to the pathogen. Such knowledge may allow the development of novel immune therapies against active disease, which are urgently required in the era of drug resistance.

3. HOST RESISTANCE TO *M. TUBERCULOSIS:* EXPERIMENTAL STUDIES

Host defense to tuberculosis depends primarily on cells of the monocyte lineage and T lymphocytes. Thus, most research has focused on these cell types, although it is likely that other cell types have an important and probably underestimated accessory role in host resistance (Table I).

3.1. Monocytes and Macrophages

Cytokines derived from monocytic cells have a pivotal role in host resistance. More is known about cytokine responses in *M. tuberculosis*-infected monocytes than other aspects of host resistance, although the data are by no means complete. Other potentially important components of immunity depend on intercellular adhesion mechanisms and release of enzymes from cellular stores, but relevant experimental investigations have been scarce.

3.1.1. Proinflammatory Cytokines

Fever, weight loss (consumption was the original name for tuberculosis), and a prolonged acute phase protein response with an elevated plasma C-reactive protein and erythrocyte sedimentation rate are the classic features of tuberculosis.

TABLE I
Cellular Components of Host Resistance to *M. tuberculosis* Infection

Cell type	Function	Example
Monocytes/macrophages	Phagocytose *M. tuberculosis*	
	Secrete proinflammatory cytokines	TNF-α, IL-1
	Secrete chemokines	IL-8, MCP-1
	Secrete downregulatory cytokines	IL-10
	Process antigen via MHC	
	Express accessory molecules	B7-1
	Upregulate adhesion molecules	ICAM-1
	Secrete cellular enzymes	Cathepsin D, MMP-1
	Downregulate enzyme release	TIMP-1
	Kill pathogen	
T lymphocytes	Help macrophages	Th1 cytokines
(αβ and γδ)	Recognize antigen in MHC +	
	accessory signals	
	Cytotoxicity	
	Immunological memory	
Epithelial cells	Physical barrier to infection	
	Secrete chemokines	IL-8, RANTES
Other accessory cells	Secrete cytokines	TNF-α, IL-8
(fibroblasts, etc.)	Express adhesion molecules	

These are also the consequence of extended secretion of either of the early proinflammatory cytokines TNF and interleukin-1 (IL-1). Hence, initial studies focused on these cytokines. However, IL-6, which stimulates the acute phase protein response directly, and chemokines, which are critical in cellular recruitment to sites of granuloma formation, all have important roles in successful host resistance to *M. tuberculosis*.

3.1.1a. Studies on Live M. tuberculosis. Phagocytosis of the pathogen by monocytes and fixed-tissue macrophages is the major stimulus to upregulation of cytokine gene expression and secretion. Phagocytosis of *M. tuberculosis* by human monocytes upregulated TNF gene expression within 15 min and secretion followed.[12] Interestingly, in view of the fact that vitamin D receptor polymorphisms may influence susceptibility to tuberculosis, vitamin D_3 regulated such TNF-α secretion. It has been proposed that more virulent strains of mycobacteria escape the host response and stimulate less TNF-α secretion. Data from studies with murine macrophages support this hypothesis. However, neither strain virulence nor preinfection of cells with HIV influenced TNF-α secretion by human monocytic cells in response to *M. tuberculosis*.[13] IL-1, IFN-γ, and IL-6 secretion are also rapidly stimulated following phagocytosis. The magnitude of monocyte IL-6 secretion is also similar following phagocytosis of strains of *M. tuberculosis* of differing virulence.[14] Early proinflammatory cytokines such as TNF-α are also involved in activating autocrine and paracrine secretion of IL-12, a cytokine that has a major role in driving the development of CD4+ Th1 response (see ref. 15 and below).

It has been shown that early proinflammatory cytokines may have direct antibacterial activity. In the murine system, both TNF-α and IFN-γ inhibited replication of *M. tuberculosis* although this was dependent on the mycobacterial strain being investigated.[16] The generation of reactive nitrogen intermediates appeared to be important in such mycobacterial killing. However, in human monocytes and macrophages, a significant role for reactive nitrogen intermediates in killing of intracellular pathogens has not been convincingly demonstrated, although inducible nitric oxide synthase is expressed in alveolar macrophages from patients with tuberculosis.[17] Most data suggest that TNF-α does not have mycobacteriostatic or -cidal actions in human monocytes infected by *M. tuberculosis*. Cell lysis artefacts may be misinterpreted as direct antimycobacterial activity in tuberculosis-infected macrophages.[18] Although controversy remains, it is more likely that proinflammatory cytokines mainly drive secondary monocyte cytokine secretion and activate other immune cells.

There is no doubt that phagocytosis of *M. tuberculosis* by human monocytes activates transcription of chemokine (chemotactic cytokine) genes, which are critical in cellular recruitment to sites of granuloma formation. The process of phagocytosis nonspecifically stimulated gene expression and secretion of the monocyte chemotactic protein-1 (MCP-1) from the human phagocytic monocytic cell line THP-1 after phagocytosis of either otherwise inert latex beads or yeast-derived zymosan or virulent *M. tuberculosis*.[19] Other data have indicated that MCP-1 secretion after phagocytosis of *M. tuberculosis* is greater than after LPS (lipopolysaccharide) stimulation of monocytes.[20] MCP-1 is a member of the β-chemokine family characterized by a C–C structural motif that act principally as attractants for and activators of monocytes. Phagocytosis of *M. tuberculosis*, but not of other pathogens such as *Toxoplasma gondii*, was a particularly potent stimulus to IL-8 gene expression and secretion.[13,21] IL-8 and α-chemokine that is both a neutrophil and a T-cell chemoattractant, appears to be selectively important in recruitment of T cells previously exposed to *M. tuberculosis*.[22] In addition, IL-8 may directly enhance nonoxidative killing mechanisms.[23]

   3.1.1b. Studies on Lipoarabinomannans and Heat-Shock Proteins. Certain structural components of *M. tuberculosis* have been identified as having a critical role in eliciting the proinflammatory response. Cell wall lipoarabinomannan (LAM), which is in many ways the mycobacterial functional equivalent of bacterial lipopolysaccharide, is also a potent stimulus to TNF-α production by both human and murine macrophages. LAM is a compound molecule of arabinan and mannan residues bound to a phosphatidylinositol structure that is the principal stimulus to proinflammatory responses. LAM can upregulate gene expression and stimulate secretion of a wide variety of macrophage-derived cytokines. For example, chemokine secretion from both murine and human macrophages may also be upregulated by LAM.[24,25] These effects of LAM are mediated by pathways involving the transcriptional regulators NF-κB and NF-IL-6.[26] However, sulfatide, another lipid in the mycobacterial cell wall, may antagonize the effects of LAM by downregulating protein kinase C activity, which would tend to reduce NF-κB activation.[27]

As well as lipids, proteins from *M. tuberculosis* have the potential to stimulate gene expression and secretion of proinflammatory cytokines. Specific proteins such as the 30-kDa antigen of *M. tuberculosis* may be involved in regulation of TNF-α secretion.[28] There has been particular interest in heat-shock proteins (hsp), which are molecular chaperones involved in protein folding and assembly. Immune responses to the mycobacterial 65-kDa hsp are sufficient to confer significant protection against virulent *M. tuberculosis* in a murine model.[29] A number of studies have shown that the 65-kDa mycobacterial hsp can stimulate proinflammatory and chemotactic cytokine secretion from human monocytic cells.[30-32] The host proinflammatory response to specific components and whole *M. tuberculosis* is clearly complex and more data are needed before specific components, which may allow targeted development of new treatments and vaccines, can be definitely identified.

3.1.2. Downregulation of the Immune Response

Successful host resistance requires that the antimycobacterial proinflammatory response is downregulated. Uncontrolled inflammation is likely to be an important component of tissue distruction in extensive tuberculosis infection. Less is known about this critical aspect of the immune response to tuberculosis. IL-10 is a major antiinflammatory macrophage-derived cytokine and LAM as well as mycobacterial proteins upregulates monocyte IL-10 gene expression.[33,34] LAM also increases secretion from human monocytes of another important downregulatory cytokine, TGF-β (transforming growth factor-β). Ongoing studies in my laboratory indicate that monocyte-derived IL-10 has a critical role in the regulation of chemokine gene expression and secretion. One potentially deleterious consequence of secretion of downregulatory cytokines, at least in murine infection, is antagonism of proinflammatory cytokine-dependent inhibition of replication of *M. tuberculosis*. The balance and timing of pro- and antiinflammatory responses is likely to be critical in host resistance to any infection including tuberculosis.

3.1.3. Cell–Cell Interactions

It is likely that signals mediated via direct intercellular contact represent the other major influence, apart from cytokine-mediated signaling, that determines whether or not the host immune response to *M. tuberculosis* is successful. Elevated concentrations of intercellular adhesion molecule-1 (ICAM-1) are found in plasma of patients with serious, disseminated tuberculosis.[35] Such findings are probably only an indirect reflection of expression of adhesion molecules at sites of infection, but they do indicate the great extent to which adhesion is upregulated. However, cellular studies confirm that ICAM-1 appears to be a major adhesion molecule that is upregulated on human monocytic cells phagocytosing *M. tuberculosis*.

There are also direct interactions between adhesion mediated events and proinflammatory cytokine secretion. For example, adhesion to fibronectin augments the ability of the 30-kDa mycobacterial antigen to upregulate TNF-α secretion.[36] Cell–cell contact may also be critical in controlling macrophage antimycobacterial mechanisms, which are mediated by proinflammatory cytokines, in tuberculosis. Finally, adhesion between monocytes and T lymphocytes, partly mediated by accessory molecules such as B7, is critical in the development of appropriate T-cell responses and this area is considered in more detail in Section 4.

3.1.4. Other Cellular Responses

From the moment *M. tuberculosis* makes contact with the monocyte membrane, a complex series of interactions are initiated, many of which influence the immune response. Little is known about many of these processes or their importance in host resistance to tuberculosis. Complement and mannose receptors appear to be central in the process of phagocytosing *M. tuberculosis*.[37] Once inside the cell, mycobacteria appear to control the microenvironment within the phagosome and regulate its pH to maintain it at about 6.5.[38] Inhibition of phagosome–lysosome fusion is a further key mechanism by which the pathogen avoids host killing mechanisms, although the process of phagocytosis does activate a number of important signal transduction pathways such as those involving phospholipase D. However, returning to the theme of host as opposed to pathogen resistance, the secretion of cellular enzymes may be a very important aspect of the immune response to tuberculosis.

High concentrations of cathepsin D are associated with liquefaction of the caseous material that is characteristic of tuberculous granulomas.[39] The specific roles of different proteases have not been worked out in detail. However, it is likely that the balance between secretion of matrix metalloproteinases (MMPs) and the endogenous tissue inhibitors of metalloproteinases (TIMPs) from monocytes may be important in facilitating migration of leukocytes across tissues (by tissue remodeling). However, excess MMP production has the potential to cause excessive host tissue damage. More data are needed in this area and ongoing studies in my laboratory are investigating the role of MMPs in *M. tuberculosis* infection.

Even the mode of death of monocytes infected with *M. tuberculosis* may be important in host resistance to infection. In monocytes that undergo apoptosis, there may be associated killing of intracellular mycobacteria.[40] In general, it is clear that there are many mechanisms in place in monocytic cells that are necessary for control of tuberculosis. Although monocytes initiate immune responses by phagocytosing *M. tuberculosis*, they are not the only cell type involved in host defense. The T lymphocyte is the other principal cell found in the granuloma and its role is now considered.

3.2. T Lymphocytes

CD4$^+$ T lymphocytes are divided into subgroups on the basis of the cytokines that they secrete. Th1 cells produce IFN and IL-2 whereas Th2 cells secrete IL-4, IL-5, IL-6, IL-10, and IL-13. Such divisions work best in murine systems but also have broad application in human T-cell immune responses. Th1 cells appear to be critical in control of *M. tuberculosis* infection. Much of the data come from *in vivo* studies, which are considered in Section 4. If cultured human peripheral or alveolar T cells from subjects previously exposed to mycobacteria are stimulated with mycobacterial antigens, they predominantly secrete IL-2 and IFN. IFN is likely not only to drive primary Th1 responses but also to activate macrophages that have phagocytosed *M. tuberculosis*. Both $\gamma\delta$ and $\alpha\beta$ T lymphocytes contribute to the Th1-type of cytokine section. However, the situation is complex and peripheral T lymphocytes taken from patients with active tuberculosis may actually have depressed cytokine production rather than a Th1 phenotype.[41-43] In the later stages of human infection, cells can be recovered with either Th0 or Th2 phenotypes and marked IL-4 secretion has frequently been reported. One possibility is that the pattern of cytokine secretion switches between the different T-cell phenotypes during the immune response to tuberculosis.[44]

Studies on peripheral T cells may be less valuable than investigations at the sites of infection by *M. tuberculosis*. Thus, T lymphocytes from pleural fluid had more of a Th1 phenotype than those found in peripheral T cells. In this study, the IL-10 mRNA that was detected was associated mainly with macrophages and not the T cells in the pleural fluid. Further evidence of the importance of Th1 cells is derived from studies in HIV coinfected patients who are more susceptible to tuberculosis. Such individuals do not seem to have an increased Th2 response but rather a reduced Th1 response.[43] It is interesting that even T cells from patients who are mounting a Th2 response to infection with schistosomiasis still exhibit a primarily Th1 phenotype on exposure to purified protein derivative of *M. tuberculosis*.[45] It seems that Th1 cells are necessary for effective host resistance to tuberculosis. Subsequent development of a Th2 response may partly account for the fact that, although *M. tuberculosis* is successfully contained by granuloma, viable organisms may persist in the host for many years.

3.3. Other Cells of the Immune System

The role of other cells in immunity to tuberculosis has generally been overlooked. The concentration of research on the cells comprising the granuloma has inadvertently ignored the importance of cytokine networks in early stages of infection. Such networks will probably involve epithelial cells and supporting cells such as fibroblasts. Thus, in the lung, the first cells encountered by *M. tuberculosis* will be the alveolar macrophage and respiratory epithelial cells which are present in much greater numbers. The potential involvement of such cells is obvious from experiments that have shown that respiratory epithelial cells, for example, are able to secrete chemokines in response to other pathogens. *M. tuberculosis* can certainly invade and replicate within type 2 alveolar cells.

Neutrophils and natural killer cells are leukocytes that are not normally associated with the immune response to tuberculosis. However, because very high concentrations of IL-8 are secreted by monocytes infected with *M. tuberculosis*, it is likely that this leads to some neutrophil recruitment as well as a T-cell influx. Indeed, in patients it is well recognized that in tuberculous meningoencephalitis examination of the cerebrospinal fluid may reveal neutrophils early in the course of disease rather than the more typical mononuclear cell infiltrate. Although neutrophils may be involved in mycobacterial killing,[23] they may have a more important role in amplifying the immune response and recruiting further monocytes and T lymphocytes. The involvement of NK (natural killer) cells in host resistance to tuberculosis is equally poorly characterized. IL-12, which is produced by *M. tuberculosis*-infected monocytes, was first defined as a natural killer cell stimulatory factor.[15] This cytokine was subsequently shown to have the potential to activate the cytolytic activity of NK cells toward *M. tuberculosis*-infected monocytes.[46] In summary, future research into the area of regulation of cellular immune networks in both up- and downregulation of immune responses is likely to provide interesting information that will increase the understanding of host resistance to tuberculosis. In particular, understanding of early events at epithelial cell surfaces may be vital in the future development of genetically modified vaccine strains of *M. tuberculosis* designed to elicit protective immunity at epithelial surfaces.

4. *IN VIVO* HOST RESISTANCE TO *M. TUBERCULOSIS*

Cellular models of tuberculosis have been extremely useful in dissecting out the facets of host resistance to *M. tuberculosis*. Many findings have since been confirmed in animal infection. However, the situation in human disease is less well defined.

4.1. Animal Models of Tuberculosis

Most studies relevant to tuberculosis have used murine models often infected with *M. bovis*, BCG strain, which is genetically and structurally very similar to *M. tuberculosis* but relatively infrequently a pathogen in man. The importance of TNF-α in host resistance and granuloma formation was demonstrated by injecting mice with anti-TNF-α. The antibody both prevented granuloma development and allowed unrestricted mycobacterial growth in tissues.[47] Using a different approach, adenovirus vectors expressing the TNF-α 55-kDa receptor exacerbated disease, providing further evidence for the importance of this cytokine.[48] IFN-γ appears as effective as TNF-α in increasing murine resistance to virulent *M. tuberculosis*. This has been confirmed in murine knockout animals lacking either the IFN-γ or the IFN-γ receptor gene.[40–51] This reflects the fact that reactive nitrogen intermediates are important in murine disease and IFN-γ upregulates the interferon γ regulatory factor-1 (IRF-1) gene which in turns switches on the inducible nitric oxide synthase gene.[52] Murine studies have also confirmed the importance of IL-12 in resistance to tuberculosis.[53]

In addition, IFN-γ receptor knockout mice have aberrant regulation of expression of class II major histocompatibility antigens and both class 1 and II MHC responses are required in immunity to tuberculosis. Third, IFN-γ together with TNF-α is required for *in vivo* generation of IL-12[54] and administration of IL-12 has been shown to increase survival of *M. tuberculosis*-infected BALB/c mice. IL-6 and chemokines have also been detected in murine infection but functional investigations are difficult to interpret, as murine chemokines have poor functional homology to human ones. However, experiments using neutralizing antibodies to IL-8 indicate that this cytokine is critical during granuloma formation in the delayed-type hypersensitivity (DTH) reaction to mycobacterial antigens.[55]

Numerous studies have confirmed the importance of Th1 responses in murine resistance to *M. tuberculosis*. In murine *M. bovis* infection the upregulation of IL-10, which is important in controlling inflammatory responses, does not appear adequate to shift the T-cell response from a Th1 to Th2 type.[56] This suggests that there is a strong host immune bias to Th1 responses in mycobacterial infections. Both αβ and γδ T cells are involved in the successful *in vivo* immune response to tuberculosis in murine models. However, the participation of CD8+ T cells in immunity to *M. tuberculosis* is more controversial, although there are experimental data supporting a potential role.[57] In addition, there are double-negative T lymphocytes lacking CD4 and CD8 that recognize mycobacterial lipoglycan antigens presented via CD1 proteins, which have distant homology to the MHC.[58]

4.2. Human Tuberculosis

Investigations in patients are both vital and difficult. One problem is that such investigations occur at a poorly defined time point during the immune response to infection. Furthermore, it is frequently not ethical to obtain sufficient tissue for extensive investigation and hence many studies focus on peripheral blood leukocytes. TNF, IL-1, and IL-6 have all been demonstrated to have roles in human infection, which is consistent with animal studies. As well as being detected in blood and released from patient leukocytes, these cytokines have been found in pleural effusions and biopsies and cerebrospinal fluid of tuberculosis patients. Similar data have been generated for IL-12, although the functional significance of such observations is always uncertain. Studies on human T-lymphocyte-derived cytokines have been discussed earlier.

The chemokines that have important functions in cellular and animal studies are also found in human disease. IL-8 and MCP-1 were detected in pleural and bronchoalveolar lavage fluid from patients with tuberculosis.[59,60] Additional studies have shown that mRNA for another chemokine RANTES, attractant for memory T cells, is present in tuberculous lymph nodes.[61] Leukocytes from patients with fatal tuberculosis have an inability to secrete IL-8, which is partly due to the presence of a circulating inhibitor in plasma and this may be important in determining outcome.[62] In survivors, leukocyte IL-8 secretion was dysregulated even 9 months after clinical presentation.[63] Downregulatory cytokines such as TGF-β have been detected *in vivo*[64] but the whole area of *in vivo* regulation of regulation of proinflammatory cytokine secretion in humans awaits detailed examination.

5. CONCLUSIONS

It is clear that host resistance to *M. tuberculosis* is a complex multifaceted process modified by genetic and environmental influences. The pivotal cells in this process are those of the macrophage/monocyte lineage and the T lymphocyte, but the role of accessory cells has probably been underestimated. Many different aspects of cellular activity are involved in development of granulomas and containment of the pathogen. The greatest focus to date has been on the involvement of secreted cytokines and cell-contact mediated events although much detail on the important area of regulation of such processes remains to be elucidated. Dissection of the role of cell enzymes such as matrix metalloproteinases is just one area where further research is needed.

An important concept is that normally the immune system prevents infection by *M. tuberculosis* from becoming established. Only in those instances in which there is some impairment of host resistance does disease supervene. The factors that influence this may range from minor genetic ones to the obvious immune suppression that is associated with advanced HIV infection. Once there is understanding of how the host contains *M. tuberculosis*, then how the organism takes advantage of a relative immune deficiency will become more apparent with consequent insight into how clinical disease develops. In this context, it is critical that research is supported both in the field and in the clinic. Then, there will be every prospect that novel adjuvant therapies for or vaccination against tuberculosis will be developed.

REFERENCES

1. Ravilione, M. C., Snider, D. E., and Kochi, A. 1995, Global epidemiology of tuberculosis: Morbidity and mortality of a worldwide epidemic, *JAMA* **273:** 220–226.
2. Newport, M. J., Huxley, C. M., Huston, S., Hawrylowicz, C. M., Oostra, B. A., Williamson, R., and Levin, M., 1996, A mutation in the interferon-γ-receptor gene and susceptibility to mycobacterial infection, *N. Engl. J. Med.* **335:**1941–1949.
3. Jouanguy, E., Altare, F., Lamhamedi, S., Revy, P., Emile, J., Newport, M. J., Levin, M., Blanche, S., Seboun, E., Fischer, A., and Casanova, J.-L., 1996, Interferon-γ-receptor deficiency in an infant with fatal Bacille Calmette-Guerin infection, *N. Engl. J. Med.* **335:** 1956–1961.
4. Shirakawa, T., Enomoto, T., Shimazu, S., and Hopkin, J. M. 1997, The inverse association between tuberculin responses and atopic disorder, *Science* **275:**77–79.
5. Allen, S., Batungwanayo, J., Kerlikowske, K., Lifson, A. R., Wolf, W., Granich, R., Taelman, H., van de Perre, P., Serufilira, A., Bogaerts, J., Slutkin, G., and Hopewell, P. C., 1992, Two-year incidence of tuberculosis in cohorts of HIV-infected and uninfected urban Rwandan women, *Am. Rev. Respir. Dis.* **146:**1439–1444.
6. Goletti, D., Weissman, D., Jackson, R. W., Graham, N. M. H., Vlahov, D., Kein, R. S., Munsiff, S. S., Ortona, L., Cauda, R., and Fauci, A. S., 1996, Effect of *Mycobacterium tuberculosis* on HIV replication: Role of immune activation, *J. Immunol.* **157:**1271–1278.
7. Shattock, R. J., Friedland, J. S., and Griffin, G. E., 1994, Phagocytosis of *Mycobacterium tuberculosis* enhances HIV transcription in human monocytic cells, *J. Gen. Virol.* **75:**849–856.
8. Zhang, Y., Nakata, K., Weiden, M., and Rom, W. N., 1995, *Mycobacterium tuberculosis* enhances human immunodeficiency virus-1 replication by transcriptional activation of the long terminal repeat, *J. Clin. Invest.* **95:**2324–2331.
9. Clerici, M., and Shearer, G. M., 1994, The Th1-Th2 hypothesis of HIV infection: New insights, *Immunol. Today* 15:575–581.
10. Hall, C. M., Willcox, P. A., Swanepoel, C. R., Kahn, D., and Smit, R., 1994, Mycobacterial infection in renal transplant recipients, *Chest* **106:**435–439.
11. Miller, R. A., Lanza, L. A., Kline, J. N., and Geist, L. J., 1995, *Mycobacterium tuberculosis* in lung transplant recipients, *Am. J. Respir. Crit. Care. Med.* **152:**374–376.
12. Rook, G. A. W., Taverne, J., Leverton, C., and Steele, J., 1987, The role of gamma-interferon, vitamin D3, metabolites and tumour necrosis factor in the pathogenesis of tuberculosis, *Immunology* **62:**229–234.
13. Friedland, J. S., Remick, D. G., Shattock, R., and Griffin, G. E., 1992, Secretion of interleukin-8 following phagocytosis of *Mycobacterium tuberculosis* by human monocyte cell lines, *Eur. J. Immunol.* **22:**1373–1378.
14. Friedland, J. S., 1993, Phagocytosis, cytokines and *Mycobacterium tuberculosis*, *Lymphokine Cytokine Res.* **12:**127–133.

15. D'Andrea, A., Rengaraju, M., Valiante, N. M., Chemini, J., Kubin, M., Aste, M., Chan, S. H., Kobayashi, M., Young, D., Nickbarg, E., Chizzonite, R., Wolf, S. F., and Trinchieri, G., 1992, Production of natural killer stimulatory factor (interleukin 12) by peripheral blood mononuclear cells, *J. Exp. Med.* **176:**1387–1398.

16. Flesch, I., and Kaufmann, S. H. E., 1987, Mycobacterial growth inhibition by Interferon-γ-activated bone marrow macrophages and differential susceptibility among strains of *Mycobacterium tuberculosis*, *J. Immunol.* **138:**4408–4413.

17. Nicholson, S., Bonecini-Almeida, M., Lapa e Silva, J. R., Nathan, C., Xie, Q., Mumford, R., Weidner, J. R., Calaycay, J., Geng, J., Boechat, N., Linhares, C., Rom, W., and Ho, J. L., 1996, Inducible nitric oxide synthase in pulmonary alveolar macrophages from patients with tuberculosis, *J. Exp. Med.* **183:**2293–2302.

18. Warwick-Davies, J., Dhillon, J., O'Brien, L., Andrew, P. W., and Lowrie, D. B., 1994, Apparent killing of *Mycobacterium tuberculosis* by cytokine-activated human monocytes can be an artefact of a cytotoxic effect on the monocytes, *Clin. Exp. Immunol.* **96:**214–217.

19. Friedland, J. S., Shattock, R., and Griffin, G. E., 1993, Phagocytosis of *M. tuberculosis* or particulate stimuli by human monocytic cells induces equivalent monocyte chemotactic protein 1 gene expression, *Cytokine* **5:**150–156.

20. Kasahara, K., Tobe, T., Tomita, M., Mukaida, N., Shao-Bo, S., Matsushima, K., Yoshida, T., Sugihara, S., and Kobayashi, K., 1994, Selective expression of monocyte chemotactic and activating factor/monocyte chemoattractant protein 1 in human blood monocytes by *Mycobacterium tuberculosis*, *J. Infect. Dis.* **170:**1238–1247.

21. Friedland, J. S., Shattock, R., Johnson, J., Remick, D. G., Holliman, R. M., and Griffin, G. E., 1993, Differential cytokine gene expression and secretion after phagocytosis by a human monocyte cell line of *Toxoplasma gondii* and *Mycobacterium tuberculosis*, *Clin. Exp. Immunol.* **91:**282–286.

22. Wilkinson, P. C., and Newman, I., 1992, Identification of IL-8 as a locomotor attractant for activated human lymphocytes in mononuclear cell cultures with anti-CD3 or purified protein derivative of *Mycobacterium tuberculosis*, *J. Immunol.* **149:**2689–2694.

23. Nibbering, P. H., Pos, O., Stevenhagen, A., and van Furth, R., 1994, Interleukin-8 enhances nonoxidative killing of *Mycobacterium fortuitum* by human granulocytes, *Infect. Immun.* **61:**3111–3116.

24. Roach, T. I. A., Barton, C. H., Chatterjee, D., and Blackwell, J. M., 1993, Macrophage activation: Lipoarabinomannan from avirulent and virulent strains of *Mycobacterium tuberculosis* differentially induces the early genes c-*fos*, KC, JE and tumor necrosis factor-α, *J. Immunol.* **150:**1886–1896.

25. Zhang, Y., Broser, M., Cohen, H., Bodkin, M., Law, K., Reibman, J., and Rom, W. N., 1995, Enhanced interleukin-8 release and gene expression in macrophages after exposure to *Mycobacterium tuberculosis* and its components, *J. Clin. Invest.* **95:**586–592.

26. Zhang, Y., and Rom, W. N., 1993, Regulation of the Interleukin-1β (IL-1β) gene by mycobacterial components and lipopolysaccharide is mediated by two nuclear factor-IL-6 motifs, *Mol. Cell Biol.* **13:**3831–38317.

27. Bronza, J. P., Horan, M., Rademacher, J. M., Pabst, K. M., and Pabst, M. J., 1991, Monocyte responses to sulfatide from *Mycobacterium tuberculosis:* Inhibition of priming for enhanced release of superoxide associated with increased secretion of interleukin-1 and tumor necrosis factor alpha and altered protein phosphorylation, *Infect. Immun.* **59:**2542–2548.

28. Averill, L., Toossi, Z., Aung, H., Boom, W. H., and Ellner, J. J., 1995, Regulation of production of tumor necrosis factor alpha in monocytes stimulated by the 30-kilodalton antigen of *Mycobacterium tuberculosis*, *Infect. Immun.* **63:**3206–3208.

29. Silva, C. L., and Lowrie, D. B., 1994, A single mycobacterial protein (hsp 65) expressed by a transgenic antigen-presenting cell vaccinates mice against tuberculosis, *Immunology* **82:**244–248.

30. Friedland, J. S., Shattock, R., Remick, D. G., and Griffin, G. E., 1993, Mycobacterial 65kD heat

shock protein induces release of TNF, IL-6, and IL-8 from human monocytic cells, *Clin. Exp. Immunol.* **91:**58–62.

31. Petermans, W. E., Raats, C. J. I., Langermans, J. A. M., and van Furth, R., 1994, Mycobacterial heat-shock protein 65 induces proinflammatory cytokines but does not activate human mononuclear phagocytes, *Scand. J. Immunol.* **39:**613–617.

32. Retzlaff, C., Yamamoto, Y., Hoffman, P. S., Friedman, H., and Klein, T. W., 1994, Bacterial heat shock proteins directly induce cytokine mRNA and IL-1 secretion in macrophage cultures, *Infect. Immun.* **62:**5689–5693.

33. Roach, T. I. A., Barton, C. H., Chatterjee, D., Liew, F. Y., and Blackwell, J. M., 1995, Opposing effects of interferon-γ on iNOS and interleukin-10 expression in lipopolysaccharide- and mycobacterial lipoarabinomannan-stimulated macrophages, *Immunology* **85:**106–113.

34. Toossi, Z., Young, T., Averill, L. E., Hamilton, B. D., Shiratsuchi, H., and Ellner, J. J., 1995, Induction of transforming growth factor β1 by purified protein derivative of *Mycobacterium tuberculosis*, *Infect. Immun.* **63:**224–228.

35. Sjijubo, N., Imai, K., Nakanishi, F., Yachi, A., and Abe, S., 1993, Elevated concentrations of circulating ICAM-1 in far advanced and miliary tuberculosis, *Am. Rev. Respir. Dis.* **148:**1298–1301.

36. Aung, H., Toossi, Z., Wisnieski, J. J., Wallis, R. S., Culp, L. A., Phillips, N. B., Phillips, M., Averill, L. E., Daniel, T. M., and Ellner, J. J., 1996, Induction of monocyte expression of tumor necrosis factor α by the 30kD α antigen of *Mycobacterium tuberculosis* and synergism with fibronectin, *J. Clin. Invest.* **98:**1261–1268.

37. Schlesinger, L. S., 1993, Macrophage phagocytosis of virulent but not attenuated strains of *Mycobacterium tuberculosis* is mediated by mannose receptors in addition to complement receptors. *J. Immunol.* **150:**2920–2930.

38. Sturgill-Koszycki, S., Schlesinger, P. H., Chakraborty, P., Haddix, P. L., Collins, H. L., Fok, A. K., Allen, R. D., Gluck, S. L., Heuser, J., and Russell, D. G., 1994, Lack of acidification in *Mycobacterium* phagosomes produced by exclusion of the vesicular proton-ATPase, *Science* **263:**678–681.

39. Converse, P. J., Dannenberg, A. M., Estep, J. E., Sugisaki, K., Abe, Y., Schofield, B. H., and Pitt, M. L. M., 1996, Cavitary tuberculosis produced in rabbits by aerosolized virulent tubercle bacilli, *Infect. Immun* **64:**4776–4787.

40. Molloy, A., Laochumroonvorapong, P., and Kaplan, G., 1994, Apoptosis but not necrosis of infected monocytes is coupled with killing of intracellular Bacillus Calmette-Guerin, *J. Exp. Med.* **180:**1499–1509.

41. Schauf, V., Rom, W. N., Smith, K. A., Sampaio, E. P., Meyn, P. A., Tramontana, J. M., Cohn, Z. A., and Kaplan, G., 1993, Cytokine gene activation and modified responsiveness to interleukin-2 in the blood of tuberculosis patients, *J. Infect. Dis.* **168:**1056–1059.

42. Johnson, B. J., and McMurray, D. N., 1994, Cytokine gene expression by cultures of human lymphocytes with autologous *Mycobacterium tuberculosis*-infected monocytes, *Infect. Immun.* **62:**1444–1450.

43. Zhang, M., Lin, Y., Iyer, D. V., Gong, J., Abrams, J. S., and Barnes, P. F., 1995, T-cell cytokine responses in human infection with *Mycobacterium tuberculosis*, *Infect. Immun.* **63:**3231–3234.

44. Sander, B., Skansen-Saphir, U., Damm, O., Hakansson, L., Andersson, J., and Andersson, U., 1995, Sequential production of Th1 and Th2 cytokines in response to live bacillus Calmette-Guerin, *Immunology* **86:**512–518.

45. Sarono, E., Kruize, Y. C. M., Kurniawan, A., Maizels, R. M., and Yazdanbakhsh, M., 1996, In Th2-biased lymphatic filarial patients, responses to purified protein derivative of *Mycobacterium tuberculosis* remain Th1, *Eur. J. Immunol.* **26:**501–504.

46. Denis, M., 1994, Interleukin-12 (IL-12) augments cytolytic activity of natural killer cells towards *Mycobacterium tuberculosis*-infected human monocytes, *Cell. Immunol.* **156:**529–536.

47. Kindler, V., Sappino, A., Grau, G. E., Piguet, P., and Vassalli, P., 1989, The inducing role of tumor necrosis factor in the development of bactericidal granulomas during BCG infection, *Cell* **56:**731–740.

48. Adams, L. B., Mason, C. M., Kolls, J. K., Scollard, D., Krahenbuhl, J. L., and Nelson, S., 1995, Exacerbation of acute and chronic murine tuberculosis by administration of a tumor necrosis factor receptor-expressing adenovirus, *J. Infect. Dis.* **171:**400–405.

49. Cooper, A. M., Dalton, D. K., Stewart, T. A., Griffin, J. P., Russell, D. G., and Orme, I. M., 1993, Disseminated tuberculoisis in Interferon γ gene-disrupted mice, *J. Exp. Med.* **178:**2243–2247.

50. Flynn, J. L., Chan, J., Triebold, K. J., Dalton, D. K., Stewart, T. A., and Bloom, B. R., 1993, An essential role for Interferon γ in resistance to *Mycobacterium tuberculosis* infection, *J. Exp. Med.* **178:**2249–2254.

51. Kamijo, R., Le, J., Shapiro, D., Havell, E. A., Huang, S., Aguet, M., Bosland, M., and Vilcek, J., 1993, Mice that lack the interferon-γ receptor have profoundly altered responses to infection with Bacillus Calmette-Guerin and subsequent challenge with lipopolysaccharide, *J. Exp. Med.* **178:**1425–1440.

52. Kamijo, R., Harada, H., Matsuyama, T., Bosland, M., Gerecitano, J., Shapiro, D., Le, J., Koh, S. I., Kimura, T., Green, S. J., Mak, T. W., Taniguchi, T., and Vilcek, J., 1994, Requirement for transcription factor IRF-1 in NO synthase induction in macrophages, *Science* **263:**1612–1615.

53. Flynn, J. L., Goldstein, M. M., Triebold, K. J., Sypek, J., Wolf, S., and Bloom, B. R., 1995, IL-12 increases resistance of BALB/c mice to *Mycobacterium tuberculosis* infection, *J. Immunol.* **155:**2515–2524.

54. Flesch, I. E. A., Hess, J. H., Huang, S., Aguet, M., Rothe, J., Bluthemann, H., and Kaufmann, S. H. E., 1995, Early interleukin-12 production by macrophages in response to mycobacterial infection depends on interferon γ and tumor necrosis factor α, *J. Exp. Med.* **181:**1615–1621.

55. Larsen, C. G., Thomsen, M. K., Gesser, B., Thomsen, P. D., Deleuran, B. W., Nowak, J., Skodt, V., Thomsen, H. K., Deleuran, M., Therstrup-Pedersen, K., Harada, A., Matsushima, K., and Menne, T., 1995, The delayed-type hypersensitivity reaction is dependent on IL-8, *J. Immunol.* **155:**2151–2157.

56. Flesch, I. E. A., and Kaufmann, S. H. E., 1994, Role of macrophages and αβ T lymphocytes in early interleukin 10 production during *Listeria monocytogenes* infection, *Int. Immunol.* **6:**463–468.

57. Flynn, J. L., Goldstein, M. M., Triebold, K. J., Koller, B., and Bloom, B. R., 1992, Major histocompatibility complex class 1-restricted T cells are required for resistance to *Mycobacterium tuberculosis* infection, *Proc. Natl. Acad. Sci. USA* **89:**12013–12017.

58. Sieling, P. A., Chatterjee, D., Porcelli, S. A., Prigozy, T. I., Mazzaccaro, R. J., Soriano, T., Bloom, B. R., Brenner, B. R., Kronenberg, M., Brennan, P. J., and Modlin, R. L., 1995, CD1-restricted T cell recognition of microbial lipoglycan antigens, *Science* **269:**227–230.

59. Antony, V. B., Godbey, S. W., Kunkel, S. L., Hott, J. W., Hartman, D. L., Burdick, M. D., and Strieter, R. M., 1993, Recruitment of inflammatory cells to the pleural space, *J. Immunol.* **151:**7216–7223.

60. Grunewald, T., Schuler-Mane, W., and Ruf, B., 1993, Interleukin-8 and granulocyte colony-stimulating factor in bronchoalveolar lavage fluid and plasma of human immunodeficiency virus-infected patients with *Pneumocytis carinii* pneumonia, bacterial pneumonia or tuberculosis, *J. Infect. Dis.* **168:**1077–1078.

61. Devergne, O., Marfaing-Koka, A., Schall, T. T., Leger-Ravet, M., Sadick, M., Peuchmaur, M., Crevon, M., Kim, T., Galanaud, P., and Emilie, D., 1994, Production of the RANTES chemokine in delayed-type hypersensitivity reactions: Involvement of macrophages and endothelial cells, *J. Exp. Med.* **179:**1689–1694.

62. Friedland, J. S., Hartley, J. C., Hartley, C. G. C., Shattock, R. J., and Griffin, G. E., 1995, Inhibition of *ex vivo* proinflammatory cytokine secretion in fatal *Mycobacterium tuberculosis* infection, *Clin. Exp. Immunol.* **100:**233–238.

63. Friedland, J. S., Hartley, J. C., Hartley, C. G. C., Shattock, R. J., and Griffin, G. E., 1996, cytokine secretion *in vivo* and *ex vivo* following chemotherapy of *Mycobacterium tuberculosis* infection, *Trans. R. Soc. Trop. Med. Hyg.* **90:**199–203.

64. Toossi, Z., Gogate, P., Shiratsuchi, H., Young, T., and Ellner, J. J., 1995, Enhanced production of TGF-β by blood monocytes from patients with active tuberculosis and presence of TGF-β in tuberculous granulomatous lung lesions, *J. Immunol.* **154:**465–473.

4

The Influence of Adrenal Steroids on Macrophage and T-Cell Function in Tuberculosis

GRAHAM A. W. ROOK and ROGELIO
HERNANDEZ-PANDO

1. INTRODUCTION

It is no longer possible to consider the immune and endocrine systems in isolation. There is a continuous dialogue between the two. The hypothalamo–pituitary–adrenal (HPA) axis continuously responds to signals it receives from the immune system via cytokines and the vagus nerve.[1] After integrating these signals with inputs from other sources such as the cerebral cortex, the HPA axis regulates production of adrenal steroids. These steroids, even in healthy individuals, exert continuous and clearly demonstrable background effects on the functions of macrophages and T cells, and play a very significant role during chronic inflammatory states.

There are very clear examples of the crucial immunoregulatory role of physiological levels of endogenous adrenal steroids generated by the HPA axis in response to the activity of the immune system. Attempts to induce streptococcal cell wall arthritis[2] or experimental autoallergic encephalitis (EAE)[3] in rats have

GRAHAM A. W. ROOK • Department of Bacteriology, University College London Medical School, London, England. ROGELIO HERNANDEZ-PANDO • Department of Pathology, Instituto Nacional de la Nutricion, Salvador Zubrian, Delegacion Tlalpan, 14000 Mexico DF.

Opportunistic Intracellular Bacteria and Immunity, edited by Lois J. Paradise *et al.* Plenum Press, New York, 1999.

been successful in some rat strains, but not in others. The outcome depends upon the size of the corticosterone peak at a critical time point during disease induction. Strains that give a sufficient corticosterone peak, terminate the Th1-mediated inflammatory response, and, as has been demonstrated more recently, divert it toward Th2.[4] This concept is shown in Fig. 1. It is of fundamental interest for the discussion that follows. It suggests that genetic diversity at any point within the cytokine–HPA axis may contribute to a balance between a tendency to develop autoimmune disease and a tendency to develop chronic infection. Thus a failure to terminate Th1-mediated inflammation may predispose to autoimmunity, but conversely, premature termination or premature incapacitation of Th1 responses to pathogens such as *M. tuberculosis* may contribute to chronic infection.

In this chapter tuberculosis is used to illustrate the ways in which glucocorticoids (GCs; cortisol in man, and corticosterone in rodents) and steroids with "antiglucocorticoid" activity [dehydroepiandrosterone (DHEA)] affect cell-mediated immunity. The dicussion includes the actions of these steroids on T cells and macrophages, and the ways in which their actions are regulated in the periphery. Other adrenal steroids (such as sex steroids) also affect the immune system, but this chapter is confined to the two that play a dominant role in individuals of either sex. It is argued that there are abnormalities in the handling of these steroids in tuberculosis patients (and tuberculous rodents) and that these abnormalities play a major role in the dysregulated immune response that accompanies the disease. These concepts have a general relevance to other situations in which there is chronic unresolved cell-mediated inflammation.

2. THE MODE OF ACTION OF GLUCOCORTICOIDS

GC hormones bind to intracellular receptors that exist complexed to the 90-kDa heat-shock protein (hsp90) and to other proteins of lower molecular weight

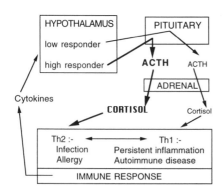

FIGURE 1. The size of the corticosterone peak that results from activation of the cytokine–hypo-thalamo–pituitary–adrenal axis varies in different rat strains. Those with a weak corticosterone response to immunization are more susceptible to induction of persistent Th1-mediated autoimmune inflammation. In strains with large corticosterone responses, the Th1 response is terminated and probably deviated toward Th2. In chronic infections, this early termination of the Th1-mediated inflammation would be a disadvantage rather than an advantage.

(Fig. 2). Dissociation of the receptor–GC complex from hsp90 then occurs, and receptor dimers are formed. In the nucleus these then interact with "glucocorticoid response elements" (GREs) that are involved in the regulation of expression of numerous genes including some that encode cytokines and other genes involved in the regulation of inflammation and immunity (Fig. 2).

This relatively simple picture, however, is complicated by other factors. Those factors operating at the receptor level include interaction of GC–receptor complexes with other transcription factors such as activator protein-1 (AP-1), nuclear factor-κB (NF-κB), and Janus kinase-signal transducer and activator of transcription (JAK STAT),[5] and modulation of GC action via alternative receptors for GCs. These include the mineralocorticoid receptors[6] (dicussed further later) and an alternative splicing of the glucocorticoid receptor yielding the β isoform that may act as a physiological inhibitor.[7] Little is known about the role of the latter, which is not considered further.

2.1. Interaction of GCs with Other Agonists

In vivo T cells are exposed to GCs in the presence of multiple agonists that can modulate or even reverse the effects of the GCs. For instance, low concentrations of dexamethasone or prostaglandin E_2 that did not inhibit the responsive

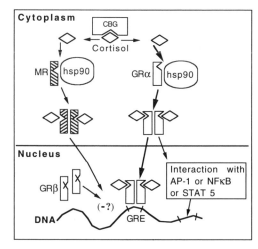

FIGURE 2. Most cortisol (represented as diamonds) is normally bound to cortisol-binding globulin (CBG). Once it has dissociated from the CBG it can enter cells, and in the cytoplasmic compartment it causes dissociation of the glucocorticoid receptor (GRα or type 2 receptor) and mineralocorticoid receptor (MR or type 1 receptor) from the 90-kDa heat-shock protein (hsp90). Receptor dimers are formed and these travel to the nucleus and bind to glucocorticoid response elements (GREs) that regulate transcription of the associated genes. MR dimers can act as functional antagonists of the GRs, and an alternative transcript of the GR (GRβ) may also act as a physiological inhibitor. The receptor dimers can also interact with and modulate the function of several other transcription factors such as AP-1, NF-κB, and STAT5.

ness of human T cells to stimulation by anti-CD3 acted synergistically to inhibit both interleukin-2 (IL-2) secretion and subsequent proliferation.[8]

The interaction of GCs with other mediators is particularly apparent when GCs are considered as inducers of T-cell apoptosis. Thus GC-induced apoptosis of T cells can be inhibited by ligands for CD44. Similarly peripheral blood T cells show sensitivity to GC-induced apoptosis soon after the proliferative response to mitogen stimulation, but they can be protected from apoptosis by several cytokines such as IL-2 and IL-4.

An important modulator of the effects of GCs on macrophages is migration inhibition factor (MIF). This was one of the first cytokines to be demonstrated, but only recently has its role begun to be understood. It modulates release of pro-inflammatory cytokines from macrophages by reducing the downregulatory effects of GCs.[9,10] This is discussed in greated detail in the section on GCs and macrophages.

2.2. The Diurnal Rhythm of Cortisol Production and T-Cell Function

In normal individuals there is a diurnal rhythm of serum cortisol level, which peaks in the morning and then declines throughout the day. Since cortisol has a 10-fold higher affinity for the mineralocorticoid receptor (MR) than it has for the glucocorticoid receptor (GR), this rhythm tends to result in occupation of the MR *and* GR in the morning, but only the MR later in the day. T cells in the thymus and peripheral blood express mostly or exclusively GR. These tend to mediate a lymphocyte suppressive effect, so these T cells alternate between steroid-suppressed and non-steroid-suppressed states in each 24-cycle.

In other organs such as spleen the situation can be more complex. The rat spleen expresses MR as well as GR, so the trough in the diurnal cycle of GC levels can result not just in diminished GC effects, but even in their replacement with contrary effects mediated via the MR. In this model, effects mediated via the MR can stimulate T-cell function.[6]

Similarly human monocytes are said to express MR as well as GR, and aldosterone is able to inhibit lipopolysaccharide (LPS)-induced IL-1ra secretion by monocytes *in vitro*.[11] The balance of MR- and GR-mediated effects on the immune system must therefore vary naturally during the 24-h cycle.

There is evidence suggesting that this physiological cycle is sufficient to cause a corresponding cyclical variation in lymphocyte function in humans.[12,13] For instance, release of interferon-γ (IFN-γ) in response to tetanus toxoid or purified protein derivative (PPD),[12] and the proliferative response of peripheral blood T cells to tetanus toxoid,[13] both show an inverse correlation with plasma cortisol levels. Diurnal rhythms can also be shown *in vivo*, and there is cyclical variation in the response to challenge with oxazolone, a contact sensitizing agent, in sensitized rats.[14]

The results emphasize the role of GCs, as even the normal physiological variations appear to be significant for T-cell function.

2.3. Abnormalities of the Diurnal Rhythm in Tuberculosis and HIV

Tuberculosis patients are reported to have a striking loss of this diurnal rhythm.[15] This effect is not disease specific. The rhythm can be lost during chronic or subacute stress or chronic infection and it can also be lost during HIV infection.[16] This lack of disease specificity does not detract from the probability that it has important immunological consequences. We have emphasized the possibility that GCs contribute to the loss of CD4[+] T lymphocytes in HIV infection, and to a lesser extent in tuberculosis.[17] There is an unconfirmed claim that HIV-seropositive individuals benefit from treatment with single early morning doses of prednisolone.[18] If true, this may be attributable to a beneficial effect of an artifically imposed prednisolone diurnal rhythm, replacing the faulty endogenous cortisol rhythm associated with the disease.[16] This may be beneficial because it stops the exposure of the patients' T cells to a 24-h GC influence.

3. REGULATION OF TISSUE CONCENTRATIONS OF CORTISOL

The local concentration of cortisol in any cell or tissue is not dependent only on the concentration reaching that tissue from the circulation. In most tissues local concentrations are regulated in response to the particular requirements of the tissue. The major mechanism for this involves interconversion of active cortisol and inactive cortisone (cortisol–cortisone shuttle).

Most interconversion of cortisol and cortisone is thought to occur in two sites, the kidney and the liver. In the kidney the enzyme 11β-hydroxysteroid dehydrogenase type 2 (11βHSD-2) converts cortisol into inactive cortisone, and so stops the MR from binding cortisol.[19] This allows mineralocorticoid functions to be mediated almost exclusively by aldosterone in spite of the facts that this hormone is present at much lower levels than GCs, and GCs have a high affinity for MR. In normal individuals an oxidoreductase in the liver known as 11βHSD-1 then rapidly converts the resulting cortisone back to cortisol, so that the circulating cortisol is maintained 5 to 10 times higher than the circulating cortisone.

The importance of these observations has been highlighted by studies of infection with *Listeria monocytogenes* in mice. Treating the animals with an inhibitor of 11βHSD was equivalent to treating them with dexamethasone, and resulted in increased bacterial counts, decreased production of IFN-γ, and increased production of IL-10.[20] Moreover these effects could be blocked with RU486, a potent antagonist of GC receptors. Thus although the 11βHSD inhibitor actually resulted in *lowered* plasma corticosterone levels (due to increased feedback), failure of inactivation of endogenous GCs in lymphoid tissue was sufficient to mimic administration of exogenous GCs. A very similar phenomenon appears to occur spontaneously in tuberculosis, as described in the following section.[21]

3.1. Abnormalities of the Cortisol–Cortisone Shuttle in Tuberculosis

In tuberculosis patients the ratio of metabolites of cortisol to metabolites of cortisone is heavily biased toward cortisol.[21] This clearly cannot be due to failure of conversion to cortisone in the kidney, because such a failure would lead to hypertension and salt retention. Recent studies of changes in cortisol levels after oral intake of cortisone indicate that it is in fact due to accelerated "single-pass" conversion of cortisone to cortisol (Baker *et al.*, in preparation). This may be happening in the liver, but the lung is clearly another alternative.

Most tissues, in addition to lung and liver mentioned earlier, possess enzymes that can interconvert cortisol and cortisone, and can therefore adjust the local GC concentration. In the context of tuberculosis the crucial organs are the lymph nodes and the lungs, both of which contain fascinating 11βHSD activities.

The enzyme in the lung may be particularly relevant to tuberculosis. It resembles the one in the liver, though in the lungs of normal donors it is running in reverse, converting cortisol into inactive cortisone.[22] Therefore the type 1 enzyme is clearly a reversible and regulated oxidoreductase. It has been observed that in granulosa cell preparations, removal of contaminating T cells alters the activity of the enzyme, suggesting that it may be regulated by cytokines.[23] We postulate therefore that in the cytokine-rich environment of the tuberculous lung, the 11β-HSD-1 may convert cortisone back to cortisol. This hypothesis is accessible to investigation.

4. DEHYDROEPIANDROSTERONE AS AN ANTIGLUCOCORTICOID

There is a further category of regulatory pathways that modulate the functions of GC in the periphery. These are mediated by "antiglucocorticoid" effects of dehydroepiandrosterone sulfate (DHEAS), or of metabolites of this steroid. The mechanisms are not understood, but the effects are striking and experimental data in murine models and correlations in man, outlined later, suggest that DHEA is important in tuberculosis.

DHEA is the most abundant product of the human adrenal after adrenarche. The adrenal secretes 10 to 15 mg of DHEAS/day in healthy young adults, but serum levels then fall steadily with increasing age. It is strongly bound to albumin and undergoes renal tubular reabsorption. In young adults it is present at concentrations close to 4 μg/ml. Eventually most of it is converted to DHEA. Thus in humans the major source of DHEA is DHEAS. Most DHEA circulates freely but some is weakly bound to albumin.

4.1. Mechanism of Action of DHEA on the Immune System

It is not known how DHEA exerts its antiglucocorticoid effects. It is not a competitive antagonist of the GC receptor. There is a report of a specific DHEA-binding protein (? receptor) in T lymphocytes but this remains unconfirmed. DHEAS bind to some receptors on cell membranes in the brain, but there is no evidence for such membrane receptors in the periphery.

Another intriguing possibility has emerged from the discovery that DHEAS acts as a peroxisome proliferator. This results in upregulation of expression of enzymes responsible for lipid homoeostasis, fatty acid degradation, and destruction of leukotriene B4 (LTB4). This action of DHEAS requires the presence of peroxisome proliferator-activated receptor-α (PPAR-α). There is no direct evidence that DHEAS is a ligand for this receptor, but it is interesting that there is a protein that binds DHEAS in liver, and PPAR-α is expressed at particularly high levels in this organ and in the immune system (reviewed elsewhere).[24,25] The PPARs are a family of transcription factors analogous to the steroid receptors. They form heterodimers with RXR, the receptor for 9-*cis*-retinoic acid, and bind to DNA motifs known as PPAR-response elements. It has been suggested that its role as a peroxisome proliferator could explain the restoration of immunological competence by DHEAS in old animals, via changes in cell membrane fluidity, phospholipid-dependent cell signaling pathways, and arachidonate-dependent mediators.[24,25]

Alternatively DHEA may be metabolized to unidentified effector steroids acting through one of the "orphan" steroid receptors, but there is no direct evidence for this.

4.2. DHEA and Immune Response in Rodents

The physiology of DHEA in rodents, in which most of the experimental work has been done, is different from its physiology in man, and this must be taken into account when interpreting the available data. Thus whereas there are about 4 μg/ml of DHEAS in adult human plasma, rat plasma contains < 1 ng/ml of this hormone.[26] Unexpectedly, in rodents the brain is the site where concentrations of DHEAS (and at a lower level, DHEA) are highest. Thus rat brain contained an average of 3.5 ng/g of tissue over a 24-h period.[26] DHEAS in brain has clear neurological functions that are outside the scope of this chapter. The DHEAS in brain is thought to be locally synthesized, and it is possible that it is not synthesized at all in rodent adrenals because this organ lacks 17α-hydroxylase. Nevertheless DHEAS and fatty acid esters of DHEA were found in the adrenals of rats at 5.1 ± 2.6 and 16.1 ± 6.4 ng/g of tissue, respectively.[26] If the rodent adrenal does make DHEA it must use an unusual pathway. Alternatively in rodents the immunological functions of DHEA may be performed by some other derivative that can be reached via a different route.

In view of the points outlined in the previous paragraph, it is clear that much of the literature on the effects of DHEA or DHEAS in rodents should be interpreted with caution, or discounted altogether, because quantities as high as 1 g/kg have been used in species with physiological levels < 1 ng/ml of plasma or gram of tissue! At more appropriate, but still high dose levels, three daily injections of 1.2 mg of DHEA (i.e., 50 to 60 mg/kg/day) were found to stop dexamethasone from rendering peripheral lymphocytes of mice unresponsive to mitogens, or causing involution of the thymus.[27] In fact even this dose is neither required nor optimal, and doses in the microgram range are more effective. Larger doses actually diminish the effect in the thymus protection assay used by Blauer and colleagues, probably because of conversion to testosterone which decreases thymic bulk. As an example of the efficacy of lower doses, optimal inhibition of GC-induced thymic involution in mice requires only 10 to 20 μg/mouse of DHEA or of its derivative 3,17-androstenediol (i.e., ~ 0.5 mg/kg; see Ref. 27a).

In summary, DHEA, using acceptable doses in the low microgram range opposes GCs, and promotes a Th1 cytokine pattern in rodents. It has also been shown to restore immune functions in aged mice, and to correct the dysregulated spontaneous cytokine release seen in old animals.[28,29] It also enhances production of Th1 cytokines such as IL-2 and IFN-γ.[30] This is the reverse of the effect of GCs, which often enhance Th2 activity and synergize with Th2 cytokines, and as described later, drive newly recruited T cells toward Th2.

DHEA also enhances IL-2 secretion from human peripheral blood T cells,[31] and we have found that DHEA or 3β, 17β-androstenediol (AED) will enhance mitogen-stimulated production of IFN-γ from murine or human T cells in the range 10^{-7} to 10^{-8} M (Al-Nakhli et al., in preparation).

4.3. Abnormalities of DHEAS Production and Metabolism in Tuberculosis

The overall ratio of DHEA to cortisol is decreased in tuberculosis.[21] This can be shown by measuring DHEAS metabolites in 24-h urine collections. This is not a disease-specific effect, and similar changes can be induced by extreme physical and mental stress,[32] or other severe illness.

The pattern of metabolism of DHEA also changes in tuberculosis, so that less than usual is reduced to androsterone or aetiocholanolone, while more of it is converted to 16α-hydroxylated derivatives (even in the absence of antituberculosis therapy; this is not an effect induced by rifampicin, though rifampicin can activate the relevant enzyme, CYP 3A7).[21] Because we do not know which metabolites exert the anti-GC effects, interpretation of this change is difficult, but it may be significant that these 16α-hydroxylated derivatives are not active *in vivo* as anti-GCs (Al-Nakhli *et al.*, in preparation). Moreover the same 16α-hydroxylated derivatives are formed during pregnancy and by premature neonates.[33] Our hypothesis is that this represents one of several mechanisms that tend to drive the immune response towards Th2 in pregnancy,[34] as Th1 responses to placental antigens are associated with abortion.[35] Perhaps tuberculosis is "attempting" to do the same thing.

5. MODULATION OF MACROPHAGE FUNCTIONS BY *GLUCOCORTICOIDS*

GCs can inhibit many macrophage functions, but the precise effects seen depend upon dose and time of exposure. The literature is biased by the fact that most workers use unrealistically high concentrations of synthetic and very potent GC agonists such as dexamethasone. Moreover, *in vitro* systems do not mimic the diurnal rhythm discussed earlier. For instance dexamethasone can inhibit both phagocytosis and tumor necrosis factor-α (TNF-α) release by rat macrophages.[36] However, short-term exposure of rat alveolar macrophages to dexamethasone, or longer exposure to low-dose dexamethasone, *increase* subsequent LPS-induced NO and IL-1β secretion. Suppression is seen only with higher doses or longer exposure.[37]

Many effects of GC on macrophages are secondary to induction of other antiinflammatory molecules. For instance, lipocortin-1 may be involved in dexamethasone-mediated suppression of LPS-triggered release of TNF-α and prostaglandin E_2 from peripheral blood mononuclear cells.[38] Similarly it was found that administration of GCs to patients undergoing cardiopulmonary bypass prevented release of IL-8, but caused a 10-fold increase in IL-10 release.[39] In view of the antiinflammatory roles of this cytokine, and its ability to influence Th1/Th2 balance, this is a potentially important observation, and parallels the increased IL-10 production seen in the *Listeria* model when the inactivation of GCs was blocked with an inhibitor of 11βHSD,[20] as discussed in Section 3. Moreover GC-treated macrophages are said to secrete other novel antiinflammatory activities.[40]

5.1. Modulation of the Effects of GCs on Macrophages by MIF

As mentioned earlier, the effects of GC on macrophages are modified by MIF. Thus LPS-triggered macrophages pretreated with low doses of MIF became refractory to GC-mediated inhibition of release of IL-1β, IL-6, IL-8, and TNF-α.[9,10]

However, MIF is not only released locally by inflammatory cells. It is an abundant preformed constituent of the anterior pituitary where it is found in granules with adrenocorticotropic hormone (ACTH) or thyroid-stimulating hormone (TSH).[41] Moreover, corticotropin-releasing hormone (CRH) is a potent secretagogue for MIF. Thus while ACTH is being released in response to stimulation of the cytokine–hypothalamo–pituitary–adrenal axis, MIF can also be released and can then oppose the effect of GCs on macrophages in the periphery. This effect appears to be physiologically relevant. For instance, MIF potentiates LPS-mediated shock, as can be demonstrated directly by the administration of recombinant MIF. Similarly, neutralizing antibody to MIF is protective in the same model.[10] It is therefore probable that in tuberculosis MIF is playing a role in the regulation of GC-mediated suppression of proinflammatory cytokine release, and this is central to the pathogenesis of the disease. Unfortunately, we currently know nothing about its abundance in tuberculosis, or how its release from the pituitary is affected by the changes in diurnal rhythm previously outlined.

5.2. GCs and Apoptosis of Myeloid Cells

A further important role of GCs is the regulation of apoptosis in myeloid cells. Neutrophils express both Fas and Fas ligand which may indicate a constitutive commitment to apoptosis. This apoptosis is blocked by granulocyte-colony-stimulating factor (G-CSF), granulocyte-macrophage-colony-stimulating factor (GM-CSF), IFN-γ, TNF-α, or dexamethasone.[42] In contrast, treatment of asthma with GC leads to eosinophil apoptosis, and to the appearance of eosinophil-derived material in macrophages.[43] Thus GCs inhibit neutrophil apoptosis, but induce eosinophil apotosis.

5.3. GCs, Macrophages, MIF, and Tuberculosis

The ability of human and murine macrophages to control the growth of *M. tuberculosis* is severely compromised by GCs *in vitro*.[44] Similarly the ability of restraint stress to enhance mycobacterial growth *in vivo* was shown to be directly attributable to GCs.[45] Interestingly this ability of GC to enhance mycobacterial growth in murine macrophages *in vitro* is seen using macrophages from *Bcg^s* mice but not from *Bcg^r* mice.[45] *Bcg^s* and *Bcg^r* are alleles of an autosomal dominant gene, *Nramp1*, that affects innate resistance of mice to mycobacteria and to several other intracellular pathogens.

It will be interesting to know whether this effect of GCs can be abrogated by MIF, though this has not yet been studied. It is known that in a murine model of delayed-type hypersensitivity (DTH) to tuberculin, where MIF mRNA and protein were shown to be abundant (mostly in macrophages), a neutralizing antibody to MIF inhibited the DTH response.[46] We have argued elsewhere that proinflammatory cytokines contribute significantly to tissue damage in this infection.[47,48]

6. MODULATION OF T-CELL FUNCTION BY GLUCOCORTICOIDS

The fundamental importance of GCs as regulators of T-lymphocyte function is highlighted by the discovery that radioresistant thymic epithelial cells contain steroidogenic enzymes.[49] These cells actively secrete steroids that may play crucial role in thymic T-lymphocyte repertoire selection.[49]

However, GCs also influence the types of function that T cells develop, and their Th1/Th2 bias. For instance, T cells were sorted by fluorescence activated cell sorter into CD4+CD45RO− (naive) and CD4+CD45RO+ (memory) subsets, and then primed with anti-CD3 (solid phase) in the presence of IL-2 for 9 days, resulting in considerable clonal expansion. The cells were then washed, put into fresh medium, and restimulated for 72 h with anti-CD3 and IL-2. GCs were added to these cultures, either in the priming phase or during the restimulation. Then supernatants from the restimulation phase were assayed for cytokines.[50] The results were quite different with naive and primed cells, and also depended critically on whether the GCs were present during priming or during restimulation. Memory (CD45RO+) T cells switched to exclusive IL-10 production if the GCs were present during the priming phase, but if present during *restimulation*,the only cytokine produced was IFN-γ.[50] This type of observation tends to be misinterpreted. Much more significant is the observation that the naive (CD45RO−) cells cultured with GCs always tended to switch toward Th2. They eventually secreted IL-10 if the GCs were present during the priming phase, and both IL-4 and IL-10 if GCs were present during the restimulation phase.

These results are in accordance with the finding that if an immune response in naive cells is allowed to develop in the presence of GC, a Th2 line will develop. This has been rather clearly shown with spleen cells from "clean" laboratory rodents,[4] which have few memory cells under normal circumstances. Overall the "bottom line" may be that GC favor the *development* of a Th2 cytokine profile from naive cells, although cytokine secretion by established Th2 cells is readily inhibited. The ability of some Th1 cells to continue to secrete Th1 cytokines after exposure to GCs does not alter the fact that Th1 *function* is blocked by GCs. This is partly due to other GC effects such as blockage of macrophage function and enhanced expression of TGF-β and IL-10, and partly due to the fact that in a dynamic *in vivo* situation what is important is the diversion of subsequently recruited T cells toward Th2. Thus conventional treatments for Th2-mediated diseases such as eczema, asthma, and hay fever may work via antiinflammatory effects, and by reducing cytokine production by Th2 cells, and by apoptosis of eosinophils[43] and yet at the same time encourage perpetuation of the underlying problem by driving newly recruited T cells toward Th2.

6.1. T-Cell Function in Tuberculosis; Possible Effects of GCs

Late progressive murine tuberculosis is accompanied by a clearcut switch to a Th2-dominated pattern of cytokine production.[51] In humans the switch is less complete but there is overwhelming evidence for inappropriate activation of a Th2 component that coexists with a dominant Th1 pattern. Tuberculosis patients have IgE antibody to *M. tuberculosis*.[52] The IL-4 gene is expressed in peripheral blood mononuclear cells, and there is a deficit in IL-2 expression.[53] They also have relatively large numbers of circulating T cells that can be activated *in vitro* to express IL-4 after culture with phorbol myristate acetate and calcium ionophore. Such cells are not found in normal peripheral blood (Thapa *et al.*, manuscript in preparation). All of the changes in the production and metabolism of GCs and DHEA that have been identified in tuberculosis patients would be expected to increase the net exposure of T cells to GC-mediated effects (Fig. 3), and so cause

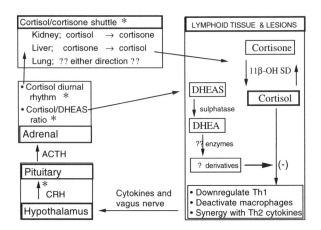

*abnormalities shown in tuberculosis

FIGURE 3. Factors that determine the effective cortisol function in lymphoid tissue. Cytokines and signals arriving via the vagus nerve cause the hypothalamus to send signals to the pituitary, particularly corticotropin-releasing hormone (CRH). The pituitary releases adrenocorticotropic hormone (ACTH), which increases steroid production by the adrenal. However, the diurnal rhythm of this steroid production and the ratio of DHEAS to cortisol secreted are important variables that are controlled in ways we do not fully understand. The cortisol/cortisone shuttle then modulates the actual delivery of cortisol to the tissues. Finally, within lymphoid tissues and the target organs, both DHEAS and cortisol are subject to regulated local metabolism. The pathway of conversion of DHEA to the putative active antiglucocorticoid is unknown. The action of this antiglucocorticoid is indicated with (-).

the development of Th2 cells, and premature termination or dysregulation of the Th1 response (Fig. 1).

Stress, which increases GC production, can contribute to these effects. The incidence of tuberculosis increases in war zones and in areas of poverty. Similarly, moving cattle from one farm to another in trucks is sufficient to cause reactivation of latent bovine tuberculosis. This point can be demonstrated in a more controlled manner in laboratory animals. Stress due to crowding or restraint can increase mycobacterial growth in tuberculous mice.[54,55]

At present the contention that GCs are fundamental to these swings toward Th2 remains speculative. However, recent studies in a mouse model reinforce this concept. Murine tuberculosis provides a model that is acutely sensitive to the presence of even a small Th2 component.[48]

7. MURINE TUBERCULOSIS AND THE ROLE OF THE ADRENALS

When mice were infected with virulent *Mycobacterium tuberculosis* H37Rv by the intratracheal route, there was an early phase of adrenal hyperplasia, histologically resembling the ACTH driven changes seen in Cushing's disease. This was followed at 3 weeks by progressive atrophy until the weight of the adrenals was ~ 50% of that seen in control uninfected mice, in spite of the fact that the adrenals were not infected (Fig. 4a). All layers of the adrenal cortex were affected, but the medulla was normal. Electron microscopic studies revealed apoptosis.[48,56]

7.1. Changes in Adrenal Size and the Th1/Th2 Balance

The switch from adrenal hyperplasia to adrenal atrophy correlated with a switch from a Th1-dominated to a mixed Th1 + Th2 cytokine profile. Thus after an early peak (days 3 to 7 after infection), the numbers of cells positive for IL-2 in inflammatory sites (by immunocytochemistry) decreased progressively, while the percentage of IL-4 positive cells rose abruptly between days 21 and 28.[27a]

This relationship between increasing Th2 activity and adrenal atrophy could also be demonstrated by preimmunizing the mice so that they had a Th2 component even before infection with *M. tuberculosis*. If 2 months before mice received the intratracheal infection, they were preimmunized with a very large dose of *M. vaccae* (10^9 autoclaved bacilli) known to prime a mixed pattern of cytokine release (IFN-γ and IL-4),[57] the adrenal atrophy began within 4 days of infection, and was complete by day 14 (Fig. 5).[48,56] In contrast, if the mice were preimmunized with 10^7 autoclaved *M. vaccae*, a stimulus previously shown to induce an exclusively Th1 pattern of response, the early increase in adrenal weight was attenuated and delayed, and the subsequent atrophy did not occur (Fig. 5).[48,56]

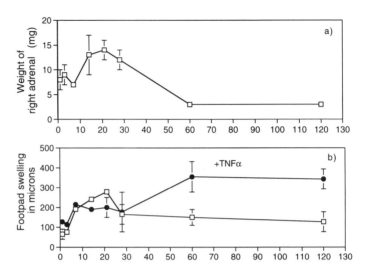

FIGURE 4. Events in murine pulmonary tuberculosis that correlate with changes in adrenal weight. Following intratracheal infection with *M. tuberculosis*, the adrenals increase in weight for 21 days (a). During this phase DTH to tuberculin is increasing (b, □) and DTH sites are not sensitive to TNF-α (b, ●). After 21 days, the adrenals start to atrophy (a). Simultaneously DTH decreases (b, □), and the DTH sites become sensitive to TNF-α (b, ●). (From ref. 48, with permission.) Recent studies show that these events between day 21 and day 28 also correlate with the sudden appearance of large numbers of lymphocytes with a Th2 cytokine profile.[51,56,57]

7.2. Changes in Adrenal Size and the Toxicity of Cytokines

A further important correlate of the late phase of murine tuberculosis (when the adrenals are atrophic and the immune response characterized by a mixed Th1 + Th2 cytokine profile) is increased toxicity of TNF-α. DTH responses to tuberculin were seen throughout the infection, but differed in their sensitivity to TNF-α in a manner that correlated closely with adrenal size. Thus if TNF-α was injected at 24 h into DTH sites elicited during the phase of adrenal hyperplasia, there was no increment in swelling at 48 h. However, similar injections of TNF-α resulted in a doubling of the swelling in DTH sites elicited during the phase of adrenal atrophy (Fig. 4b). It may be relevant that the toxicity of cytokine such as TNF-α is closely regulated by rapid feedback from the cytokine–hypothalamo–pituitary–adrenal axis (cytokine–HPA axis). Failure of this feedback enhances toxicity.[58] Studies in this[47] and other laboratories[59] have led us to argue that although TNF-α has essential protective macrophage-activating roles in certain Th1 responses to mycobacteria in mice, it nevertheless has important toxic roles in the *disease* where immunity is failing, and when an inappropriate Th2 component is present.[57] We do not know whether the adrenal in tuberculosis is capable

FIGURE 5. The consequences for the adrenals of preimmunisation to preset the Th1 / Th2 balance before infection with *M. tuberculosis*. Mice were immunized so as to evoke a Th1 response (△) or a mixed Th1 + Th2 response (●) or injected with saline (○). Two months later they were given intratracheal *M. tuberculosis*. The adrenals of control (saline) mice (○) showed changes similar to those in Figure 4a. The adrenals of mice with mixed Th1 + Th2 responses started to atrophy within 3 days (●). In contrast, the changes were attenuated in mice with Th1 responses (△). (From ref. 48, with permission.)

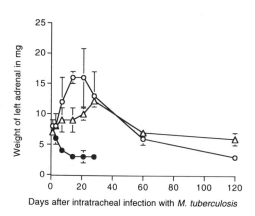

Days after intratracheal infection with *M. tuberculosis*

of responding appropriately to a sudden "acute-on-chronic" cytokine-mediated stimulus, though this is testable.

7.3. The Scope for Endocrinological Manipulations of Murine Tuberculosis

These observations make the murine model of pulmonary tuberculosis particularly accessible to experiments designed to clarify the role of GC levels and of GC/DHEA ratios in this infection. For example, preliminary studies indicate that administration of DHEA is protective if it is given during the early phase of progressive adrenal hypertrophy.[60] In contrast, administration of DHEA later in the disease, when the adrenals have atrophied, leads to accelerated death. However, DHEA is known to be toxic to mice in the absence of adequate adrenal function, presumably because of its anti-GC actions. Therefore in further pilot studies, mice in this late Th2-dominated phase of the disease (day 60, Fig. 4a) were treated with both a DHEA derivative and GC supplements. This had led to prolonged survival, although either hormone used alone was detrimental.[61] In this system, therefore, the balance of GC to DHEA appears to be critical. Further experiments are in progress, and it is hoped that they will lead not only to increased understanding of the immunoendocrine interactions in tuberculosis, but also to novel therapies.

8. CONCLUSIONS

In tuberculosis patients there are several changes in the production, diurnal rhythm, and peripheral metabolism of GCs and of DHEA that will result in an increase in the total impact of GCs on T cells and macrophages in each 24-h period. The long-term effect of increased GC-mediated gene regulation is to terminate Th1 activity and deviate the immune system toward a Th2 cytokine profile. In tuberculosis even a minor Th2 component is sufficient to undermine the efficacy of immunity. Preimmunization to establish a Th2 component before infection results in animals that are more susceptible to the disease than are nonimmunized controls.[48] In progressive human tuberculosis the Th1 response remains dominant, but there is conclusive evidence for the simultaneous presence of an inappropriate Th2 component. This may represent an attempt by the HPA axis to cause premature termination of the Th1 response. Recent attempts to manipulate murine tuberculosis by purely endocrine means lend support to this concept, and suggest that endocrine-based therapies may become a reality.

ACKNOWLEDGMENTS. We are grateful to the Wellcome Trust for supporting R. B.'s studies of the endocrinology of tuberculosis and to the National University of Mexico and the CONACYT for supporting Dr. R. Hernandez-Pando's visits to the U. K. and laboratory work in Mexico.

REFERENCES

1. Layé, S., Bluthé, R. M., Kent, S., Combe, C., Médina, C., Parnet, P., Kelley, K. W., and Dantzer, R., 1995, Subdiaphragmatic vagotomy blocks the induction of interleukin-1β mRNA in the brain of mice in response to peripherally administered lipopolysaccharide, *Am. J. Physiol.* **268:**R1327–R1331.
2. Sternberg, E. M., Young, W. S., Bernardini, R., Calogero, A. E., Chrousos, G. P., and Gold, P. W., and Wilder, R. L., 1989, A central nervous system defect in the biosynthesis of CRH is associated with susceptibility to streptococcal cell wall-induced arthritis in Lewis rats, *Proc. Natl. Acad. Sci. USA,* **86:**4771–4775.
3. MacPhee, I. A. M., Antoni, F. A., and Mason, D. W., 1989, Spontaneous recovery of rats from experimental allergic encephalomyelitis is dependent on regulation of the immune system by endogenous adrenal corticosteroids, *J. Exp. Med.* **169:**431–445.
4. Ramirez, F., Fowell, D. J., Puklavec, M., Simmonds, S., and Mason, D., 1996, Glucocorticoids promote a Th2 cytokine response by CD4+ T cells *in vitro, J. Immunol.* **156:**2406–2412.
5. Stöcklin, E., Vissler, M., Gouilleux, F., and Groner, B., 1996, Functional interactions between Stat5 and the glucocorticoid receptor, *Nature* **383:**726–728.
6. Wiegers, G. J., Reul, J. M., Holsboer, F., and de Kloet, E. R., 1994, Enhancement of rat splenic lymphocyte mitogenesis after short term preexposure to corticosteroids in vitro, *Endocrinology* **135:**2351–2357.
7. Oakley, R. H., Sar, M., and Cidlowski, J. A., 1996, The human glucocorticoid receptor beta isoform. Expression, biochemical properties, and putative function, *J. Biol. Chem.* **271:**9550–9559.
8. Elliott, L. H., Levay, A. K., Sparks, B., Miller, M., and Roszman, T. L., 1996, Dexamethasone and prostaglandin E2 modulate T-cell receptor signaling through a cAMP-independent mechanism, *Cell. Immunol.* **169:**117–124.

9. Calandra, T., Bernhagen, J., Mitchell, R. A., and Bucala, R., 1994, The macrophage is an important and previously unrecognized source of macrophage migration inhibitory factor, *J. Exp. Med.* **179:**1895–1902.

10. Calandra, T., Bernhagen, J., Metz, C. N., Spiegel, L. A., Bacher, M., Donnelly, T., Cerami, A., and Bucala, R., 1995, MIF as a glucocorticoid-induced modulator of cytokine production, *Nature* **377:**68–71.

11. Sauer, J., Castren, M., Hopfner, U., Holsboer, F., Stalla, G. K., and Arzt, E., 1996, Inhibition of lipopolysaccharide-induced monocyte interleukin-1 receptor antagonist synthesis by cortisol: Involvement of the mineralocorticoid receptor, *J. Clin. Endocrinol. Metab.* **81:**73–79.

12. Petrovsky, N., McNair, P., and Harrison, L. C., 1994, Circadian rhythmicity of interferon-gamma production in antigen-stimulated whole blood, *Chronobiologia* **21:**293–300.

13. Hiemke, C., Brunner, R., Hammes, E., Muller, H., Meyer, z. B. K., and Lohse, A. W., 1995, Circadian variations in antigen-specific proliferation of human T lymphocytes and correlation to cortisol production, *Psychoneuroendocrinology* **20:**335–342.

14. Pownall, R., Kabler, P. A., and Knapp, M. S., 1979, The time of day of antigen encounter influences the magnitude of the immune response, *Clin. Exp. Immunol.* **36:**347–354.

15. Sarma, G. R., Chandra, I., Ramachandran, G., Krishnamurthy, P. V., Kumaraswami, V., and Prabhakar, R., 1990, Adrenocortical function in patients with pulmonary tuberculosis, *Tubercle* **71:**277–282.

16. Lortholary, O., Christeff, N., Casassus, P., Thobie, N., Veyssier, P., Trogoff, B., Torri, O., Brauner, M., Nunez, E. A., and Guillevin, L., 1996, Hypothalamo–pituitary–adrenal function in human immunodeficiency virus-infected men, *J. Clin. Endocrinol. Metab.* **81:**791–796.

17. Rook, G. A. W., Onyebujoh, P., and Stanford, J. L., 1993, TH1 → TH2 switch and loss of CD4 cells in chronic infections; an immuno-endocrinological hypothesis not exclusive to HIV, *Immunol. Today* **14:**568–569.

18. Andrieu, J. M., Lu, W., and Levy, R., 1995, Sustained increases in CD4 cell counts in asymptomatic human immunodeficiency virus type 1-seropositive patients treated with prednisolone for 1 year, *J. Infect. Dis.* **171:**523–530.

19. Walker, B. R., 1994, Organ-specific actions of 11 beta-hydroxysteroid dehydrogenase in humans: Implications for the pathophysiology of hypertension, *Steroids* **59:**84–89.

20. Hennebold, J. D., Mu, H.-H., Poynter, M. E., Chen, X.-P., and Daynes, R. A., 1997, Active catabolism of glucocorticoids by 11β-hydroxytseroid dehydrogenase *in vivo* is a necessary requirement for natural resistance to infection with *Listeria monocytogenes*, *Int. Immunol.* **9:**105–115.

21. Rook, G. A. W., Honour, J., Kon, O. M., Wilkinson, R. J., Davidson, R., and Shaw, R. J., 1996, Urinary steroid metabolites in tuberculosis; a new clue to pathogenesis, *Q. J. Med.* **89:**333–341.

22. Hubbard, W. C., Bickel, C., and Schleimer, R. P., 1994, Simultaneous quantitation of endogenous levels of cortisone and cortisol in human nasal and bronchoalveolar lavage fluids and plasma via gas chromatography-negative ion chemical ionization mass spectrometry, *Anal. Biochem.* **221:**109–117.

23. Evangelatou, M., Antoniw, J., and Cooke, B. A., 1996, The effect of leukocytes on 11β-HSD activity in human granulosa cell cultures, *J. Endocrinol.* **148** (Suppl.):Abstract P55.

24. Spencer, N. F. L., Poynter, M. E., Henebold, J. D., Mu, H. H., and Daynes, R. A., 1995, Does DHEAS restore immune competence in aged animals through its capacity to function as a natural modulator of peroxisome activities?, *Ann. NY Acad. Sci.* **774:**201–216.

25. Devchand, P. R., Keller, H., Peters, J. M., Vasquez, M., Gonzalez, F. J., and Wahli, W., 1996, The PPARα-leukotriene B4 pathway to inflammation control, *Nature* **384:**39–43.

26. Robel, P., and Baulieu, E. E., 1995, Dehydroepiandrosterone (DHEA) is a neuroactive neurosteroid, *Ann. NY Acad. Sci.* **774:**82–110.

27. Blauer, K. L., Poth, M., Rogers, W. M., and Bernton, E. W., 1991, Dehydroepiandrosterone

antagonises the suppressive effects of dexamethasone on lymphocyte proliferation, *Endocrinology* **129**:3174–3179.

28. Daynes, R. A., Araneo, B. A., Ershler, W. B., Maloney, C., Li, G.-Z., and Ryu, S.-Y., 1993, Altered regulation of IL-6 production with normal aging; possible linkage to the age-associated decline in dehydroepiandrosterone and its sulphated derivative, *J. Immunol.* **150**:5219–5230.

29. Garg, M., and Bondada, S., 1993, Reversal of age-associated decline in immune response to Pnuimune vaccine by supplementation with the steroid hormone dehydroepiandrosterone, *Infect. Immun.* **61**:2238–2241.

30. Daynes, R. A., Araneo, B. A., Hennebold, J., Enioutina, J., and Mu, H. H., 1995, Steroids as regulators of the mammalian immune response, *J. Invest. Dermatol.* **105**:14S–19S.

31. Suzuki, T., Suzuki, N., Daynes, R. A., and Engleman, E. G., 1991, Dehydroepiandrosterone enhances IL2 production and cytotoxic effector function of human T cells, *Clin. Immunol. Immunopathol.* **61**:202–211.

32. Bernton, E., Hoover, D., Galloway, R., and Popp, K., 1995, Adaptation to chronic stress in military trainees. Adrenal androgens, testosterone, glucocorticoids, IGF-1 and immune function, *Ann. NY Acad. Sci.* **774**:217–231.

33. Kitada, M., Kamataki, T., Itahashi, K., Rikihisa, T., and Kanakubo, Y., 1987, P-450 HFLa, a form of cytochrome P-450 purified from human foetal livers, is the 16α-hydroxylase of dehydroepiandrosterone 3-sulphate, *J. Biol. Chem.* **262**:13534–13537.

34. Wegmann, T. G., Lin, H., Guilbert, L., and Mosmann, T. R., 1993, Bidirectional cytokine interactions in the maternal–fetal relationship: Is succesful pregnancy a Th2 phenomenon?, *Immunol. Today* **14**:353–356.

35. Hill, J. A., Polgar, K., and Anderson, D. J., 1995, T-helper 1-type immunity to trophoblast in women with recurrent spontaneous abortion, *JAMA* **273**:1933–1936.

36. Nakamura, Y., Murai, T., and Ogawa, Y., 1996, Effect of in vitro and in vivo administration of dexamethasone on rat macrophage functions: Comparison between alveolar and peritoneal macrophages, *Eur. Respir. J.* **9**:301–306.

37. Broug-Holub, E., and Kraal, G., 1996, Dose- and time-dependent activation of rat alveolar macrophages by glucocorticoids, *Clin. Exp. Immunol.* **104**:332–336.

38. Sudlow, A. W., Carey, F., Forder, R., and Rothwell, N. J., 1996, The role of lipocortin-1 in dexamethasone-induced suppression of PGE2 and TNF alpha release from human peripheral blood mononuclear cells, *Br. J. Pharmacol.* **117**:1449–1456.

39. Tabardel, Y., Duchateau, J., Schmartz, D., Marecaux, G., Shahla, M., Barvais, L., Leclerc, J. L., and Vincent, J. L., 1996, Corticosteroids increase blood interleukin-10 levels during cardiopulmonary bypass in men, *Surgery* **119**:76–80.

40. Hamann, W., Floter, A., Schmutzler, W., and Zwadlo-Klarwasser, G., 1995, Characterization of a novel anti-inflammatory factor produced by RM3/1 macrophages derived from glucocorticoid treated human monocytes, *Inflamm. Res.* **44**:535–540.

41. Nishino, T., Bernhagen, J., Shiiki, H., Calandra, T., Dohi, K., and Bucala, R., 1995, Localization of macrophage migration inhibitory factor (MIF) to secretory granules within the corticotrophic and thyrotrophic cells of the pituitary gland, *Mol. Med.* **1**:781–788.

42. Liles, W. C., Kiener, P. A., Ledbetter, J. A., Aruffo, A., and Klebanoff, S. J., 1996, Differential expression of Fas (CD95) a Fas ligand on normal human phagocytes: Implications for the regulation of apoptosis in neutrophils, *J. Exp. Med.* **184**:429–440.

43. Woolley, K. L., Gibson, P. G., Carty, K., Wilson, A. J., Twaddell, S. H., and Woolley, M. J., 1996, Eosinophil apoptosis and the resolution of airway inflammation in asthma, *Am. J. Respir. Crit. Care Med.* **154**:237–243.

44. Rook, G. A., Steele, J., Ainsworth, M., and Leveton, C., 1987, A direct effect of glucocorticoid hormones on the ability of human and murine macrophages to control the growth of *M. tuberculosis*, *Eur. J. Respir. Dis.* **71**:286–291.

45. Brown, D. H., LaFuse, W., and Zwilling, B. S., 1995, cytokine-mediated activation of macrophages from *Mycobacterium bovis* BCG-resistant and -susceptible mice: Differential effects of corticosterone on antimycobacterial activity and expression of the *Bcg* gene (candidate *Nramp*), *Infect. Immun.* **63**:2983–2988.

46. Bernhagen, J., Bacher, M., Calandra, T., Metz, C. N., Doty, S. B., Donnelly, T., and Bucala, R., 1996, An essential role for macrophage migration inhibitory factor in the tuberculin delayed-type hypersensitivity reaction, *J. Exp. Med.* **183**:277–282.

47. Rook, G. A. W., and Bloom, B. R., 1994, Mechanisms of pathogenesis in tuberculosis, in: *Tuberculosis; Pathogenesis, Protection and Control* (B. R. Bloom, ed.), ASM Press, Washington, D.C., pp. 485–501.

48. Rook, G. A. W., and Hernandez-Pando, R., 1996, The pathogenesis of tuberculosis, *Annu. Rev. Microbiol.* **50**:259–284.

49. Vacchio, M. S., Papdopoulos, V., and Ashwell, J. D., 1994, Steroid production in the thymus: Implications for thymocyte selection, *J. Exp. Med.* **179**:1835–1846.

50. Brinkmann, V., and Kristofic, C., 1995, Regulation by corticosteroids of Th1 and Th2 cytokine production in human CD4+ effector T cells generated from CD45RO− and CD45RO+ subsets, *J. Immunol.* **155**:3322–3328.

51. Hernandez-Pando, R., Orozco, H., Sampieri, A., Pavón, L., Velasquillo, C., Larriva-Sahd, J., Alcocer, J. M., and Madrid, M. V., 1996, Correlation between the kinetics of Th1/Th2 cells and pathology in a murine model of experimental pulmonary tuberculosis, *Immunology* **89**:26–33.

52. Yong, A. J., Grange, J. M., Tee, R. D., Beck, J. S., Bothamley, G. H., Kemeny, D. M., and Kardjito, T., 1989, Total and anti-mycobacterial IgE levels in serum from patients with tuberculosis and leprosy, *Tubercle* **70**:273–279.

53. Schauf, V., Rom, W. N., Smith, K. A., Sampaio, E. P., Meyn, P. A., Tramontana, J. M., Cohn, Z. A., and Kaplan, G., 1993, Cytokine gene activation and modified responsiveness to interleukin-2 in the blood of tuberculosis patients, *J. Infect. Dis.* **168**:1056–1059.

54. Tobach, E., and Bloch, H., 1956, Effect of stress by crowding prior to and following tuberculous infection, *Am. J. Physiol.* **187**:399–402.

55. Brown, D. H., Miles, B. A., and Zwilling, B. S., 1995, Growth of *Mycobacterium tuberculosis* in BCG-resistant and -susceptible mice: Establishment of latency and reactivation, *Infect. Immun.* **63**:2243–2247.

56. Hernandez-Pando, R., Orozco, H., Honour, J. P., Silva, J., Leyva, R., and Rook, G. A. W., 1995, Adrenal changes in murine pulmonary tuberculosis; a clue to pathogenesis?, *FEMS Immunol. Med. Microbiol.* **12**:63–72.

57. Hernandez-Pando, R., and Rook, G. A. W., 1994, The role of TNFα in T cell-mediated inflammation depends on the Th1/Th2 cytokine balance, *Immunology* **82**:591–595.

58. Bertini, R., Bianchi, M., and Ghezzi, P., 1988, Adrenalectomy sensitizes mice to the lethal effects of interleukin 1 and tumor necrosis factor, *J. Exp. Med.* **167**:1708–1712.

59. Kaplan, G., 1994, Cytokine regulation of disease progression in leprosy and tuberculosis, *Immunobiology* **191**:564–568.

60. Hernandez-Pando, R., de la Luz Streber, M., Orozco, H., Arriaga, K., Pavon, L., Al-Nakhli, S. A., and Rook, G. A. W., 1998, The effects of androstenediol and dehydroepiandrosterone on the course and cytokine profile of tuberculosis in Balb/c mice, *Immun:* in press.

61. Hernandez-Pando, R., de la Luz Streber, M., Orozco, H., Arriaga, K., Pavon, L., Marti, O., Lightman, S. L., and Rook, G. A. W., 1998, Emergent therapeutic properties of a combination of glucocorticoid and anti-glucocorticoid steroids in tuberculosis Balb/c mice, *Quart. Journ. Med:* in press.

5

Mycobacterium leprae as an Opportunistic Pathogen

JAMES L. KRAHENBUHL and LINDA B. ADAMS

1. INTRODUCTION

Armauer Hansen described *Mycobacterium leprae*, the first human bacterial pathogen, in 1873. In 1985 there were an estimated 10 to 12 million cases in the world predominantly distributed in Asia, Africa, and South America. Today the World Health Organization (WHO) estimates only a few million registered cases in existence as prevalence is decreased by the implementation of multidrug therapy (MDT) in WHO's intensive effort to eliminate leprosy as a public health problem by the end of the millennium.[1] It is noteworthy that the incidence of leprosy in the world remains at >500,000 new cases per year.

One hundred and twenty-five years after identification of the leprosy bacillus we still cannot cultivate it *in vitro* nor are we certain of the route of transmission in man. Expulsion of enormous numbers of organisms in the nasal discharge of lepromatous patients and depositions of bacilli in the nasal mucosa of susceptible individuals is widely accepted as the likely route. The incubation period for leprosy is also unclear; 2 to 4 or more years is commonly cited,[2] but longer periods of incubation have been observed.

Among the different mycobacterial species *M. leprae* has not received as much attention as widely known killers such as *M. tuberculosis* and it is not widely recognized as a stealthy pathogen like *M. avium-intracellulare*, waiting until the

JAMES L. KRAHENBUHL and LINDA B. ADAMS • G. W. Long Hansen's Research Center, Laboratory Research Branch, Louisiana State University, Baton Rouge, Louisiana 70803.

Opportunistic Intracellular Bacteria and Immunity, edited by Lois J. Paradise *et al.* Plenum Press, New York, 1999.

host's defenses are down. The leprosy bacillus is a quiet, well-adapted, obligate intracellular pathogen that causes a chronic, slowly evolving disease unique in its clinical and immunopathological spectrum.[3,4] The inclusion of *M. leprae* in this volume on opportunistic pathogens may seem strange to most readers. However, the human immunodeficiency virus (HIV) pandemic and AIDS are raging through leprosy endemic areas, especially in Africa and Southeast Asia and the question is indeed being addressed of whether individuals infected with HIV or patients with AIDS are more susceptible to leprosy. A related question also being addressed is whether existing clinical leprosy is exacerbated in individuals when they become coinfected with HIV. Finally, there are reasons to address the question of whether leprosy increases susceptibility to HIV infection.

Because of the unusual clinical/histopathological spectrum of leprosy and the immunologically specific anergy in cell-mediated immunity (CMI) to *M. leprae* antigens in lepromatous disease, leprosy already represents a unique model to the immunologist. The possible influence of coinfection with HIV and progression of AIDS on clinical leprosy represents a further unique opportunity to explore immunoregulation in a human disease.

2. THE LEPROSY SPECTRUM

Unlike any other infectious disease, there is great variability in the course of clinically apparent leprosy.[2,4,5] Leprosy patients can be classified in a five-stage clinical immunohistopathological spectrum[3,6] ranging from paucibacillary disease (PB), in which few if any bacilli are found in the tissues, to multibacillary disease (MB), in which skin lesions teem with billions of organisms. Leprosy is predominantly a disease of skin, mucous membranes of the upper respiratory tract, and peripheral nerves. Nerve damage is the hallmark of leprosy, both in PB and MB disease. *M. leprae* is the only bacterial pathogen to have a predilection for peripheral nerves. In PB disease, nerve damage seems attributable to the localized host immune response to the presence of relatively few bacilli in areas of the dermis adjacent to peripheral nerves. In MB disease overwhelming bacterial proliferation in the nerves underlies nerve damage.

The natural history of leprosy is depicted in Fig. 1. As is the case with most infectious diseases (unfortunately, not including HIV infections), not all individuals infected with the leprosy bacillus develop clinical disease. Understanding the evolution of leprosy from infection to clinically manifested disease is central to our consideration of *M. leprae* as a (possible) opportunistic pathogen.[2,3]

2.1. Indeterminant Leprosy

Indeterminant leprosy often is unrecognized, consisting of a single or a few hypopigmented lesions, perhaps with some sensory loss and minimal histological

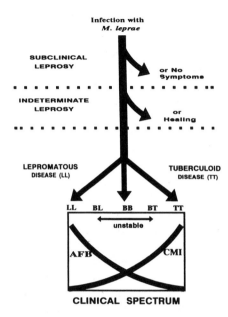

FIGURE 1. Natural history and clinical spectrum of leprosy.

changes. Spontaneous healing usually occurs but some patients may progress to one of the established forms of leprosy.

2.2. Lepromatous Leprosy

Polar lepromatous leprosy (LL) is the widespread, anergic form of the disease. Proliferation of *M. leprae* results in skin lesions of a variety of types ranging from diffuse generalized skin involvement to nodules (called lepromas) in a widespread, usually symmetrical distribution. These skin lepromas in advanced LL may contain 10^{10} *M. leprae* per gram of tissue. Characteristically, the cooler parts of the body surface are involved due, it is thought, to *M. leprae*'s preference for temperatures cooler than core body temperature.[7] Thus, in addition to the skin, the anterior third of the eye (but not the warm, posterior two thirds) and the nasal mucosa (but usually not the oral mucosa) may be involved. During periods of bacillemia, which occur primarily in MB disease, *M. leprae* can be carried to different organs and tissues.[3] Sensory nerve loss due to dermal nerve fiber involvement has a characteristic pattern in advanced LL.[8] Despite the intense burden of *M. leprae* in polar LL, there are remarkably few symptoms other than those of the lesions themselves. LL lesions are characterized by a massive accumulation of macrophages (MΦs) filled with large numbers of acid-fast bacilli and often containing large amounts of lipids, creating a foamy appearance on hematoxylin and eosin staining. These foamy MΦs may occupy 90% of the dermis and are separated from the epidermis by a clear zone. Few T lymphocytes are found in the LL lesions. There is a potent antibody response in LL and, strikingly a clearly identified progressive anergy in T-cell response that is limited to specific antigens of the leprosy bacillus. Several hypotheses are under investigation to explain specific CMI (cell-mediated immunity) anergy in LL, including a genetic predisposition, clonal deletion of *M. leprae*-specific T cells, and a role for specific suppressor T cells. LL can develop from indeterminant leprosy or from the downgrading of borderline disease (see below). Thus LL presents to the immunologist the opportunity to investigate defective T cell interactions in a chronic nonfatal human immunodeficiency disease.

2.3. Tuberculoid Leprosy

Polar tuberculoid leprosy (TT) is more localized than LL. Also unlike LL disease, in which bacterial proliferation results in signs and symptoms, much of the clinical picture in TT is due to the immunological responses of the host to a relatively few bacilli. One or, at most, a few well-circumscribed skin lesions with profound anesthesia of the skin lesion itself characterize TT. Peripheral nerves in the vicinity of the skin lesions(s) may be enlarged. Histopathologically, there are very few, if any, demonstrable acid-fast bacilli. Well-organized granulomas consist of epithelioid cells, multinucleated Langhans giant cells, and a discrete organization of CD4+ and CD8+ cells.[9-12] Individuals with TT manifest a strong delayed type hypersensitivity (DTH) to antigens but produce relatively low levels of antibody. Nerve damage in TT may be due to CMI to *M. leprae* in sites adjacent to nerves. TT leprosy can develop from indeterminant leprosy or from the upgrading of borderline tuberculoid disease (see below).

2.4. Borderline Leprosy

Borderline leprosy encompasses those types of disease between polar LL and polar TT and, unlike the highly stable LL and TT points of the spectrum, it is unstable and may shift. Mid-borderline is rare because it is the most unstable. A patient with borderline leprosy can develop clinical, bacteriological, and histopathological features of more tuberculoid disease with time, and this shift is termed upgrading. A shift from the borderline area to more lepromatous disease is called downgrading. As in TT, the signs and symptoms of borderline leprosy tend to be due to a combination of bacterial multiplication and the host CMI response to *M. leprae*. Borderline tuberculoid leprosy (BT) resembles tuberculoid disease but with more skin lesions with well defined edges. Satellite lesions tend to develop near the edges of the larger lesions, and individual-lesions tend to be larger. Peripheral nerve damage tends to be more prevalent and more severe in BT than in TT. This nerve damage is largely on the basis of the immune response of the host to the bacilli. BT skin lesions resemble the histopathology of TT except that the granuloma does not extend up to involve the basal layer of the epidermis. The numbers of *M. leprae* vary in lesions from undetectable to a few. Borderline lepromatous (BL) leprosy resembles lepromatous disease except that at least some of the skin lesions are selectively anesthetic and are less distinct in their borders. Peripheral nerve trunk involvement (due to host CMI) is more widespread than in LL, but proliferation of bacilli in the mucous membranes is less than in LL. Skin lesions of BL leprosy contain predominantly MΦs with far more lymphocytes than in LL. The numbers of acid-fast bacilli are usually somewhat less than in LL. BL leprosy can develop from indeterminate leprosy or by downgrading from BB or (rarely) from BT.

2.5. Reactions

Reactions in leprosy are clinically apparent, immunologically mediated inflammatory host responses to *M. leprae* that occur during the disease in about half the patients.[3,5] Reactions are described here because they may represent movement in the classification scheme. Reactions only occur in the unstable (borderline) and LL area of the spectrum. There are two types of reactions.

2.5.1. Type 1 (Reversal) Reactions

Reversal reactions appear as the result of DTH and affect patients classified in the BB to BT areas of the spectrum. Type 1 reactions are characterized by edema and erythema of preexisting lesions. There is a tendency for the classification to upgrade (move toward TT). Type 1 reactions histologically consist of edema in the acute phase on a BT or BB background. If a type 1 reaction upgrades, lymphocyte numbers may increase. In intense type 1 reactions, necrosis may occur accompanied by severe nerve damage.

2.5.2. Type 2 (Erythema Nodosum Leprosum [ENL]) Reactions

ENL reactions have long been considered as manifestations of an Arthus type of hypersensitivity reaction. Type 2 reactions affect BL and LL patients and are characterized by the development of crops of tender, erythematous skin nodules and fever. Because type 2 reactions can involve any tissue containing *M. leprae* antigens, ENL lesions are not confined to the skin, but can involve the eye, joints, nasal mucosa, etc. Type 2 reactions are characterized by an influx of neutrophils on a BL or LL background. A vasculitis involving arterioles or venules is demonstrable in about half of the cases in type 2 reactions.

3. PREDISPOSITION TO LEPROSY AND LOCAL IMMUNOREGULATION

Genetic and epidemiological studies have suggested that these disparate responses to *M. leprae* can be partially explained by a genetic predisposition in the HLA system, especially the class II alleles, of the host. For example, TT is often linked to HLA-DR3, whereas LL is associated with HLA-DQ1. Interestingly, no association has been found between HLA genes and acquisition of leprosy *per se*. Thus, it has been proposed that while susceptibility to leprosy is controlled by some non-HLA gene, HLA alleles control the type of CMI and immunopathology which ensues.[12a]

A unique feature of leprosy is the rare demonstration of systemic features of the disease in contrast to the localized nature of the skin lesions and the limitation of certain immunoregulatory mechanisms to the microenvironment of the granuloma.

Distinct differences across the leprosy spectrum have been demonstrated upon immunohistological examination of biopsies using monoclonal antibodies that distinguish CD4 and CD8 T-cell subsets.[11,12] T-cell makeup in the peripheral blood was unremarkable across the leprosy spectrum where CD4+/CD8+ ratios of 2:1 were observed. However, LL lesions displayed a striking paucity of T cells with a predominance of the CD8+ suppressor/cytotoxic subset yielding a CD4+/CD8+ ratio of 0.6:1. In TT lesions more T cells were evident and exhibited mostly CD4+ helper/inducer cells with a CD4+/CD8+ ratio of 1.9:1. A similar profile has been found in borderline leprosy lesions, with CD4+ T cells predominating in BT lesions and CD8+ T cells predominating in BL.

Even more interesting was the distribution of the cells in the microenvironment of the granuloma. In TT lesions, CD4+ cells were distributed throughout the lesion in close proximity to the granuloma MΦs, whereas cytotoxic CD8+ cells were located in the periphery of the granuloma.[11,12] In addition, Cooper *et al.*[13] examined leprosy biopsies for serine esterase, an indicator of cytotoxic T cells. Expression of serine esterase mRNA was increased fourfold in reversal reaction and TT lesions above that observed in LL lesions. These serine esterase-positive cells were microanatomically distributed throughout the tuberculoid granuloma, coinciding with the CD4+ cells. In contrast, CD8+ cells were dispersed throughout LL lesions near the *M. leprae*-laden MΦs.[10-12] Because the CD8+ cells in LL lesions are predominantly of the T suppressor phenotype, they may serve to down regulate MΦ activation and CMI.

Within the lesions T cells elaborate cytokines, protein messengers which regulate immune reactivity by coordinating antibody and cell mediated immune system interactions. Helper CD4+ T cells can be divided into two major groups based on their cytokine profiles. Th1 cells produce primarily interferon gamma (IFN-γ), interleukin 2 (IL-2), and lymphotoxin and are largely responsible for activating MΦ for microbicidal and tumoricidal activity. Conversely, Th2 cells synthesize IL-4, IL-5 and IL-10 which promote antibody production. Cytokines from one group can downregulate the opposing response. The first human demonstration of this Th1/TH2 paradigm has been reported in human leprosy[13a] where the polar forms demonstrate strikingly different cytokine profiles, closely correlating with either a Th1 (TT) or Th2 (LL) type response.

4. OTHER IMMUNOREGULATORY CELLS IN THE LEPROSY LESION

Regardless of the classification of a lesion, the most prominent cell present is the mononuclear phagocyte, present as either the epithelioid MΦ in the TT granuloma, or the foamy and/or bacilli-gorged MΦ of the LL lesion. The failure of the MΦ to cope with *M. leprae* is the most conspicuous characteristic of LL and is an issue central to understanding the mechanisms of host resistance to the leprosy bacillus.[14,15] Accumulating data suggest that, independent of specific T cell anergy, *M. leprae* and certain of its cell wall or secreted constituents may be able to subvert MΦ function and contribute to the downregulation of CMI associated with LL.

4.1. Successful Macrophage Function

Mouse MΦs, primed with interferon-γ (IFN-γ) and triggered with a second signal,[16] can be activated to kill or inhibit leprosy bacilli *in vitro*[15] as shown in studies in which *M. leprae* viability was measured by radiorespirometry[17] or when phagosome/lysosome fusion was examined.[18] The arginine-dependent production of nitric oxide, a reactive nitrogen intermediate, was shown to be a major effector mechanism of activated MΦ killing of M. leprae.[19] In contrast to the mouse system, human monocyte-derived MΦs could not be activated to kill or inhibit *M. leprae*,[15] a paradoxical finding observed with *M. tuberculosis* by others.[20] *M. leprae*-infected MΦs also release PGE_2 (prostaglandin E_2), a mediator that may profoundly suppress MΦ-mediated microbicidal capacity within the LL lesion (see below).

MΦs infected with leprosy bacilli[21] or treated with *M. leprae* constituents[22] release tumor necrosis factor α (TNF-α), a potent immunoregulatory molecule that can afford protection or be detrimental to host defenses in mycobacterial diseases.[23] *In vitro*, TNF-α production will serve as the second signal to achieve IFN-γ-induced MΦ activation in mouse cells.[16]

4.2. Defective Macrophage Function

In contrast to the toxic nature of relatively few intracellular tubercle bacilli,[14,15,24] *M. leprae* is relatively nontoxic for the MΦ; hundreds of viable organ-

isms will exist in lepromatous MΦs with little or no adverse effect on certain
MΦ functions. Lepromatous MΦs from the footpads of *M. leprae*-infected *nu/nu*
mice (see below) are gorged with bacilli yet retain their capacity to adhere and
phagocytize.[25] These cells, however, are completely refractory to the ability of
IFN-γ to enhance MΦ afferent and efferent effector functions, including microbicidal activity for the leprosy bacillus. Unresponsiveness to IFN-γ could be
induced in MΦs *in vitro* with a heavy burden of viable *M. leprae*. IFN-γ (+ LPS)
failed to induce enhanced efferent (oxidative burst, microbicidal capacity, and
cytotoxicity for tumor target cells) and afferent (enhanced Ia expression) effector
function in *M. leprae*-infected MΦs.[26] A high intracellular burden of *M. leprae*
was required (>50:1) and only viable bacilli induced the defect. Alternatively
exogenous lipoarabinomannan, secreted in copious amounts by viable *M. leprae*,[25,27,28] and other mycobacteria,[29] also rendered mouse and human MΦs
refractory to IFN-γ activation. The development of defective activation was
closely correlated with elevated PGE_2 production by MΦ, infected with live *M.
leprae*. This effect was reversible with indomethacin,[30] PGE_2 is a potent immunoregulatory molecule, especially in the microenvironment of a granuloma
where it may markedly downregulate a number of T-cell and MΦ functions,
including T-cell proliferation, MHC class II expression, and MΦ cytotoxicity
for tumor cells.[31]

5. LESSONS FROM ANIMAL MODELS OF LEPROSY

An ideal animal model for leprosy that displays the clinical spectrum, reactions, and peripheral neuritis[32] has not been demonstrated. Certain exotic species
offer promise but the unavailability of routine immunological reagents or the
rarity of the species present major obstacles to their development. Nevertheless, as
necessitated by the inability to cultivate *M. leprae in vitro*, considerable progress has
been made in animal studies.

5.1. Immunocompetent Animals

In 1960 the late Charles Shepard demonstrated at the CDC the limited
multiplication of *M. leprae*, from human origin, in the footpads of BALB/c
mice.[33] This milestone in leprosy research permitted the evaluation of new antileprosy drugs,[33,34] rudimentary evaluation of leprosy vaccine preparations,[35] and
the detection of primary and secondary drug resistance that developed in patients
receiving dapsone monotherapy for leprosy.[36,37] Growth plateaued at
1×10^6 per footpad and Shepard was able to calculate a doubling time for the
leprosy bacillus of approximately 14 days.[38] Localized growth of *M. leprae* in the
mouse footpad and disseminated growth in the nine-banded armadillo, *Dasypus*

novemcinctus,[39,40] supports Binford's hypothesis[41] that the leprosy bacillus prefers the cooler sites of the body (armadillo core temperature is 32 to 35°C).

5.2. Immunocompromised Animals

M. leprae indeed appears to be an opportunist in immunocompromised animals. Unlike the limited footpad growth of *M. leprae* in immunocompetent BALB/c mice, in neonatally thymectomized and irradiated (NTLR) mice growth in the footpads was greatly enhanced with dissemination to distant (cool) sites (ears, nose).[41,42] NTLR rats also supported enhanced growth of *M. leprae*, yielding $>10^8$ organisms.[43,44] Because larger inocula could be employed, these models permitted detection of small numbers of human "persisters," viable, drug-sensitive bacilli isolated from treated patients.

Studies with congenitally athymic (nude) mice also resulted in greatly advanced infections ($>10^{10}$ bacilli per foot) with dissemination to the opposite foot, ears, and tail.[45] This model permitted the comparison of short- and long-term drug regimens for LL,[46] the study of transmission via nasal mucosa and abraded skin,[47,48] studies of turnover and traffic of bone marrow MΦs into the footpad granulomas,[49] and investigation of immunoregulation by infected MΦs in the microenvironment of the footpad granulomas described previously. Experiments with *M. leprae*-infected *nu/nu* mice also provided recent direct *in vivo* evidence for the demonstrated *in vitro* role[25,26,28] of PGE_2 in regulating MΦ microbicidal function.[50] PGE_2 is synthesized from arachidonic acid (AA) generated from an essential fatty acid (EFA), linoleic acid, via the cyclooxygenase (COX) pathway. Ablation of AA synthesis and PGE_2 production by feeding infected *nu/nu* mice EFA-deficient diets induced permissive conditions in the microenvironment of the lepromatous footpad for the apparent activation of MΦs and killing of leprosy bacilli subsequent to the adaptive transfer of sensitized T cells from the lymph nodes of *M. leprae* immunized donor mice. Adaptive transfer in control infected *nu/nu* had no effect. These data,[50] coupled with our *in vitro* findings[25,26,28] and the demonstration that there is a high rate of bone-marrow-derived MΦ turnover in mouse lepromatous lesions,[49] support the hypothesis that any upgrading (spontaneous or induced by local immunotherapy[51-54]) in a MB lesion would be the consequence of MΦ activation in transit from the bone marrow to the lesion or immediately upon arrival.

6. LEPROSY IN IMMUNOSUPPRESSED HUMAN DISEASES

Clearly, findings with immunocompromised mice and rats show that depleted or ablated T-cell function is associated with enhanced growth of *M. leprae* in the cooler body sites. Whether there is a counterpart for these findings in human immunosuppressive diseases is not so clear. A number of well-characterized immunosuppressive human diseases and conditions have been described that are associated with opportunistic infections, but is the course of leprosy altered if the leprosy patient becomes immunosuppressed, that is, develops a lymphoma, receives immunosuppressive therapy for cancer or an organ transplant, or acquires HIV infection that progresses to AIDS?

There are isolated reports of renal transplantation in leprosy patients[55,56] in which underlying LL disease appeared to be exacerbated or reactivated, suggesting that, given the chance, *M. leprae* can exploit a compromise in host CMI defenses. But opportunities to explore leprosy in recipients of organ transplantation and/or immunosuppressive chemotherapy are rare as these are medical luxuries restricted to populations where leprosy is rarely encountered. Finding widespread numbers of HIV-related immunosuppressed individuals living in leprosy endemic areas is not a problem.

7. LEPROSY AND HIV COINFECTION

Because the incidence of HIV infection is rising at an alarming rate in countries where leprosy is endemic and because HIV infection and progression to AIDS is associated with a profound decrease in T-cell function, the implications of the AIDS pandemic on leprosy is highly relevant to the management of both diseases. In addition, because of the disorders in CMI that characterize each of these diseases, investigation of coinfection affords the opportunity to explore human immunoregulation further.

Before considering downgrading of clinical leprosy in HIV-positive individuals, the opposing image must be considered. Leprosy itself (LL) has immunocompromising features and a protracted course and might render a patient more susceptible to HIV infection. It is important to stress that LL patients are not, themselves, generally immunocompromised hosts. The immunological anergy of LL is highly specific for antigens of *M. leprae*. LL patients are not cancer-prone or susceptible to infection with the opportunistic intracellular pathogens that plague patients with immunodeficiency diseases. The PPD skin test and course of pulmonary tuberculosis is unremarkable in LL patients. There are conflicting reports that clinical leprosy affects the serological detection of anti-HIV antibodies,[57-59] but no available evidence suggests leprosy patients are more susceptible to HIV infection or AIDS.

Clearly, individuals infected with HIV are more susceptible to infection with *M. tuberculosis*[60] or *M. avium*.[61] What are the possible influences of HIV infection and AIDS on leprosy? Shifts in a patient's classification within the leprosy clinical/histopathological spectrum often occur in the normal course of the disease,[2] but it is important to reemphasize that mobility within the leprosy spectrum is limited to those patients whose clinical disease is unstable, that is, classified as BL, BB, or BT (Fig. 1). Upgrading is unlikely to occur under immunosuppressive conditions. More likely the course of clinical disease would be expected to worsen as T-cell counts and CMI diminishes.[62] Polar TT patients do not downgrade, which is even uncommon in BT leprosy. Downgrading reactions in BB or BL are more gradual and insidious and are normally associated with inadequate or irregular antileprosy chemotherapy.

An increased incidence of clinical leprosy per se might be observed as subclinical disease progresses in HIV-infected individuals. In HIV or AIDS-related immunosuppression, polar LL could become detectably more severe, manifested by new or larger lesions, or develop more rapidly. Or a higher incidence of the lepromatous form of the disease might be expected. A more subtle effect could be seen where the response to antileprosy chemotherapy might be less effective in AIDS patients in whom drug adsorption presents additional problems. As CMI is progressively lost in HIV infection, antibody production could be affected, resulting in an increase in incidence of ENL reactions. Finally, it is conceivable that epidemic AIDS in a leprosy endemic area could induce the accelerated decline of leprosy as potentially contagious LL patients die before the onset of clinical symptoms.

As discussed previously and shown in Fig. 1, downgrading of leprosy to a more multibacillary form of disease is restricted to individuals classified in the unstable borderline (BL and occasionally BB) points on the spectrum. Thus a downgrading shift of TT, or even BT, lesions from the tuberculoid end of the spectrum would be the most remarkable manifestation of HIV-/AIDS-related immunosuppression because polar TT leprosy, like polar LL, is a very stable position on the clinical/histopathological spectrum.

As summarized by Ponnighaus, *et al.*,[63] there are no published reports of enhancement of multibacillary disease in association with HIV coinfection. Their own investigation of HIV as a possible risk factor for leprosy was carried out in a large, thoroughly documented study population in the context of an ongoing leprosy vaccine trial in northern Malawi.[64] In contrast to validating data showing a strong association between HIV infection and tuberculosis they reported no evidence for an increased incidence of leprosy in HIV-infected individuals nor did they see a shift to multibacillary disease. Some evidence for relapsed leprosy was obtained in a sample of HIV-positive individuals too small for statistical analysis. They qualify their findings by pointing out that HIV infection was relatively recent at the time of this study and the proportion of severely immunosuppressed individuals may increase with time.

A thorough study of the CMI response to *M. leprae* in HIV-positive individuals was recently reported from Brazil[65] in three BL and eight BT coinfected patients. Coinfected patients showed impaired CMI to *M. leprae in vitro* and *in vivo*. Impaired CMI responses were observed in coinfected patients in lymphocyte blast transformation (LBT) responses of peripheral blood cells to *M. leprae* antigens. LBT was negative for *M. leprae* in all BT/HIV-positive patients (57% positive in BT/HIV-negative controls). Production of IFN-γ was less affected by HIV status than LBT. *In vivo*, lepromin skin test activity was uniformly negative in BT/HIV-positive patients as opposed to 92% positive in BT/HIV-negative individuals. There were no differences seen in the lesional histopathology of BT/HIV-positive and BT/HIV-negative subjects. Of great interest, immunohistopathology showed a normal distribution of CD4+ and CD8+ cells in the lesions in spite of greatly reduced CD4+ counts in the peripheral blood of all coinfected BT and two of three BL patients. Finally, no acid-fast bacilli were seen in the lesions of BT/HIV-positive individuals. Overall these findings suggest that, in spite of evidence for impaired CMI to *M. leprae* in BT patients, there were no indications of a downgrading shift from paucibacillary to multibacillary disease.

8. SUMMARY AND CONCLUSIONS

Ten years ago many immunologists would have bet that coinfection with HIV would result in downgrading of borderline disease, perhaps even TT, and an increase in the incidence of LL. Data to date suggest no interaction between the two diseases that would increase susceptibility to leprosy or accelerate its clinical features.

There is overwhelming evidence that leprosy in humans is a localized disease, involving primarily the skin and the nasal mucous membranes, probably because of temperature restrictions of the bacilli. The microenvironment of LL disease would appear to be under potent local (down) regulatory control and is already associated with the lack of (specific) T-cell CMI and a paucity of CD4+ cells in the lesions. At the level of the granuloma, the CD4+ and CD8+ ratio and the distribution of these cells at the tuberculoid end of the spectrum reflect neither the decrease in antigen-specific LBT response to *M. leprae* antigen nor the depletion of CD4+ cells in the peripheral blood which are the hallmarks of AIDS. The local control of PB lesions by CMI appears to be sufficient even though the T-cell picture in the peripheral blood is diminishing in HIV infection.

The prolonged incubation period before clinical leprosy appears and the protracted chronic course of the disease and doubling time of the leprosy bacillus are perhaps the most key factors of all. *M. leprae* grows very slowly. Even in animals completely ablated of CMI many months, a second "blind passage" is often required to detect the growth of small footpad inocula of bacilli. Developing countries, where leprosy is endemic and HIV infection is epidemic, are the only areas where sufficient numbers of coinfected individuals can be studied. Treatment for HIV and management of AIDS patients is minimal in these areas. It is likely that these individuals die of other AIDS-related opportunistic infections before any downgrading of leprosy can occur. But the verdict may still be out. As treatment for HIV infection improves and becomes available in developing countries, longer term survival of HIV patients will be observed. The intriguing question of whether HIV infection is associated with downgrading of clinical leprosy will undoubtedly continue to be investigated.

REFERENCES

1. Nordeen, S. K., 1996, Eliminating leprosy as a public health problem—is the optimism justified?, *World Health Forum* **17:**109–144.
2. Harboe, M., 1994, Overview of host–parasite relations, in: *Leprosy*, 2nd Ed. (R. C. Hastings, ed.), Churchill Livingstone, Edinburgh, p. 470.
3. Job, C. K., 1994, Pathology of leprosy, in: *Leprosy*, 2nd Ed. (R. C. Hastings, ed.), Churchill Livingstone, Edinburgh, pp. 193–224.
4. Adams, L. B., and Krahenbuhl, J. L., 1996, Granulomas induced by *Mycobacterium leprae*, *Methods: A companion to Methods in Enzymology* **9:**220–232.
5. Hastings, R. C., Gillis, T. P., Krahenbuhl, J. L., and Franzblau, S. G., 1988, Leprosy, *Clin. Microbiol. Rev.* **1:**330–348.
6. Ridley, D. S., and Jopling, W. H., 1966, Classification of leprosy according to immunity—a five-group system, *Int. J. Lepr.* **34:**255–273.
7. Hastings, R. C., Trautman, J. R., Enna, C. D., and Jacobson, R. R., 1968, Bacterial density in the skin in lepromatous leprosy as related to temperature, *Lepr. Rev.* **39:**71–74.
8. Sabin, T. D., 1969, Temperature-linked sensory loss: A unique pattern in leprosy, *Arch. Neurol.* **20:**257–262.
9. Modlin, R. L., Hofman, F. M., Taylor, C. R., and Rea, T. H., 1983, T lymphocyte subsets in the skin lesions of patients with leprosy, *J. Am. Acad. Dermatol.* **8:**182–189.
10. Modlin, R. L., Gebhard, J. F., Taylor, C. R., and Rea, T. H., 1983, In situ characterization of T lymphocyte subsets in the reactional states of leprosy, *Clin. Exp. Immunol.* **53:**17–24.
11. Modlin, R. L., and Rea, T. H., 1988, Immunopathology of leprosy granulomas, *Springer Semin. Immunopathol.* **10:**359–374.
12. Modlin, R. L., Melancon-Kaplan, J., Young, S. M. M., Pirmez, C., Kino, H., Convit, J., Rea, T. H., and Bloom, B. R., 1988, Learning from lesions: Patterns of tissue inflammation in leprosy, *Proc. Natl. Acad. Sci. USA* **85:**1213–1217.
12a. de Vries, R. P., and Ottenhoff, T. H. M., 1994, Immunogenetics of Leprosy, in: *Leprosy*, 2nd, (R. C. Hastings, ed.) pp. 113–121. Churchill Livingstone: Edinburgh.
13. Cooper, C. L., Mueller, C., Sinchaisri, T.-A., Pirmez,, C., Chan, J., Kaplan, G., Young, S. M. M., Weissman, I. L., Bloom, B. R., Rea, T. H., and Modlin, R. L., 1989, Analysis of naturally occurring delayed-type hypersensitivity reactions in leprosy by in situ hybridization, *J. Exp. Med.* **169:**1565–1581.
13a. Yamamura, M., Uyemura, K., Deans, R. J., Weinberg, K., Rea, T. H., Bloom, B. R., and Modlin, R. L., 1991. Defining protective responses to pathogens: Cytokine profiles in leprosy lesions. *Science* **254:**277–279.
14. Krahenbuhl, J. L., 1994, Role of the macrophage in resistance to leprosy, in: *Leprosy*, 2nd Ed. (R. C. Hastings, ed.), Churchill Livingstone, Edinburgh, p. 137.

15. Krahenbuhl, J. L., and Adams, L. B., 1994, The role of the macrophage in resistance to the leprosy bacillus, in: *Macrophage–Pathogen Interactions* (B. S. Zwilling and T. K. Eisenstein, eds.), Marcel Dekker, New York, pp. 281–302.

16. Sibley, L. D., Adams, L. B., Fukutomi, Y., and Krahenbuhl, J. L., 1991, Tumor necrosis factor-alpha triggers antitoxoplasmal activity of IFN-gamma primed macrophages, *J. Immunol.* **147:**2340–2345.

17. Ramasesh, N., Adams, L. B., Franzblau, S. G., and Krahenbuhl, J. L., 1991, Effects of activated macrophages on *Mycobacterium leprae, Infect. Immun.* **59:**2864–2869.

18. Sibley, L. D., Franzblau, S. G., and Krahenbuhl, J. L., 1987, Intracellular fate of *Mycobacterium leprae* in normal and activated mouse macrophages, *Infect. Immun.* **55:**680–685.

19. Adams, L. B., Franzblau,, S. G., Vavrin, Z., Hibbs, J. B., Jr., and Krahenbuhl, J. L., 1991, 1-Arginine-dependent macrophage effector functions inhibit metabolic activity of *Mycobacterium leprae, J. Immunol.* **147:**1642–1646.

20. Rook, G. A. W., Steele, J., Fraher, L., Barker, S., Karmali, R., O'Riordan, J., and Stanford, J., 1986, Vitamin D3, gamma interferon, and control of proliferation of *Mycobacterium tuberculosis* by human monocytes, *Immunology* **57:**159–163.

21. Fukutomi, Y., Adams, L. B., and Krahenbuhl, J. L., 1991, Tumor necrosis factor in experimental leprosy, *Int. J. Lepr.* **59:**711–712.

22. Adams, L. B., Fukutomi, Y., and Krahenbuhl, J. L., 1993, Regulation of murine macrophage effector functions by lipoarabinomannan from mycobacterial strains with different degrees of virulence, *Infect. Immun.* **61:**4173–4181.

23. Rook, G. A., Al Attiyah, R., and Filley, W., 1991, New insights into the immunopathology of tuberculosis, *Pathobiology* **59:**148–152.

24. Rook, G. A. W., 1988, Role of activated macrophages in the immunopathology of tuberculosis, *Br. Med. Bull.* **44:**611–625.

25. Sibley, L. D., and Krahenbuhl, J. L., 1987, *Mycobacterium leprae*-burdened macrophages are refractory to activation by gamma-interferon, *Infect. Immun.* **55:**446–450.

26. Sibley, L. D., and Krahenbuhl, J. L., 1988, Induction of unresponsiveness to gamma interferon in macrophages infected with *Mycobacterium leprae, Infect. Immun.* **56:**1912–1919.

27. Hunter, S. W., Gaylord, H., and Brennan, P. J., 1986, Structure and antigenicity of the phosphorylated lipopolysaccharide antigens from the leprosy and tubercle bacilli, *J. Biol. Chem.* **261:**12345–12351.

28. Sibley, L. D., and Krahenbuhl, J. L., 1988, Defective activation of granuloma macrophages from *Mycobacterium leprae*-infected nude mice. *J. Leukoc. Biol.* **43:**60–66.

29. Russell, D. G., 1994, Immunoelectron microscopy of endosomal trafficking in macrophages infected with microbial pathogens, in: *Microbes as Tools for Cell Biology* (D. G. Russell, ed.), Academic Press, New York, pp. 277–288.

30. Sibley, L. D., Adams, L. B., and Krahenbuhl, J. L., 1990, Inhibition of interferon-gamma-mediated activation in mouse macrophages treated with lipoarabinomannan, *Clin. Exp. Immunol.* **80:**141–148.

31. Lee, S. H., Sooyoola, E., Chanmugam, P., Hart, S., Sun, W., Zhong, H., Liou, S., Simmons, D., and Hwang, D., 1992, Selective expression of mitogen-inducible cyclooxygenase in macrophages stimulated with lipopolysaccharide, *J. Biol. Chem.* **267:**25934–25938.

32. Meyers, W. M., Gormus, B. J., and Walsh, G. P., 1994, Experimental leprosy, in: *Leprosy*, 2nd Ed. (R. C. Hastings, ed.), Churchill Livingstone, London, pp. 385–408.

33. Shepard, C. C., 1960, The experimental disease that follows the injection of human leprosy bacilli into footpads of mice. *J. Exp. Med.* **112:**445–454.

34. Shepard, C. C., 1971, A survey of drugs with activity against *M. leprae* in mice. *Int. J. Lepr.* **39:**340–348.

35. Shepard, C. C., Walker, L. L., and Van Landingham, R., 1978, Heat stability of *M. leprae* immunogenicity, *Infect. Immun.* **22:**87–93.

36. Pettit, J. H. S., and Rees, R. J. W., 1964, Sulphone resistance in leprosy. An experimental and clinical study, *Lancet* **ii:**673–674.

37. Hastings, R. C., 1977, Growth of sulfone-resistant *M. leprae* in the footpads of mice fed dapsone, *Proc. Soc. Exp. Biol. Med.* **156:**544–545.

38. Shepard, C. C., and MacRae, D. H., 1968, A method for counting acid-fast bacteria, *Int. J. Lepr.* **36:**78–82.

39. Kirchheimer, W. F., and Storrs, E. E., 1971, An attempt to establish the armadillo (*Dasypus novemcinctus*, Linn) as a model for the study of leprosy. I. Report of lepromatoid leprosy in an experimentally infected armadillo, *Int. J. Lepr.* **39:**693–702.

40. Kirchheimer, W. F., Storrs, E. E., and Binford, C. H., 1972, Attempts to establish the armadillo *Dasypus novemcinctus* as a model for the study of leprosy. II. Histopathologic and bacteriologic post mortem findings in lepromatoid leprosy in the armadillo, *Int. J. Lepr.* **40:**229–242.

41. Binford, C. H., 1956, Comprehensive program for the inoculation of human leprosy into laboratory animals, *US Public Health Rep.* **71:**995–996.

42. Rees, R. J. W., Waters, M. F. R., Weddell, A. G. M., and Palmer, E., 1967, Experimental lepromatous leprosy, *Nature* **215:**599–602.

43. Fieldsteel, A. H., and Levy, L., 1976, Neonatally thymectomized Lewis rats infected with *Mycobacterium leprae:* Response to primary infection, secondary challenge and large inocula, *Infect. Immun.* **14:**736–741.

44. Dawson, P. J., Colston, M. J., and Fieldsteel, A. H., 1983, Infection of the congenitally athymic rat with *Mycobacterium leprae, Int. J. Lepr.* **51:**336–346.

45. Colston, M. J., and Kohsaka, K., 1982, The nude mouse in studies of leprosy, in: *The Nude Mouse in Experimental and Clinical Research*, 2nd Ed. (J. Fogh and B. C. Giovanella, eds.), Academic Press, New York, pp. 247–266.

46. Ji, B., Perani, E. G., Petinom, C., and Grosset, J. H., 1996, Bactericidal activities of combinations of new drugs against *Mycobacterium leprae* in nude mice, *Antimicrob. Agents Chemother.* **40:**393–399.

47. Chehl, S., Job, C. K., and Hastings, R. C., 1985, Transmission of leprosy in nude mice, *Am. J. Trop. Med. Hyg.* **34:**1161–1166.

48. Job, C. K., Chehl, S., and Hastings, R. C., 1990, New findings on the mode of entry of *Mycobacterium leprae* in nude mice, *Int. J. Lepr.* **58:**726–729.

49. Krahenbuhl, J. L., Sibley, L. D., and Chae, G.-T., 1990, γ-Interferon in experimental leprosy, *Diagn. Microbiol. Infect. Dis.* **13:**405–409.

50. Adams, L. B., Gillis, T. P., Hwang, D. H., and Krahenbuhl, J. L., 1997, Effects of essential fatty acid deficiency on prostaglandin E_2 production and cell-mediated immunity in a mouse model of leprosy, *Infect. Immun.* **65:** 1152–1157.

51. Nathan, C. F., Kaplan, G., Levis, W. R., Nusrat, A., Witmer, M. D., Sherwin, S. A., Job, C. K., Horowitz, C. R., Steinman, R. M., and Cohn, Z. A., 1986, Local and systemic effects of intradermal recombinant interferon-gamma in patients with lepromatous leprosy, *N. Engl. J. Med.* **315:**6–15.

52. Kaplan, G., Mathur, N. K., Job, C. K., Nath, I., and Cohn, Z. A., 1989, Effect of multiple interferon gamma injections on the disposal of *Mycobacterium leprae, Proc. Natl. Acad. Sci. USA* **86:**8073–8077.

53. Sampaio, E. P., Moreira, A. L., Sarno, E. N., Malta, A. M., and Kaplan, G., 1992, Prolonged treatment with recombinant interferon gamma induces erythema nodosum leprosum in lepromatous leprosy patients, *J. Exp. Med.* **175:**1729–1737.

54. Kaplan, G., Britton, W. J., Hancock, G. E., Theuvenet, W. J., Smith, K. A., Job, C. K., Roche,

P. W., Molloy, A., Burkhardt, R., Barker, J., *et al.*, 1991, The systemic influence of recombinant interleukin 2 on the manifestations of lepromatous leprosy, *J. Exp. Med.* **173:**993–1006.

55. Teruel, J. L., Liano, F., del Hoyo, M., Rocamora, A., Gomez-Mampaso, E., Quereda, C., and Ortuno, J., 1985, Successful kidney transplantation in leprosy and transitory recurrence of the disease, *Int. J. Lepr.* **53:**410–411.

56. Adu, D., Evans, D. B., Millard, P. R., Calne, R. Y., Shwe, T., and Jopling, W. H., 1973, Renal transplantation in leprosy, *Br. Med. J.* **2:**280–281.

57. Malkovsky, M., and Dilger, P., 1989, Failure to detect antibodies to HIV-1 in sera from patients with mycobacterial infections, *Int. J. Lepr.* **57:**866–867.

58. ShivRaj, L., Patil, S. A., Girdhard, A., Sengupta, U., Desikan, K. V., and Srnivasan, H., 1988, Antibodies to HIV-1 in sera from patients with mycobacterial infections, *Int. J. Lepr.* **56:**546–551.

59. Andrade, V. L., Avelleira, J. C., Marques, A., and Vianna, F. R., !991, Leprosy as cause of false positive results in serological assays for the detection of antibodies to HIV-1, *Int. J. Lepr.* **59:** 125–126.

60. Daley, C. L., Small, P. M., Schecter, F., Schoolnik, G. K., McAdam, R. A., Jacobs Jr, W. R., and Hopewell, P. C., 1992, An out-break of tuberculosis with accelerated progression among persons infected with the human immunodeficiency virus, *N. Engl. J. Med.* **326:**2131–2135.

61. Benson, C. A., and Ellner, J. J., 1993, *Mycobacterium avium* complex infection and AIDS: Advances in theory and practice, *Clin. Infect. Dis.* **17:**7–20.

62. Turk,, J. L., and Rees, R. J. W., 1988, AIDS and leprosy, *Lepr. Rev.* **59:**193–194.

63. Ponnighaus, J. M., Mwanjasi, L. J., Fine, P. E. M., Shaw, M.-A., Turner, A. C., Oxborrow, S. M., Lucas, S. B., Jenkins, P. A., Sterne, J. A. C., and Bliss, L., 1991, Is HIV infection a risk factor for leprosy? *Int. J. Lepr.* **59:**221–228.

64. Fine, P. E. M., and Ponnighaus, J. M., 1988, Background, design, and prospects of the Karonga Prevention Trial, a leprosy vaccine trial in northern Malawi, *Trans. R. Soc. Trop. Med. Hyg.* **82:**810–817.

65. Sampaio, E. P., Caneshi, J. R. T., Nery, J. A. C., Duppre, N. C., Pereira, G. M. B., Vieira, L. M. M., Moreira, A. L., Kaplan, G., and Sarno, E. N., 1995, Cellular immune response to *Mycobacterium leprae* infection in human immunodeficiency virus-infected individuals, *Infect. Immun.* **63:**1848–1854.

6

Immunology and Immunopathology of Mycobacterial Infections

TOM H. M. OTTENHOFF, ERIC SPIERINGS,
PETER H. NIBBERING, ROLIEN DE JONG,
and RENÉ R. P. DE VRIES

1. TUBERCULOSIS AND LEPROSY

Mycobacterial pathogens are major causes of morbidity and mortality worldwide. A third of the world's population is infected with *Mycobacterium tuberculosis*. Each year 8 to 10 million new active pulmonary tuberculosis cases arise and over 3 million patients die of the disease, which is higher than the death rate attributable to any other single infectious organism.[1] The incidence of tuberculosis is rising also in Western countries and virulent multidrug-resistant strains are emerging.[1] The second mycobacterial pathogen, *Mycobacterium leprae*, causes leprosy. Leprosy remains an important health care problem particularly as a result of its striking pathology and immune-mediated tissue destruction during acute leprosy reactions. Other mycobacteria such as *Mycobacterium avium / intracellulare* are opportunistic pathogens in immunocompromised, for example, human immunodeficiency virus (HIV)-infected, or genetically susceptible individuals.

TOM H. M. OTTENHOFF, ERIC SPIERINGS, ROLIEN DE JONG, and RENÉ R. P. DE VRIES • Department of Immunohematology and Blood Bank, Leiden University Medical Center, 2333 ZA Leiden, The Netherlands.   PETER H. NIBBERING • Department of Infectious Diseases, Leiden University Medical Center, 2333 ZA Leiden, The Netherlands.

Opportunistic Intracellular Bacteria and Immunity, edited by Lois J. Paradise *et al.* Plenum Press, New York, 1999.

During infection with *M. tuberculosis*, bacilli reach the lung's alveoli, where they are phagocytosed by macrophages. Infection is initially contained in small granulomas called tubercles. These tubercles are highly dynamic and show strong influx of macrophages and T lymphocytes, the predominant cells mediating protection.[2] Protective immunity can arrest the lesion permanently at this point. If immunity is insufficient, however, bacilli escape from the granuloma and disseminate into the lung, followed by delayed-type hypersensitivity (DTH)-mediated lung tissue destruction and rupturing of liquefied lesions into the airways. At this stage highly contagious, open lung tuberculosis has developed.[2] Tuberculosis may further progress to fatal meningitis or miliary disease by hematogenous dissemination throughout the body.

M. leprae bacilli are probably also transmitted by airborne particles. *M. leprae* may infect the bronchopulmonary mucosal epithelium, but perhaps also directly affects peripheral skin. *M. leprae* displays a strong preference for macrophages and Schwann cells. The latter form myelinated sheets around peripheral nerves. It is unknown exactly how *M. leprae* reaches these neural niches but presumably this is by hematogenous dissemination or *per continuitatem*.

2. PROTECTIVE IMMUNITY TO MYCOBACTERIA IS DEPENDENT ON CD4+ Th1, CD8+ T CELLS, AND TYPE 1 CYTOKINES

CD4+ T helper (Th) cells can be classified in at least three subsets according to their functional program. Th1 type cells typically secrete high amounts of interleukin (IL)-2 and interferon-γ (IFN-γ) whereas Th2 type cells are characterized by their ability to produce high levels of IL-4 and IL-5 upon activation.[3,4] Th cells with shared features of Th1 and Th2 type cells are referred to as Th0 cells.[4] In several models of experimental autoimmunity, Th1 responses promote disease development and immunopathology, whereas Th2 responses are associated with disease resistance.[5-7] The most important factors controlling Th cell differentiation are IL-12 and IL-4, which drive Th1 and Th2 cell development, respectively.[8-10] The products of Th1 and Th2 type cells have a negative regulatory effect on the growth and function of the opposing subset, which may lead to a reinforcement of polarizing differentiation events particularly in chronic responses.[11,12]

In mice, adoptive cell transfer experiments and studies in gene knockout animals have clearly established that protective immunity to mycobacteria is dependent on both major histocompatibility complex (MHC) class II restricted CD4+ T cells and MHC class I dependent CD8+ T cells as well as type 1 cytokines.[13-20] Mice lacking functional genes encoding recombinase activating gene (RAG-1) (T, B cell deficient), T cell receptor-β (TCR-$\alpha\beta$ cell deficient), MHC class II H2-Aβ (CD4+ T cell deficient), or β2m (MHC class I/CD8+ T cell deficient) are much more susceptible to infections with *M. bovis* BCG and *M. tuberculosis* than control littermates.[13-20] Similarly IFN-$\gamma^{-/-}$, IFN-γR$^{-/-}$, tumor necrosis factor (TNF)-αR$^{-/-}$ gene knockout mice and animals treated with neutralizing anti-TNF-α or anti-IL-12 antibodies succumb rapidly from infection.[21-23] Conversely, susceptible mice acquire increased resistance to *M. tuberculosis* upon IL-12 treatment.[24] Thus, MHC class II restricted CD4+ Th1 cells, MHC class I dependent CD8+ T cells, and type 1 cytokines play a crucial role in protection against mycobacteria in mice. TCR-$\gamma\delta$ T cells[19] as well as Th1-dependent opsonizing antibodies[14] may play an accessory role in protection, whereas the contribution of CDI restricted immunity to protection remains to be established.

In humans, mycobacteria also selectively induce CD4+ Th1 cells.[25-27] These CD4+ Th1 cells produce high levels of IFN-γ and are highly cytotoxic for infected target cells.[25-27] The crucial role of human Th1 cells in protection against mycobacterial infections is supported by several lines of evidence. First, lepromatous leprosy patients who suffer from progressive disease display a specific defect in Th1 cell responsiveness to *M. leprae* (reviewed in 28). Second, acquired immunodeficiency syndrome (AIDS) patients with low numbers of CD4+ T cells are dramatically more susceptible to mycobacteria and fulminant tuberculosis is a major cause of death in AIDS. The HIV pandemic has greatly amplified the resurgence of tuberculosis. Third, patients with defective IFN-γ and/or IL-12 production capacity are highly susceptible to mycobacterial infections, often with fatal outcome.[29-31] Several of these patients could be rescued by recombinant IFN-γ immunotherapy.[29-30] Other patients have genetic defects in the IFNγRI, IFNγR2, or IL-12RβI expression as recently reported.[32,33]

Besides inducing CD4+ Th1 cells, mycobacteria also trigger CD8+ T cells. These CD8+ T cells kill mycobacterium-infected macrophages in an HLA class I restricted fashion.[20,34] CD8+ T cells were preferentially induced by particulate or live bacilli but not by soluble antigen, suggesting differences in antigen processing between live and dead bacilli. Leprosy and tuberculosis lesions also contain CD4+ and CD8+ cells, suggesting the involvement of both subsets in anti-mycobacterial immunity in humans. The precise protective effector mechanisms of CD8+ T cells are not yet known. Not only cytolytic activity but also type 1 cytokine production may be involved but this issue needs further investigation. Recently it was shown that *M. tuberculosis* reactive TCR-$\alpha\beta$+ human T cells can recognize alternative, nonpeptide ligands of *M. tuberculosis* such as mycolic acids and lipoarabinomannan, presented by MHC class I like CD1b molecules (e.g., 36). Also TCR-$\gamma\delta$+ T cells can recognize nonpeptide ligands such as prenyl pyrophosphate derivatives and nucleotide conjugated phospho antigens of *M. tuberculosis* (e.g., 37). The significance of these antigens to immunologically mediated protection in tuberculosis remains unknown and is under investigation in several laboratories.

Collectively these results demonstrate that both in mice and in humans CD4⁺ Th1 cells and type 1 cytokines play a crucial role in protection against mycobacteria. In addition, CD8⁺ T cells are crucial to protection in mice and most likely play an important role in humans as well.

3. HLA POLYMORPHISM REGULATES T-CELL IMMUNITY TO MYCOBACTERIA

T cells recognize antigens as peptide fragments bound to MHC molecules at the surface of infected cells. MHC genes are highly polymorphic and this polymorphism maps predominantly to the foreign peptide binding site of MHC. As a direct consequence, MHC molecules differ in the antigens and peptides they can bind and present to T cells.

We have investigated the role of HLA classes I and II genes in controlling immunity and susceptibility to mycobacterial pathogens. HLA class II haplotypes were found to segregate nonrandomly in leprosy and tuberculosis families. In addition, *HLA-DR/DQ* alleles were associated with certain types of leprosy and tuberculosis (revised in 38). *HLA-DR* alleles were also found to control the magnitude and specificity of (T-cell-dependent) skin test responses to mycobacteria *in vivo*.[39,40] Similar differences were found *in vitro*. The antigen and peptide specificity of CD4 Th1 cells is controlled by the HLA class II background;[41–43] HLA-DR3 restricted T cells, for example, recognize only a subset of the known target antigens for mycobacterium-reactive T cells [heat-shock protein (hsp)65, hsp70, hsp18, 85B][41] and recognize only a single epitope in each antigen.[43] In mice, H2 genes also control T-cell immunity to *M. tuberculosis*.[44,45]

HLA class II genes not only control the specificity and magnitude of the T-cell response but can also influence T cell differentiation and function. *Mycobacterium*-specific Ts cells that downregulate *M. leprae*-reactive Th1 cells in lepromatous leprosy[46] were found to recognize peptide/HLA complexes distinct from those seen by Th cells (hsp65 p435–449/HLA-DRB1*1503). This peptide/HLA complex exclusively induced Ts cells, whereas the same peptide presented by HLA-DR1 activated proliferative Th cells.[47]

Thus HLA genes play an important role in controlling the magnitude, specificity, and function of the human T-cell response to mycobacteria.

4. T-CELL-MEDIATED IMMUNITY AND IMMUNOPATHOLOGY IN MYCOBACTERIAL INFECTIONS

Tuberculosis and leprosy are both spectral diseases, with a localized form at one pole and a widely disseminating type of disease at the other pole for review see reference 28). This is particularly evident in leprosy as outlined in Fig. 1. In

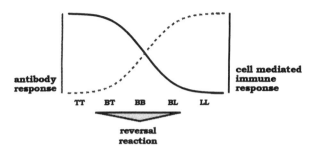

FIGURE 1. The leprosy spectrum.

tuberculoid leprosy (TT), the localized or highly resistant form of the disease, only one or few skin lesions are found, often with an involvement of peripheral nerves. The latter are often damaged and can even be completely destroyed during the course of the disease. TT lesions contain highly ordered granulomata with large numbers of CD$^+$ T lymphocytes and few CD8$^+$ T cells. Few if any bacilli can be detected in these lesions. TT patients typically show high T-cell responses to *M. leprae* antigens in skin tests as well as *in vitro*, while having low antibody titers to *M. leprae*. On the opposite pole of the leprosy spectrum lepromatous or "low-resistant" patients (LL) are found with numerous skin lesions, containing undifferentiated macrophages with massive numbers of bacilli. The few T lymphocytes present are of both the CD8$^+$ and the CD4$^+$ subsets, but are diffusely spread throughout the lesions with a seeming lack of organization. LL patients show a characteristic T-cell unresponsiveness toward *M. leprae* antigens in skin testing as well as in *in vitro* T-cell stimulation assays, but produce high levels of circulating antibodies against the bacillus. In between these two poles various intermediate forms of the disease can be found, called borderline leprosy.

Acute immunopathological reactions often occur in leprosy, particularly in borderline patients with unstable disease. Particularly damaging reactional episodes are the so-called reversal or type I reactions. These reactions are characterized by sudden clinical changes representing a shift to the tuberculoid pole of the spectrum, a rapid increase in DTH to *M. leprae*, and acute neuritis episodes, leading to profound and irreversible nerve damage. The precise mechanisms involved in reactional episodes have not been defined so far, but current evidence implicates an important role for T cells. Histologically type I reactions are associated with a local increase in CD4$^+$CD45RO$^+$ "memory" T cells and CD8$^+$CD28$^+$ "cytotoxic" T cells (for reviews, see reference 20). *In situ* hybridization and polymerase chain reaction (PCR) assisted analysis of cytokine patterns in type I reaction skin lesions have indeed revealed the predominant expression of T helper type (Th1) like cytokines such as IL-2 and IFN-γ,[48,49] confirming a role for DTH type Th cells in reactional skin lesions.

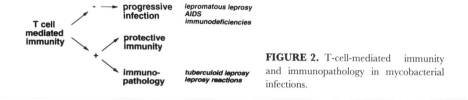

FIGURE 2. T-cell-mediated immunity and immunopathology in mycobacterial infections.

So the cellular immune response is a two-edged sword. It protects, by limiting bacillary growth, yet it also can harm. If turned on improperly, it can induce severe pathology as in tuberculoid leprosy and leprosy reactions, and if it is turned off improperly, bacteria proliferate massively and cause diffuse lepromatous pathology (Fig. 2).

5. ROLE OF SCHWANN CELLS IN IMMUNOPATHOLOGICAL TYPE I LEPROSY NERVE REACTIONS

Because Schwann cells are sites of predilection for *M. leprae*, these cells may well be involved in antigen presentation to *M. leprae*-reactive T cells. The resulting T-cell response may have detrimental effects on the Schwann cells (Fig. 3). Several reports indicate that immunological processes might indeed be involved

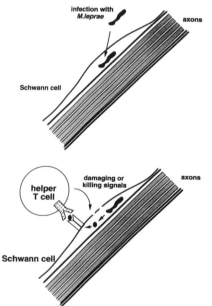

FIGURE 3. Role of Schwann cells in immunopathological type I neural leprosy reactions.

in Schwann cell damage either through specific recognition of *M. leprae* presented by the Schwann cell or through bystander effects. Studies in murine and rat Schwann cells have revealed that these cells can indeed express MHC class II antigens.[50,51] *In vitro*, rat and mouse Schwann cells are able to present exogenous antigens such as myelin basic protein,[52] P2,[53] HSP65,[54] and mycobacterial HSP70[55] to T cells. T cells recognizing HSP65 epitopes are also able to lyse IFN-γ activated murine Schwann cells that are not primed with HSP65,[56] suggesting that Schwann cells can also present self-antigens to T cells. In addition, rodent Schwann cells have been reported to produce IL-1[57] and IL-12,[58] two cytokines that play a key role in the initiation and continuation of immune responses, and IL-6,[59] possibly important in the generation of specific cytotoxic T cells.[60] Until recently human Schwann cells could not be cultured, so this issue could not be addressed in humans. We now have succeeded in culturing long-term human Schwann cell lines from sural nerves. Antigen presentation studies were performed using a CD4+ cytotoxic T-cell clone directed against a 15-kDa protein of *M. leprae*. Our preliminary data indicate that human Schwann cells are indeed capable of presenting exogenous antigens to T cells in an MHC-restricted manner (Fig. 4). These data support our hypothesis that T cells can recognize *M. leprae* presented by Schwann cells and that both cell types may therefore play a role in the immunopathology of nerve damage in leprosy.

6. PHARMACOLOGICAL MODULATION OF IMMUNOPATHOLOGICAL Th1 CELL ACTIVITY

To investigate whether immunopathology-associated Th1 activity can be modulated pharmacologically, we studied a drug that is being used in the treatment of psoriasis. Psoriasis vulgaris is a human inflammatory skin disorder, characterized by epidermal hyperplasia with cellular infiltrates of lymphocytes and

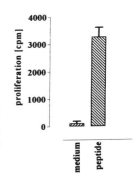

FIGURE 4. Antigen presentation by human Schwann cells. Human Schwann cells (2500 cells/well) were pulsed with a peptide from a 15-kDa protein of *M. leprae*. A CD4+ cytotoxic T-cell clone recognizing this peptide was added and proliferation was measured. Data are depicted as the mean cpm [³H]TdR incorporation ± SEM of quintuplicate determinations.

monocytes.[61] This disease is thought to be a Th1-associated autoimmune disorder.[62,63] Clinical efficacy of cyclosporin A, CD4[+] mAb, and IL-2 in psoriasis
treatment has been well established.[61,62] These compounds selectively block or
eliminate CD4[+] T-cell activation and expansion. More recently, however, clinical improvement in psoriasis vulgaris and psoriatic arthritis patients has been
observed upon therapy with Fumaderm®,[64–67] which is composed of monoethylfumarate (MEF) and dimethylfumarate (DMF). The most effective fumarate
metabolite of this drug is monomethylfumarate (MMF), which is formed in the
circulation by hydrolysis of DMF;[68] considering the possibility that these compounds may act in psoriasis by modulating Th1/Th2 subset development, we
have analyzed the ability of MMF to redirect T-cell cytokine secretion profiles.
Our data indicate that MMF is indeed able to upregulate selectively the secretion
of cytokines that are associated with type 2 immune responses.[69a]

MMF stimulated both IL-4 and IL-5 production by *M. tuberculosis*-activated
T cells, whereas untreated cells usually display a typical Th-1-type cytokine
profile (Fig. 5C, D). Neither IL-2 nor IFN-γ production or proliferation was
modulated by MMF (Fig. 5A,B and not shown). MMF was also capable of
modulating the T-cell cytokine secretion profile of (virtually) fully differentiated
cells away from their Th1 phenotype at the clonal level (not shown). These
findings show indicate that MMF can indeed reset the Th subset balance during
antigen-specific memory T-cell responses.

These results may be surprising at first sight, as modulation of established
T-cell responses by cytokines or soluble factors has been suggested to be more
difficult than modulation of primary T-cell responses. However, Perez et al.[69]
described that established murine Th1 cells can still be converted into IL-4
producers upon exposure to IL-4 whereas the Th2 phenotype could not be
altered under the influence of cytokines. Our own data further support the view
that differentiated Th1 type cells can still be modulated instead of being irreversi-
bly committed. Importantly, this opens avenues for the design of immune-inter-
vention-based therapeutic strategies directed at altering the cytokine balance. The
balance between Th1- and Th2-associated cytokines has been shown to crucially
affect the course of various immune disorders.[3,4]

An immunopathological role of polarized Th1 responses has been proposed in
organ-specific autoimmune diseases such as experimental allergic encephalomyelitis (EAE) and type 1 insulin-dependent diabetes.[6,8] Th2 cells instead may
prevent the development of disease by downregulating the activities of Th1 cells.[6,7]
In an adoptive model of murine EAE, Khoruts et al.[70] elegantly demonstrated that
subtle changes in cytokine secretion patterns may already have important consequences for the development of T-cell responses, whereas Th1 type cells are highly
pathogenic and Th2 cells do not cause EAE; incompletely skewed Th0-like cell
populations that produce both type 1 and type 2 cytokines are only weakly
pathogenic and thus largely resemble the Th2 type cells in their functional behavior.

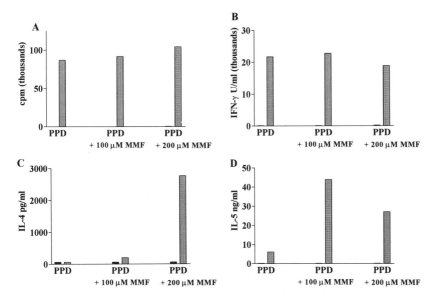

FIGURE 5. Modulation of recall antigen responses by MMF. Peripheral blood mononuclear cells (PBMCs) were stimulated in primary cultures with PPD of *M. tuberculosis* or with PPD together with 100 μ*M* or 200 μ*M* MMF. After 6 days, 20 U/ml rIL-2 was added. At day 13, cells were washed and restimulated (0.75 × 10⁶ cells/ml) with CD2 mAb and CD28 mAb (gift of Dr. R. A. W. van Lier, CLB, Amsterdam). Supernatants were harvested for cytokine analysis 3 days later. Data are representative of three separate experiments. Gray bars: restimulation with CD2/CD28 mAb. Black bars: restimulation with medium.

Thus, it is possible to redirect the functional program of activated, established Th1 cells toward a Th0/Th2 type. These observations offer the basis for the development of novel strategies to modulate immunopathological Th1 activity, in autoimmune disorders as well as during acute inflammatory reactions in infectious diseases.

7. CYTOKINE-BASED ENHANCEMENT OF Th1 CELL RESPONSIVENESS IN MYCOBACTERIAL INFECTIONS: IMPLICATIONS FOR VACCINE DEVELOPMENT

Cytokines play a central role in the expansion and differentiation of antigen-specific T lymphocytes. Several features of IL-12 that have been recognized in recent years point to a critical function of this cytokine in T-cell activation. IL-12 is a disulfide-linked heterodimeric cytokine composed of a 40-kDa (p40) and a 35-kDa (p35) subunit.[71] IL-12 is released by antigen-presenting cells, including macrophages, dendritic cells, and B cells and its production is induced by infection with intracellular parasites. Antigen-activated T lymphocytes and natural killer (NK) cells respond to IL-12 with increased levels of proliferation (reviewed in 72). In terms of differentiation, IL-12 is a powerful inducer of IFN-γ production by T cells and NK cells, thereby facilitating Th1 cell development.[73] In addition, a promoting effect of IL-12 on the cytolytic activity of Ag-specific T cells and NK cells has been well documented.[72]

Development of Th-1 immunity is of crucial importance for the elimination of intracellular microorganisms, such as mycobacteria (e.g., 34a, 74–76). As discussed earlier, TT patients develop strong antigen-specific Th1 immunity to *M. leprae*,[26,27,77] but LL patients typically fail to mount Th1 type responses and develop multibacillary, disseminated disease.[9,10] Leprosy thus provides a valuable model system for the study of the mechanism(s) that underlie immunological (un)responsiveness.

We have investigated the immunoregulatory capacity of cytokines to reverse unresponsiveness in more detail and find that rIL-2 and rIL-12 strongly synergize to overcome *M. leprae*-specific unresponsiveness in leprosy patients in terms of both T-cell proliferation and differentiation.[78a] We first demonstrated that endogenously produced IL-12 and IL-2 are crucial cytokines in the Th1 response of high responder individuals toward *M. leprae*. This was accomplished by employing neutralizing, cytokine-specific monoclonal antibodies in *in vitro* T-cell stimulation assays. We next investigated the ability of IL-2 and IL-12 to reverse T-cell unresponsiveness to *M. leprae* in non-/low-responder patients. In our experiments, rIL-2 was used at 0.5 U/ml, which was the highest concentration that could be used without exerting mitogenic activity in the absence of antigen. Addition of rIL-2 (0.5 U/ml) or rIL-12 (1 U/ml) did not significantly enhance *M. leprae*-induced proliferation in non-/low-responders. Interestingly, rIL-2, however, strongly synergized with rIL-12 in inducing proliferative responses that were comparable to those seen in cultures of high-responder patients stimulated with *M. leprae* alone (Fig. 6). These effects were cytokine specific in that *M. leprae* specific responses that were induced in the presence of either rIL-2 or rIL-12 were not modulated by either IL-4 or by rIFN-γ (not shown).

Time course experiments indicated that the synergistic effect of rIL-2 and rIL-12 was not related to a shift in the kinetics of the response because the synergistic effects of these two cytokines were detected at various time intervals following *M. leprae* stimulation (not shown). Similar observations were made regarding the induction of Th1 responses to a candidate vaccine tumor antigen (HPV 16E7, the cervical cancer associated human papilloma virus serotype 16 oncoprotein E7). These results suggest an important role for IL-2/IL-12 in Th1 promoting vaccines.

Also, a strong synergistic effect in the induction of IFN-γ production was observed in these low-/non-responder patients, showing that rIL-2/rIL-12 indeed stimulates Th1 differentiation and expansion. Our data thus show that rIL-2 or rIL-12 cannot efficiently overcome non-/low-responsiveness to *M. leprae*. In

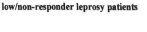

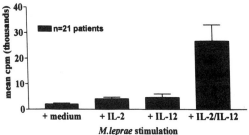

FIGURE 6. IL-2 and IL-12 synergize to reverse T-cell responsiveness. PBMCs of 21 low-/non-responder leprosy patients (7.5 × 10⁵ cells/ml) were stimulated with *M. leprae* (5 μg/ml). IL-2 (0.5 U/ml), IL-12 (1 U/ml), or the combination of cytokines were added as indicated at the initiation of the culture. Data are given as the mean cpm [³H]TdR incorporation at day 7 of these 21 patients ± SEM. Unstimulated PBMC fractions and cultures of PBMCs that were stimulated with cytokines alone contained <700 cpm.

combination, however, these cytokines appear to synergize strongly and to induce proliferative responses that are similar in magnitude to those observed in *M. leprae*-stimulated PBMCs of high-responder patients. In addition, we show that rIL-12 and rIL-2 act in synergy on Th1 cell differentiation by inducing high levels of IFN-γ production but no IL-4 in *M. leprae*-stimulated cultures.

Our data demonstrate the crucial importance of IL-2 and IL-12 in controlling and regulating *M. leprae*-specific T-cell responsiveness across the entire immunological and clinical leprosy spectrum. Because we also observed synergy between rIL-2 and rIL-12 in the induction of T-cell responses to *M. tuberculosis* as well as human papilloma virus-derived tumor antigens (data not shown), we propose that the effects of this cytokine combination are applicable in the design of antimicrobial and antitumor vaccines in general.

ACKNOWLEDGMENTS. This work was supported by the Amsterdam Leiden Institute for Immunology (ALIFI), the MACROPA Foundation, the Commission of the European Communities (CEC), the Netherlands Leprosy Relief Association (NSL), and the UNDP/World Bank/WHO Special Programme for Research and Training in Tropical Diseases.

REFERENCES

1. WHO, 1996, WHO report on the Tuberculosis epidemic, Geneva.
2. Hopewell, P. C., 1994, Overview of clinical tuberculosis, in: *Tuberculosis: Pathogenesis, Protection and Control* (B. R. Bloom, ed.), ASM Press, Washington, D.C., pp. 25–46.
3. Mosmann, T. R., Coffman, R. L., Seder, R. A., *et al.*, 1995, TH1 and TH2 cells: Different

patterns of lymphokine secretion lead to different functional properties. Acquisition of lympho-kine-producing phenotype by CD4+ T cells B7-1 and B7-2 costimulatory molecules activate differentially the Th1/Th2 developmental pathways: Application to autoimmune disease thera-py, *Annu. Rev. Immunol.* **80:**707–718.

4. Seder, R. A., and Paul, W. E., 1994, Acquisition of lymphokine-producing phenotype by CD4+ T cells, *Annu. Rev. Immunol.* **12:**635–673.

5. Kuchroo, V. K., Das, M. P., Brown, J. A., et al., 1995, Acquisition of lymphokine-producing phenotype by CD4+ T cells B7-1 and B7-2 costimulatory molecules activate differentially the Th1/Th2 developmental pathways: Application to autoimmune disease therapy, *Cell* **80:**707–718.

6. Liblau, R. S., Singer, S. M., and McDevitt, H. O., 1995, Th1 and Th2 CD4+ T cells in the pathogenesis of organ-specific autoimmune diseases, *Immunol. Today* **16:**34–38.

7. Chen, Y., Kuchroo, V. K., Inobe, J., Hafler, D. A., and Weiner, H. L., 1994, Regulatory T cell clones induced by oral tolerance: Suppression of autoimmune encephalomyelitis, *Science* **265:**1237–1240.

8. Hsieh, C. S., Macatonia, S. E., Tripp, C. S., Wolf, S. F., O'Garra, A., and Murphy, K. M., 1993, Development of TH1 CD4+ T cells through IL-12 produced by *Listeria*-induced macrophages, *Science* **260:**547–549.

9. Afonso, L. C., Scharton, T. M., Vieira, L. Q., Wysocka, M., Trinchieri, G., and Scott, P., 1994, The adjuvant effect of interleukin-12 in a vaccine against *Leishmania major*, *Science* **263:**235–237.

10. Seder, R. A., Paul, W. E., Davis, M. M., and Fazekas de St. Groth, B., 1992, The presence of interleukin 4 *in vitro* priming determines the lymphokine-producing potential of CD4+ T cells from T cell receptor transgenic mice, *J. Exp. Med.* **176:**1091–1098.

11. Paul, W. E., and Seder, R. A., 1994, Lymphocyte responses and cytokines, *Cell* **76:**241–251.

12. Powrie, F., Correa Oliveira, R., Mauze, S., and Coffman, R. L., 1994, Regulatory interactions between CD45RBhigh and CD45RBlow CD4+ T cells are important for the balance between protective and pathogenic cell-mediated immunity, *J. Exp. Med.* **179:**589–600.

13. Orme, I. M., and Collins, F. M., 1994, Mouse model of tuberculosis, in: *Tuberculosis: Pathogenesis, Protection and Control* (B. R. Bloom, ed.), ASM Press, Washington, D.C., pp. 113–134.

14. Kaufmann, S. H., 1993, Immunity to intracellular bacteria, *Annu. Rev. Immunol.* **11:**129–163.

15. Orme, I. M., Miller, E. S., Roberts, A. D., et al., 1992, T lymphocytes mediating protection and cellular cytolysis during the course of *Mycobacterium tuberculosis* infection. Evidence for different kinetics and recognition of a wide spectrum of protein antigens, *J. Immunol.* **148:**189–196.

16. Orme, I. M., 1987, The kinetics of emergence and loss of mediator T lymphocytes acquired in response to infection with *Mycobacterium tuberculosis, J. Immunol.* **138:**293–298.

17. Ladel, C. H., Daugelat, S., and Kaufmann, S. H., 1995, Immune response to *Mycobacterium bovis* bacille Calmette Guérin infection in major histocompatibility complex class I- and II-deficient knock-out mice: Contribution of CD4 and CD8 T cells to acquired resistance, *Eur. J. Immunol.* **25:**377–384.

18. Flynn, J. L., Goldstein, M. M., Triebold, K. J., Koller, B., and Bloom, B. R., 1992, Major histocompatibility complex class I-restricted T cells are required for resistance to *Mycobacterium tuberculosis* infection, *Proc. Natl. Acad. Sci. USA* **89:**12013–12017.

19. Ladel, C. H., Hess, J., Daugelat, S., Mombaerts, P., Tonegawa, S., and Kaufmann, S. H., 1995, Contribution of alpha/beta and gamma/delta T lymphocytes to immunity against *Mycobacterium bovis* bacillus Calmette Guérin: Studies with T cell receptor-deficient mutant mice, *Eur. J. Immu-nol.* **25:**838–846.

20. Ottenhoff, T. H., and Mutis, T., 1995, Role of cytotoxic cells in the protective immunity against and immunopathology of intracellular infections, *Eur. J. Clin. Invest.* **25:**371–377.

21. Cooper, A. M., Dalton, D. K., Stewart, T. A., Griffin, J. P., Russell, D. G., and Orme, I. M., 1993, Disseminated tuberculosis in interferon gamma gene-disrupted mice, *J. Exp. Med.* **178:** 2243–2247.

22. Flynn, J. L., Chan, J., Triebold, K. J., Dalton, D. K., Stewart, T. A., and Bloom, B. R., 1993, An

essential role for interferon gamma in resistance to *Mycobacterium tuberculosis* infection, *J. Exp. Med.* **178:**2249–2254.

23. Flynn, J. L., Goldstein, M. M., Chan, J., *et al.*, 1995, Tumor necrosis factor-alpha is required in the protective immune response against *Mycobacterium tuberculosis* in mice, *Immunity* 2:561–572.

24. Flynn, J. L., Goldstein, M. M., Triebold, K. J., Sypek, J., Wolf, S., and Bloom, B. R., 1995, IL-12 increases resistance of BALB/c mice to *Mycobacterium tuberculosis* infection, *J. Immunol.* **155:**2515–2524.

25. Ottenhoff, T. H., Neuteboom, S., Elferink, D. G., and De Vries, R. R., 1986, Molecular localization and polymorphism of HLA class II restriction determinants defined by *Mycobacterium leprae*-reactive helper T cell clones from leprosy patients, *J. Exp. Med.* **164:**1923–1939.

26. Haanen, J. B., de Waal Malefijt, R., Res, P. C., *et al.*, 1991, Selection of a human T helper type 1-like T cell subset by mycobacteria, *J. Exp. Med.* **174:**583–592.

27. Mutis, T., Kraakman, E. M., Cornelisse, Y. E., *et al.*, 1993, Analysis of cytokine production by *Mycobacterium*-reactive T cells. Failure to explain *Mycobacterium leprae*-specific nonresponsiveness of peripheral blood T cells from lepromatous leprosy patients, *J. Immunol.* **150:**4641–4651.

28. Ottenhoff, T. H., 1994, Immunology of leprosy: Lessons from and for leprosy, *Int. J. Lepr. Other Mycobact. Dis.* **62:**108–121.

29. Holland, S. M., Eisenstein, E. M., Kuhns, D. B., *et al.*, 1994, Treatment of refractory disseminated nontuberculous mycobacterial infection with interferon gamma. A preliminary report, *N. Engl. J. Med.* **330:**1348–1355.

30. Levin, M., Newport, M. J., D'Souza, S., *et al.*, 1995, Familial disseminated atypical mycobacterial infection in childhood: A human mycobacterial susceptibility gene?, *Lancet* **345:**79–83.

31. Frucht, D. M., and Holland, S. M., 1996, Defective monocyte costimulation for IFN-gamma production in familial disseminated *Mycobacterium avium* complex infection: Abnormal IL-12 regulation, *J. Immunol.* **157:**411–416.

32. Newport, M. J., Huxley, C. M., Huston, S., Hawrylowicz, C. M., Oostra, B. A., Williamson, R., and Levin, M., 1996, A mutation in the interferon-γ-receptor gene and susceptibility to mycobacterial infection, *N. Engl. J. Med.* **335:**1941–1961.

33. Jouanguy, E., Altare, F., Lamhamedi, S., Revy, P., Emile, J., Newport, M., Levin, M., Blanche, S., Seboun, E., Fischer, A., and Casanova, J., 1996, Interferon-γ-receptor deficiency in an infant with fatal bacille Calmette-Guérin infection. *N. Engl. J. Med.* **335:**1956–1961.

34. Turner, J., and Dockrell, H. M., 1996, Stimulation of human peripheral blood mononuclear cells with live *Mycobacterium bovis* BCG activates cytolytic CD8+ T cells *in vitro*, *Immunology* **87:**339–342.

34a. de Jong, R., Altare, F., Haagen, I.-A., *et al.*, 1998, Severe Mycobacterial and *Salmonella* infections in interleukin-12 receptor deficient patients, *Science* **280:**1435–1439.

35. Kaleab, B., Ottenhoff, T., Converse, P., *et al.*, 1990, Mycobacterial-induced cytotoxic T cells as well as nonspecific killer cells derived from healthy individuals and leprosy patients, *Eur. J. Immunol.* **20:**2651–2659.

36. Sieling, P. A., Chatterjee, D., Porcelli, S. A., *et al.*, 1995, CD1-restricted T cell recognition of microbial lipoglycan antigens, *Science* **269:**227–230.

37. Morita, C. T., Beckman, E. M., Bukowski, J. F., *et al.*, 1995, Direct presentation of nonpeptide prenyl pyrophosphate antigens to human gamma delta T cells, *Immunity* **3:**495–507.

38. Ottenhoff, T. H. M., and De Vries, R. R. P., 1987, HLA class II immune response and suppression genes in leprosy, *Int. J. Lepr.* **55:**521–534.

39. Ottenhoff, T. H. M., Torrez, P., Terencio de las Aguas, J., Van Eden, W., De Vries, R. R. P., and Stanford, J. L., 1986, Evidence for an HLA DR4 associated immune response gene for *Mycobacterium tuberculosis:* A clue to the pathogenesis of rheumatoid arthritis?, *Lancet* **ii:**310–313.

40. Van Eden, W., De Vries, R. R. P., Stanford, J. L., and Rook, G. A. W., 1983, HLA-DR3 associated genetic control of response to multiple skin tests with new tuberculins, *Clin. Exp. Immunol.* **52:**287.

41. Janson, A. A. M., Klatser, P. R., Vd Zee, R., Cornelisse, Y. E., De Vries, R. R. P.,

Thole, J. E. R., and Ottenhoff, T. H. M., 1991, A systematic molecular analysis of the T cell stimulating antigens from *M. leprae* with T cell clones of leprosy patients. Identification of a novel *M. leprae* hsp 70 fragment by *M. leprae* specific T cells, *J. Immunol.* **147:**3530–3537.

42. Geluk, A., Van Meijgaarden, K. E., Janson, A. A. M., Drijfhout, J. W., Meloen, R., De Vries, R. R. P., and Ottenhoff, T. H. M., 1992, Functional analysis of DR17 (DR3)-restricted mycobacterial T cell epitopes reveals DR17 binding motif and enables the design of allele-specific competitor peptides. *J. Immunol.* **149:**2864–2871.

43. Ottenhoff, T. H. M., Haanen, J. B. A. G., Geluk, A., Mutis, T., Kale, Ab B., Thole, J. E. R., Van Schooten, W. C. A., Van den Elsen, P. J., and De Vries, R. R. P., 1991, Regulation of mycobacterial heat shock protein reactive T cells by HLA class II molecules: Lessons from leprosy, *Immunol. Rev.* **121:**171–191.

44. Orme, I. M., and Collins, F. M., 1994, *Tuberculosis: Pathogenesis, Protection and Control* (B. R. Bloom, ed.), ASM Press, Washington, D.C., 531 pp.

45. Kaufmann, S. H. E., 1993, Immunity to intracellular bacteria, *Annu. Rev. Immunol.* **II:**129.

46. Ottenhoff, T. H. M., Klatser, P. R., Ivanyi, J., Elferink,, D. G., De Wit, M., and De Vries, R. R. P., 1986, *Mycobacterium leprae* specific protein antigens defined by cloned human helper T cells, *Nature* **319:**66–68.

47. Mutis, T., Cornelisse, Y. E., Datema, G., Van den Elsen, P. J., Ottenhoff, T. H. M., and De Vries, R. R. P., 1994, Definition of a human suppressor T cell epitope, *Proc. Natl. Acad. Sci. USA* **91:**9456–9460.

48. Cooper, C. L., Mueller, C., Sinchaisri, T. A., Pirmes, C., Chan, J., Kaplan, G., Young, S. M., Weissman, I. L., Bloom, B. R., Rea, T. H., *et al.*, 1989, Analysis of naturally occurring delayed-type hypersensitivity reactions in leprosy by in situ hybridization, *J. Exp. Med.* **169:**1565–1581.

49. Yamamura, M., Wang, X. H., Ohmen, J. D., Uyemura, K., Rea, T. H., Bloom, B. R., and Modlin, R. L., 1992, Cytokine patterns of immunologically mediated tissue damage, *J. Immunol.* **149:**1470–1475.

50. Bergsteindottir, K., Kingston, A., and Jessen, K. R., 1992, Rat Schwann cells can be induced to express major histocompatibility complex class II molecules *in vivo*, *J. Neurocytol.* **21:**382–390.

51. Lisak, R. P., and Bealmear, B., 1992, Differences in the capacity of gamma-interferons from different species to induce class I and II major histocompatibility complex antigens on neonatal rat Schwann cells in vitro, *Pathobiology* **60:**322–329.

52. Wekerle, H., Schwabb, M., Linington, C., and Meyermann, R., 1986, Antigen presentation in the peripheral nervous system: Schwann cells present endogenous autoantigens to lymphocytes, *Eur. J. Immunol.* **16:**1551–1557.

53. Argall, K. G., Armati, K. G., Pollard, J. D., Watson, E., and Bonner, J., 1992, Interactions between CD4+ T-cells and rat Schwann cells *in vitro*. 1. Antigen presentation by Lewis rat Schwann cells to P2-specific CD4+ T-cell lines, *J. Neuroimmunol.* **40:**1–18.

54. Gold, R., Toyka, K. V., and Hartung, H. P., 1995, Synergistic effect of IFN-γ and TNF-Ó on expression of immune molecules and antigen presentation by Schwann cells, *Cell. Immunol.* **165:**65–70.

55. Ford, A. L., Britton, W. J., and Armati, P. J., 1993, Schwann cells are able to present exogenous mycobacterial hsp70 to antigen-specific T lymphocytes, *J. Neuroimmunol.* **43:**151–159.

56. Steinhoff, U., Schoel, B., and Kaufmann, S. H., 1990, Lysis of IFN-γ activated Schwann cell by cross-reactive CD8+αβ T cells with specificity to the mycobacterial 65 kd heat shock protein, *Int. Immunol.* **2:**279–284.

57. Bergsteindottir, K., Kingston, A., Mirsky, R., and Jessen, K. R., 1991, Rat Schwann cells produce interleukin-1, *J. Neuroimmunol.* **34:**15–23.

58. Turka, L. A., Goodman, R. E., Rutkowski, J. L., Sima, A. A., Merry, A., Mitro, R. S., Wrone-Smith, T., Toews, G., Strieter, R. M., and Nickoloff, B. J., 1995, Interleukin 12: A potential link between nerve cells and the immune response in inflammatory disorders, *Mol. Med.* **1:**690–699.

59. Bolin, L. M., Verity, A. N., Silver, J. E., Shooter, E. M., and Abrams, J. S., 1995, Interleukin-6 production by Schwann cells and induction in sciatic nerve injury, *J. Neurochem.* **64:**850–858.

60. Fink, S., De la Barrera, S., Minnucci, F., Valdez, R., Balina,, L. M., and Sasiain, M. C., 1993, IFN-γ, IL-6 and IL-4 modulate *M. leprae-* or PPD-specific cytotoxic T cells in leprosy patients, *Scand. J. Immunol.* **38:**551–558.

61. Baker, B. S., and Fry, L., 1992, The immunology of psoriasis, *Br. J. Dermatol.* **126:**1–9.

62. Kolbach, D. N., and Nieboer, C., 1995, Fumaric acid therapy in psoriasis: Results and side effect of 2 years of treatment, *N. Engl. J. Med.* **332:**581–588.

63. Gottlieb, S. L., Gilleaudeau, P., Johnson, R., Estes, L., Woodworth, T. G., Gottlieb, A. B., and Krueger, J. G., 1995, Response of psoriasis to a lymphocyte-selective toxin (DAB389II-2) suggests a primary immune, but not keratinocyte, pathogenic basis, *Nat. Med.* **1:**442–447.

64. Thio, H. B., Van der Schroeff, J. G., Nugteren-Huying, W. M., and Vermeer, B. J., 1995, Long-term systematic therapy with dimethylfumarate and monoethylfumarate (Fumaderm) in psoriasis, *J. Eur. Acad. Dermatol. Venereol.* **4:**35–40.

65. Altmeyer, P. J., Matthes, U., Pawlak, F., Hoffmann, K., Frosch, P. J., Ruppert, P., Wassilew, S. W., Horn, T., Kreysel, H. W., Lutz, G., Barth, J., Rietzschel, I., and Joshi, R. K., 1994, Antipsoriatic effect of fumaric acid derivatives, *J. Am. Acad. Dermatol.* **30:**977–981.

66. Kolbach, D. N., and Nieboer, C., 1992, Fumaric acid derivates evoke a transient increase in intracellular free calcium concentration and inhibit proliferation of human keratinocytes, *J. Am. Acad. Dermatol.* **27:**769–771.

67. Peeters, A. J., Dijkmans, B. A. C., and Van der Schroeff, J. G., 1992, Fumaric acid therapy for psoriatic arthritis. A randomized, double blind, placebo controlled study, *Br. J. Rheumatol.* **31:**502–504.

68. Nibbering, P. H., Thio, B., Zomerdijk, T. P. L., Bezemer, A. C., Beijersbergen, R. L., and Van Furth, R., 1993, Effects of monomethylfumarate on human granulocytes, *J. Invest. Dermatol.* **101:**37–42.

69. Perez, V. L., Lederer, J. A., Luchtman, A. H., and Abbas, A. K., 1995, Stability of Th1 and Th2 populations, *Int. Immunol.* **7:**869–875.

69a. de Jong, R., Bezemer, A. C., Zomerdijk, T. P. L., *et al.*, 1996, Selective stimulation of T helper 2 cytokine responses by the anti-psoriasis agent monomethylfumarate, *Eur. J. Immun.* **26:**2067–2074.

70. Khoruts, A., Miller, S. D., and Jenkins, M. K., 1995, Neuroantigen-specific Th2 cells are inefficient suppressors of experimental encephalomyelitis induced by effector Th cells, *J. Immunol.* **155:**5011–5017.

71. Kobayashi, M., Fitz, L., Ryan, M., Hewick, R. M., Clark, S. C., Chan, S., Loudon, R., Sherman, F., Perussia, B., and Trinchieri, G., 1989, Identification and purification of natural killer cell stimulatory factor (NKSF), a cytokine with multiple biologic effects on human lymphocytes, *J. Exp. Med.* **170:**827–845.

72. Trinchieri, G., 1994, Interleukin-12: A cytokine produced by antigen-presenting cells with immunoregulatory functions in the generation of T-helper cells type 1 and cytotoxic lymphocytes. *Blood* **84:**4008–4027.

73. Hsieh, C., Macatonia, S. E., Tripp, C. S., Wolf, S. F., O'Garra, A., and Murphy, K. M., 1993, Development of Th1 CD4+ T cells through IL-12 produced by *Listeria*-induced macrophages, *Science* **260:**547–549.

74. Cooper, A. M., Dalton, D. K., Stewart, T. A., Griffin, J. P., Russell, D. G., and Orme, I. M., 1993, Disseminated tuberculosis in IFNγ gene-disrupted mice. *J. Exp. Med.* **178:**2243–2247.

75. Flynn, J. L., Chan, J., Triebold, K. J., Dalton, D. K., Stewart, T. A., and Bloom, B. R., 1993, An essential role for IFNγ in resistance to *Mycobacterium tuberculosis* infection, *J. Exp. Med.* **178:**2249–2254.

76. Flynn, J. L., Goldstein, M. M., Triebold, K. J., Sypek, J., Wolf, S., and Bloom, B. R., 1995, IL-12 increases resistance of BALB/C mice to *Mycobacterium tuberculosis* infection, *J. Immunol.* **155:**2515–2524.

77. Yamamura, M., Uyemura, K., Deans, R. J., Weinberg, K., Rea, T. H., Bloom, B. R., and Modlin, R. L., 1991, Defining protective responses to pathogens: Cytokine profiles in leprosy lesions, *Science* **254:**277–279.

78. de Jong, R., Janson, A. A. M., Faber, W. R., *et al.*, 1997, IL-2 and IL-12 act in synergy to overcome antigen-specific T cell unresponsiveness in mycobacterial disease, *J. Immun.* **159:**786–793.

7

Mycobacterium avium-Complex Infections and Immunodeficiency

FRANK M. COLLINS

1. INTRODUCTION

Pulmonary tuberculosis was shown to be caused by an infectious agent, *Mycobacterium tuberculosis*, when Robert Koch first isolated the organism in pure culture in 1882 and demonstrated that it satisfied his postulates as the causative agent of this devastating human disease.[1] Subsequently, another strain of tubercle bacillus, *M. avium* (which can infect chickens and swine), was isolated from lung and cervical lymph node infections in infants and young children.[2] Following the introduction of antituberculous chemotherapy for the treatment of pulmonary tuberculosis more than half a century later, a number of drug-resistant nontuberculous mycobacteria were isolated from adults with tuberculosis. Initially, many of these organisms had been considered to be avirulent laboratory contaminants the presence of which in clinical specimens could be safely ignored. However, as more and more of these organisms were isolated from individuals who were clearly suffering from progressive lung disease, it was realized that these atypical mycobacteria were, in fact, opportunistic human pathogens that were capable of causing progressive disease in individuals whose cellular defenses had been depressed for some reason.

FRANK M. COLLINS • Laboratory of Mycobacteria, CBER, FDA, Bethesda, Maryland 20852.

Opportunistic Intracellular Bacteria and Immunity, edited by Lois J. Paradise *et al.* Plenum Press, New York, 1999.

Many of these so-called atypical mycobacteria were originally designated simply as "Battey bacilli" (named after the TB Sanitorium of the same name). Following the detailed taxonomic studies of Runyon, Wayne, and others, the Battey bacilli were designated as members of the *M. avium–intracellulare–scrofulaceum* (MAIS) complex, largely on the basis of their cultural and biochemical characteristics.[3] Most members of this group are widely distributed in the natural environment (soil and water) and as a result, most of them were studied more for their taxonomic than their pathogenetic interest.[4] Seroagglutination tests divided the MAIS into 31 antigenically distinct serovars, the first 4 being listed as *M. avium*, the next 24 as *M. intracellulare*, with 3 *M. scrofulaceum* serovars as a separate subgroup.[5] Recent DNA homology studies carried out on these organisms suggest that 11 of these serovars (namely 1–6, 8–11, and 21) should be considered *M. avium* strains, and the remaining 17 serovars as *M. intracellulare*.[6] Because virtually all of these *M. intracellulare* serovars were originally isolated from human clinical specimens, they should also be considered to be opportunistic human pathogens. Most of them seem capable of causing progressive lung disease in immunosuppressed individuals as well as patients suffering from some form of lung disease such as silicosis, pneumoconiosis, or sarcoidosis.[2] It is likely that these organisms are also capable of colonizing (at least temporally) the nasal, oropharyngeal, or intestinal mucosae of individuals who unknowingly ingest *Mycobacterium avium* complex (MAC)-contaminated food or water.[7] However, such local involvement seldom leads to infection of the underlying tissues in normal immunocompetent adults. Once established within the tissues, their innate drug resistance makes these organisms extremely difficult to control effectively, leading to life-threatening disease, especially in elderly and debilitated patients.

The incidence of MAC disease in the United States has increased dramatically as a result of the emerging human immunodeficiency virus (HIV) epidemic. As a result, *M. avium* complex changed in less than a decade from a rare, even exotic, human pathogen to a common, life-threatening complication for many terminally ill acquired immunodeficiency syndrome (AIDS) patients.[8] As the number of AIDS patients continues to increase worldwide,[9] it seems likely that we will also be subjected to an increasingly severe tuberculosis pandemic, much of it drug-resistant.[10] In the United States, the number of AIDS cases reported to the Centers for Disease Control in Atlanta now exceeds 500,000[11] and this figure may well exceed 1 million cases by the year 2000. Several epidemiological studies indicate that as many as 60% of these AIDS patients will be infected with nontuberculous mycobacteria by the time they are examined postmortem.[12] Up to half of these patients will develop disseminated *M. avium*-complex (DMAC) disease, most of it caused by *M. avium* serovars 1, 4, and 8,[13] with smaller numbers of serovars 6, 9, and 10 being reported, especially overseas.[14] These MAC serovars are considered to be among the more "virulent" members of this group and have also been recovered from a number of cancer and transplant patients undergoing prolonged immunosuppressive chemotherapy.[15] Interesting, though for unknown reasons, the dominant MAC strains recovered from the non-AIDS patients often belong to different serovars from those found in AIDS patients. Many of these serovars have also been recovered from the hot water faucets and showerheads in homes and hospitals treating AIDS patients, suggesting that this may be a major source of such infections in the highly immunosuppressed patient.[16] However, direct demonstration of a water-borne infection route in these patients is a technically demanding task and so far has been attempted only in a handful of outbreaks.[8] Clearly, we need a great deal more, good epidemiological data before the precise distribution route for these important opportunistic pathogens can be established within the community.[17]

A number of *M. avium*-complex strains are able to colonize (at least temporarily) the bronchial and intestinal mucosae of normal individuals (especially infants and young children who develop a self-limiting lymphadenitis). It is presumed that they acquire these infections by ingestion of MAC-contaminated food or water.[2] Such water-borne organisms are more likely to be the less virulent *M. intracellulare* and *M. scrofulaceum* which are widely distributed in water and soil samples collected from the southeastern states.[18] However, epidemiological studies carried out in Sweden and Finland suggest that *M. avium* infections are not uncommon in these countries.[19,20] Despite the diversity of MAC serovars present in local soil and water samples, the majority of *M. avium* isolates from American AIDS patients fall into serovars 1, 4, and 8, suggesting that these strains possess some pathogenetic advantage over the other serovars in the environment that allows them to gain entry into the gut-associated lymphoid tissue (GALT) in a preferential manner.[21] Localized MAC infections may be more frequent in rural communities where the inhabitants are more likely to be exposed to colonization by environmental mycobacteria.[22] The existence of inapparent MAC infections in many communities can be inferred from the skin hypersensitivity responses to purified protein derivative (PPD-A) (*M. avium*-derived tuberculin) and PPD-B (*M. intracellulare*) observed in many apparently normal adults in this country.[23] When such an individual is subjected to some form of immunosuppression (whether natural or iatrogenic), the latent MAC infection will be released from its normally effective cellular constraints, leading to the development of disseminated MAC disease.[8,24] The number of MAC organisms actually present in the GALT organs of these latently infected individuals will be very low, making the early detection of this infection extremely difficult, even problematic. Recent advances in the molecular biology of these mycobacteria make it possible to detect very small numbers of mycobacteria in bone marrow and other biopsy materials and it is likely that this technical problem will be overcome in the not too distant future.[25]

There has been an ongoing debate in the literature for many years regarding the virulence of many mycobacteria, both in humans and experimental animals.[26] The problem may be due in part to the attenuation that occurs whenever

these organisms are maintained for any length of time on laboratory media. Most
M. avium-complex strains exhibit a characteristic change in colonial morphology
when cultivated on laboratory media and this can also be associated with a
substantial change in virulence and drug susceptibility.[27,28] Prior to the introduction of agar-based media, this colony change was difficult to detect and as a
consequence was seldom documented adequately, especially in virulence studies.
On first isolation, most clinical isolates of *M. avium* produce flat, smooth, translucent (SmT) colonies that are considered to be the most virulent of the different
colony variants present in the culture. As the organism is cultivated on laboratory
media, an increasing number of domed, opaque (SmD) colonies develop and
eventually this form may dominate the culture. If cultivation is continued in
media containing high concentrations of detergent, a rough (Rg) colony variant
appears and eventually this form will take over the culture completely. Once this
happens, the organism is completely avirulent for experimental animals and
virulence cannot be restored by means of animal passage. The three colony forms
can be maintained in virtually pure culture by means of direct plate-to-plate
transfer. However, these cultures revert to mixed colonies following a single
transfer through liquid culture. Inoculation of a mixed colony culture into normal
mice results in the elimination of the less virulent SmD colony variant and
eventually only the virulent SmT colony form will be recovered from splenic
homogenates (Fig. 1). Some MAC strains produce only the SmD colony variant
when cultured on Middlebrook 7H10 agar (*M. intracellulare* Yandle is one such
example) and such strains usually exhibit low mouse virulence, although they may
retain some virulence for chickens.[27] The molecular mediators of these subtle
colony variations are largely unknown,[29] although the change from the SmD to
the Rg colony form has been related to a loss of C-mycoside antigens from the cell
wall.[30] The molecular changes associated with the decline in virulence when the
SmT colony changes into the SmD form may depend on the strength of the

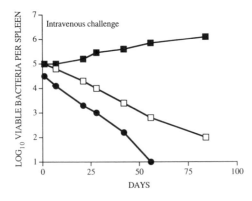

FIGURE 1. Growth of *M. intracellulare* 1405 in the spleens of C57BL/6 mice following their intravenous infection with a suspension of approximately equal numbers of SmT (■), SmD (□), and Rg (●) colony variants. The counts represent the means of five replicates with a standard error of <10%.

cytokine response induced by specific cell membrane lipids associated with the SmT strain within the host phagocyte.[31] Comparison of cell-wall lipids isolated from the translucent and opaque colony variants of *M. intracellulare* also suggest that it is a loss of specific acidic polysaccharides from the surface of the organism that is responsible for both the change in colonial morphology and drug resistance.[32]

The present chapter discusses some of the public health implications associated with *M. avium*-complex infections as the AIDS epidemic continues to develop both in the United States and overseas, elevating an obscure group of environmental mycobacteria into a major, life-threatening pathogen for these severely immunosuppressed patients. Given the continued worldwide spread of the HIV epidemic,[9] it seems that a concurrent MAC epidemic is virtually inescapable and so this once obscure group of nontuberculous mycobacteria is likely to continue to be an important public health problem for the foreseeable future.

2. *M. AVIUM*-COMPLEX INFECTIONS IN IMMUNOCOMPETENT INDIVIDUALS

The nontuberculous mycobacteria constituted something of an enigma to taxonomists and clinicians alike until Runyon devised his system of classification based on differences in colony pigmentation, biochemical activity, and growth rates in laboratory media.[33] One of the most important groups in this system were generally referred to as *M. avium–intracellulare–scrofulaceum* (MAIS), which was further differentiated into a large number of serovars by means of seroagglutination testing.[6] Although *M. avium* was clearly an overt human and animal pathogen, there was a considerable debate in the literature regarding the potential pathogenicity of the other members of this group. Most strains of *M. intracellulare* and *M. scrofulaceum* were considered to be little more than opportunistic, environmental contaminants that somehow gain entry to the tissues. This misconception probably stemmed from the fact that many MAIS strains failed to induce a detectable pathology in mice and guinea pigs infected with large numbers of the organisms. As a result, they were often accorded little or no pathological significance and were all too frequently simply ignored and discarded. However, some serovars were present in such numbers and with sufficient frequency in sputum and bronchial and gastric washings taken from tuberculosis patients that they had to be accorded the status of opportunistic pathogens.[2] However, it was generally felt that most of these organisms were nonpathogenic for normal immunocompetent individuals.[4] Regardless of the validity of this assumption, these opportunistic pathogens are capable of causing a severe, life-threatening lung disease in a proportion of tuberculosis patients, as well as some apparently immunocompetent individuals who usually develop a relatively dilatory form of the disease, in which the patient may live a more or less normal life for many years.[34,35] Many of these individuals had no known underlying or potentiating disease and the reason for the increasing number of MAC infections in these communities is unclear. Regardless of the reason for the attack, the relatively high level of drug resistance expressed by these nontuberculous mycobacteria makes them difficult to control clinically and if the patient is also receiving cancer or transplantation chemotherapy, the infection can become fulminant, rapidly progressing to a fatal conclusion.[8,13] Cancer patients seem particularly susceptible to infection by a number of *M. avium*-complex serotypes, most of which were never fully speciated or serodiagnosed.[15,21,35] The frequency of occurrence of these MAC strains in severely immunosuppressed cancer and transplant patients can be as high as 50% of all nontuberculous isolates, resulting in an annual prevalence rate of 1.3 cases per 10^5 persons. However, the true incidence of these MAC infections in the community is difficult to determine because they are not reportable to the Centers for Disease Control and most of what we know about their occurrence is based on retrospective studies that are often fragmentary and incomplete in nature.[8,15,36]

Normally, we are all exposed from time to time to oral inoculation with a variety of nontuberculous mycobacteria judging from the widespread skin hypersensitivity to PPD-A (*M. avium*) and PPD-B (*M. intracellulare*) in many parts of the United States.[38] Latent, inapparent MAC infections can also be inferred from the sharp rise in IgG antibody levels in the sera of healthy 5- to 10-year-old children tested with *M. avium* sonicate and *M. tuberculosis* LAM (lipoarabinomannan).[39] A predominantly oral route can be postulated for these infections judging from the relative ease with which these nontuberculous mycobacteria can be recovered from the stool samples of many apparently normal adults.[40] Normally, it could be expected that it would be difficult for such orally introduced mycobacteria to establish themselves within the normal intestinal tract because they will have to compete with the resident microflora for any available mucosal attachment sites. The fact that *M. avium* seems to achieve this with relative ease suggests that it possesses a cell-wall adhesin that attaches the organism to receptors on the mucosal cell surface, thus enabling the organism to take up a temporary residence within the intestinal tract.[41,42] It is possible that all members of the *M. avium* complex possess such a receptor, but only the more "virulent" members of the group (serovars 1, 4, 6, 8, 9, and 12 for instance) are able to invade the underlying submucosa and eventually colonize the draining lymph node(s). The resulting infection will be a self-limiting lymphadenitis of the type seen in infants before they have developed an effective mucosal defense against these opportunistic mycobacteria.[2,35,42] In normal immunocompetent adults, such mesenteric lymph node involvement is likely to be benign and resolves without treatment unless the patient is immunosuppressed (either naturally or iatrogenically induced). Without the normally effective cellular defenses to restrict the spread of the infection, the patient develops a disseminated form of MAC disease resembling that seen in miliary tuberculosis.

Differences in the innate virulence of several members of this group are demonstrated in the growth curves observed in intravenously infected C57BL/6 mice (Fig. 2). The mouse virulent *M. avium* (TMC 724; serotype 2) multiplies extensively in both the spleen and the lung (not shown) until it eventually reaches lethal proportions.[43] When *M. avium* was introduced into the lung, little or no indication of any cellular immune response could be detected in the heavily infected mice.[44,45] However, when adoptive transfers were carried out using spleen cells harvested from these mice, it was clear that immune T cells were nevertheless present in the chronically infected spleen which could provide detectable antituberculous immunity to naive, syngeneic recipients. No such protection was observed if the transfer was attempted using the naturally resistant A/J strain of mouse. This unexpected result was explained when the growth behavior of the primary *M. avium* (vaccinating) infection was examined. The virulent *M. avium* 724 did not multiply within the spleens of the A/J (*Bcg*[r]) mice, which as a result did not produce the sensitized T cells needed to adoptively protect the recipient mice from the subsequent challenge infection. This is another example of the earlier finding that a nonreplicating vaccine cannot induce a protective antituberculous immune response.[46]

A similar growth pattern is seen when mice are infected with *M. avium* using the aerogenic route of inoculation (Fig. 3). However, when athymic "nude" and thymectomized T-cell-depleted BALB/c mice were infected aerogenically with this organism, the severity of the resulting lung infection was greatly enhanced (Fig. 4) with most of the mice dying as a result of the widely disseminated disease. Some systemic disease developed even when the mice were challenged using the oral route, although the resulting infection developed relatively slowly and none of the mice died as a result of this massive challenge.[44] The majority of *M. avium*

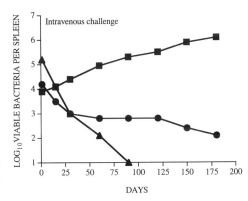

FIGURE 2. Growth of *M. avium* 724 serovar 2 (■), *M. intracellulare* 1406 serovar 16 (●), and *M. scrofulaceum* 1305 serovar 42 (▲) in the spleens of intravenously infected C57BL/6 mice.

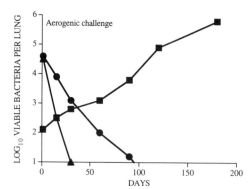

FIGURE 3. Growth of *M. avium* 724 (■), *M. intracellulare* 1406 (●), and *M. scrofulaceum* 1305 (▲) in the lungs of aerogenically infected C57BL/6 mice.

recovered from these orally challenged mice were cultured from homogenates of the Peyer's patches and mesenteric lymph nodes. However, small numbers of mycobacteria were present in the spleen by the conclusion of the experiment, indicating that some hematogenous spread did occur in these animals.

When normal lC57BL/6 mice were infected with *M. intracellulare* (TMC 1406; serotype 16) or *M. scrofulaceum* (TMC 1305; serovar 42) there was little or no sign of active disease involving either the spleen or lung, regardless of the route of infection (Figs. 2 and 3). *M. scrofulaceum* has long been known to be completely avirulent for mice and this was consistent with the rapid clearance of the inoculum from the liver and spleen even when large numbers of organisms were injected. The inability of this organism to survive in mouse tissues was seen even when inoculated into athymic (nude) BALB/c mice (Collins, unpublished data).

Initially, the apparent incidence of *M. avium*-complex infections in any given community often depended on the level of laboratory expertise available at the time. However, even when good laboratory resources were available, wide varia-

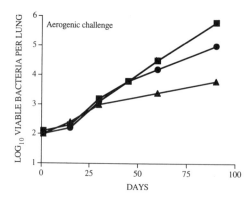

FIGURE 4. Growth of *M. avium* 724 in the lungs of aerogenically challenged athymic "nude" (■), thymectomized, bone marrow reconstituted (●) or sham-thymectomized BALB/c mice (▲).

tions in the incidence of nontuberculous disease were noted in different hospitals and even the same hospital over a period of years.[36] These infection clusters usually had no obvious common infection source, occupational hazard, or other predisposing factor to explain the outbreaks. Although the reason(s) for these cases of non-AIDS-related MAC disease is largely obscure, some form of immunodepletion or underlying disease (an old tuberculous cavity, silicosis, lymphoma) is assumed to be involved in most of the cases.[47] This situation changed dramatically with the development of the HIV epidemic in this country, so that now we face a major public health problem due to the increasing importance of these environmental mycobacteria. Some of these problems are discussed in greater detail in the following sections.

3. *M. AVIUM*-COMPLEX INFECTIONS AND IMMUNODEFICIENCY

M. avium TMC 724 multiplies freely in the lungs and spleens of intravenously (and aerogenically) infected C57BL/6 mice (*Bcg*^{S}) that show little sign of the immune response characteristic of BCG-infected mice.[48] As a result of the slow growth and low tissue toxicity of *M. avium* for these mice, even heavily infected animals show little sign of malaise or distress and may survive for remarkably long periods of time.[44] Eventually, the increasing granulomatous response within the chronically infected lung reaches the point where its functional activity is compromised and the animal dies, as much a result of the host response to the infection as of the pathogenic action of the organism on the host tissues.[49] As a result of its low tissue toxicity, *M. avium* counts in moribund mice may be many times that recovered from similar mice infected with virulent *M. tuberculosis*.[48] Interestingly, isolates of *M. avium* obtained from AIDS versus non-AIDS patients do not seem to differ appreciably in their virulence or tissue toxicity for beige (C57BL/6Bg/Bg[*Bcg*^{S}]) mice.[50] On the other hand, the innately resistant A/J (*Bcg*^{r}) mice developed a persistent, though nonlethal *M. avium* infection when challenged with equivalent numbers of this organism.[51]

Susceptibility to infection by members of the *M. avium* complex depends on a number of extraneous factors, some natural (genetic, prolonged physical or mental stress, intercurrent viral infection, terminal renal disease, cancer) others iatrogenic (whole body irradiation, systemic corticosteroid or anticancer chemotherapy). Any of these factors seem capable of exacerbating the severity of any resulting infection, presumably by depressing the normal cellular defenses of the host. In particular, several viral infections (measles, herpes, cytomegalovirus) may induce a temporary reduction in the ability of the host to express an existing cellular hypersensitivity response to specific bacterial sensitins such as tuberculin or candidin.[52] The loss of tuberculin sensitivity has important diagnostic consequences for individuals living in areas where tuberculosis is endemic and tuberculin skin testing is widely used as an indicator of exposure to mycobacterial infections. This diagnostic tool is lost when a patient becomes anergic.[37] Skin test anergy occurs in many patients suffering from the miliary form of tuberculosis, and such false-negative reactions can adversely affect the survival of the patient. The increasing incidence of AIDS in populations known to be at high risk of exposure to tuberculosis is most worrisome, as such patients are likely to be totally anergic to all skin test antigens.[53]

Other groups of patients at increased risk of developing MAC disease are those suffering terminal renal disease, or ones who have received a kidney transplant. A variety of nontuberculous mycobacteria have been isolated from these patients, even when they are living in communities where MAC disease is normally a very rare occurrence.[54] The reason for this increase in susceptibility to nontuberculous mycobacterioses is not altogether clear, but is presumed to be due to toxic effects associated with severe nephritis or to the long-term immunosuppressive therapy that must be provided to transplant patients. Repeated heavy doses of cytoxan, methotrexate, and corticosteroid therapy markedly reduce the ability of the host to mount an effective cell-mediated defense against these opportunistic pathogens.

Cancer patients are susceptible to nontuberculous mycobacterial infections, although usually at a lower frequency than that observed for *M. tuberculosis* and *M. kansasii*.[55] Interestingly, these patients are also susceptible to infections caused by such rapid growers as *M. gordonae* and *M. fortuitum*, infections that are virtually never seen in other members of the community,[14] although these species are known to be distributed in the natural environment. They can be readily recovered from the tap water supplied to many communities around the world. Presumably, people living in these areas ingest food or water contaminated with these organisms from time to time. A few organisms may gain entry to the GALTs and establish a temporary residence there, especially if the patient has been exposed to heavy radiation and/or prolonged immunosuppressive chemotherapy. When normally effective cellular defenses are depleted as a result of an ongoing HIV infection, these normally nonpathogenic mycobacteria may begin to proliferate and spread *in vivo*. This process is extremely difficult to verify experimentally and all attempts to establish *M. fortuitum* and *M. nonchromogenicum* infections in immunosuppressed mice by means of repeated oral inoculations have been uniformly unsuccessful.[56] Even attempts to infect germ-free mice orally with these organisms have been unsuccessful (Collins, unpublished data). Thus, the host–parasite interactions responsible for the establishment of an *M. gordonae* infection within the tissues of the immunosuppressed patient cannot be investigated in any detail simply because there is no suitable animal model of this human disease. Regardless of the mechanisms involved, these nominally avirulent organisms can produce severe systemic disease in these patients because their drug resistance can make them difficult to control. For this reason, the presence of even small numbers of these nontuberculous mycobacteria in bone marrow or biopsy samples must always be reviewed extremely carefully and the most appropriate chemotherapeutic regimen implemented as soon as possible.[57]

Acquired antituberculous resistance is mediated by a population of specifically sensitized T cells that release a battery of lymphokines when stimulated by the specific sensitins released by the actively growing mycobacteria within the developing lesion.[48] The spectrum of lymphokines released by actively growing cells within the host tissues will determine the predominant type of immune response, driving it into a predominantly Th1 (antibacterial) or Th2 (humoral) immune response.[58] However, antituberculous immunity is ultimately expressed by a population of interferon-γ (IFN-γ)-activated macrophages that enter into the developing lesion from the bloodstream to kill or at least prevent the further growth of the phagocytosed mycobacteria, thereby preventing the spread of the infection to other uninvolved tissues and organs.[59] Theoretically, these immunologically activated cells should be able to eliminate the infecting population altogether. However, in actual practice, a few residual mycobacteria will persist within chronic lesions *in vivo,* the resulting latent disease often lasting for the lifetime of the host.[60] Some organisms may persist even after prolonged exposure to a multidrug chemotherapeutic regimen that would normally be expected to eliminate the organisms from the tissues. Antibiotic treated mice still contained substantial amounts of mycobacterial DNA long after completion of treatment, although it was not clear whether this represented residual live or dead mycobacteria.[61] Attempts to detect small numbers of residual organisms in such animals using conventional cultural methods or by guinea pig inoculation have failed repeatedly.[60] However, a few organisms must survive in these animals because active disease will recur following heavy corticosteroid treatment. This apparent paradox has been explained by the development of filterable, cell-wall-free or dormant cell forms that later revert to the conventional bacterial form by some unknown mechanism.[62]

The nature of the factors responsible for development of the latent form of tuberculosis in a substantial proportion (50% to 95%) of individuals exposed to tuberculous infection are poorly understood, despite their obvious public health importance.[48] Such latent infections are remarkably stable, despite the presence of an immune response capable of rapidly inactivating a secondary challenge inoculum of the same organism. Presumably, the residual primary infection is sequestered in a site where the activated T-cell defenses are unable to reach them. The activated macrophages that surround the chronic lesion are normally able to prevent the spread of the infection to other uninvolved tissues. However, with the depletion of these cellular defenses as a result of stress, old age, cancer, or an intercurrent viral infection, active disease may light up once again.[63,64] Most of this reactivational tuberculous disease is caused by *M. tuberculosis* or *M. kansasii,* although some *M. avium* isolates have also been recovered from transplant and cancer patients who have been exposed to prolonged immunosuppressive chemotherapy.[13,36] Some of these infections can occur in apparently normal individuals with no previous history of clinical tuberculosis and the reason for these infections (usually seen late in life) is unclear. More research will obviously be needed to settle this matter.

Various nonspecific environmental and socioeconomic factors (senescence, malnutrition, inadequate housing, alcoholism, drug abuse) can also contribute to the development of tuberculous disease in apparently normal individuals. Some of these patients suffer from silicosis, pneumoconiosis, black lung disease, or exposure to a number of industrial solvents, all of which are known to deplete the normal macrophage defenses. Old age has traditionally been associated with reactivational tuberculosis, a proportion of which will be due to members of the *M. avium* complex.[64] The causes of this geriatric form of tuberculosis are still unclear,[65,66] although it has been widely presumed to be a consequence of the progressive immunological senescence associated with aging, poor nutrition, alcoholism, and inadequate health care. However, given the confined environment associated with nursing home life it is possible some of these cases may represent *de novo* infections originating from an unsuspected index case. More frequent infections have been reported in prisons, homeless shelters, and inner city areas where poor nutrition, overcrowding, alcoholism, and drug addiction are undoubtedly contributory factors.

4. *M. AVIUM*-COMPLEX INFECTIONS IN HIV-INFECTED INDIVIDUALS

AIDS was first described in small groups of homosexual men living in New York and San Francisco.[67] These previously healthy subjects inexplicably developed an unusually malignant form of Kaposi's sarcoma or one of several fulminant lung infections caused by such opportunistic pathogens as *Pneumocystis carinii*, *Candida albicans*, or *M. avium*.[68] These organisms had previously been isolated from the lungs of severely immunosuppressed cancer and transplant patients who went on to develop life-threatening disease caused by what had previously been considered to be virtually nonpathogenic members of the normal body microflora. HIV infection was shown to ablate the patient's CD4 T-cell defenses which normally protected the host from these opportunistic pathogens.[8] The pivotal role played by these CD4 cells in protecting the host against tuberculosis explained the dramatic increase in susceptibility by the HIV-infected patient to *M. tuberculous* infection. However, the large number of patients infected with nontuberculous mycobacteria was much more of a surprise.[21] As these isolates were serotyped, an equally unexpected pattern emerged in the distribution of the *M. avium*-complex strains isolated from AIDS patients. Virtually all of the MAC isolates were typed as serovars 4 and 8, with few representatives coming from the other 25 MAC serotypes.[8,15] This was in sharp contrast to isolates from Scandinavian AIDS patients in which serovars 6 and 9 predominated, with few 4 and 8 isolates.[14] To complicate the picture further, no *M. avium* isolates were reported for a group of Ugandan AIDS patients[69] although studies carried out in other parts of Africa reported both *M. tuberculosis* and MAC isolates.[70] It has been postulated that AIDS patients who were born overseas where tuberculosis is endemic will have been exposed to this organism early in life. The resulting latent disease may provide an effective protection against any subsequent *M. avium* infections.[71] The reasons underlying these differences in distribution in different AIDS populations may simply reflect the wide variations known to occur in the distribution of MAC strains in different localities.[20] Similarly, American AIDS patients may be less subject to *M. tuberculosis* infection than Third World patients simply because they are less likely to be exposed to tuberculous infection during early childhood. Interestingly, African and Asian born AIDS patients living in American cities do not usually develop *M. avium*-complex disease although they must be just as exposed to MAC-contaminated drinking water as their American-born counterparts.[71] Epidemiological data obtained from a large cohort of HIV-infected patients failed to detect any correlation between MAC disease and showering, water consumption, or exposure to a variety of environmental factors despite CD4+ counts <50 T cells/mm^3 blood.[72] As many as 50% of AIDS patients living in New York City and Miami are infected with one, sometimes two, MAC strains, whereas only 10% yield *M. tuberculosis* cultures.[73] This distribution ratio was reversed for Haitian AIDS patients living in the same cities, despite the fact that they must have been equally exposed to MAC infections as the American patients.[71] That MAC colonization occurs in many apparently healthy Americans can be inferred from the fact that many adults tested with PPD (*M. tuberculosis*), PPD-A (*M. avium*), or PPD-B (*M. intracellulare*) reacted positively with these reagents.[74] The close association between HIV and mycobacterial disease can be deduced from the fact that up to 60% of AIDS patients are coinfected with *M. tuberculosis* or one of the nontuberculous mycobacteria and up to one third of these patients go on to develop a life-threatening, disseminated form of the disease.[58] In Africa, two thirds of all tuberculosis patients living in some regions were reported to be HIV positive.[75]

The presence of nontuberculous mycobacteria in many AIDS patients often was not suspected until postmortem examination revealed their presence.[76] These infections are difficult to diagnose because the lung pathology is aberrant, resembling that associated with miliary tuberculosis in young children, with massive involvement of the liver, spleen, kidney, bone marrow, and brain. Such patients will not develop open cavitary lung disease and so sputum, bronchial, and gastric washings are smear and culture negative, despite the presence of enormous body loads of viable mycobacteria. Early identification of these MAC infections requires testing buffy coat and bone marrow cell cultures by means of polymerase chain reaction (PCR) expansion with specific DNA probes to identify the small number of *M. avium* present in the patient's tissues.[77]

The increasing number of AIDS patients reported to the CDC each year[11] is an ominous portent of an analogous rise in the amount of nontuberculous mycobacterial disease likely to occur in the United States in the near future (Fig. 5). The exact number of MAC-infected patients in the United States is not known at present with any certainty, as this is not a reportable disease to the CDC and there are relatively little good epidemiological data available on which to base an assessment of their probable numbers in the community at this time.[8,13,15,71] In the past, many hospital laboratories lacked the facilities to fully identify these nontuberculous mycobacteria on a routine basis, relying instead on regional public health laboratories to carry out this diagnostic chore for them. As a result of the time and technical expertise needed to serotype and test the increasing number of nontuberculous mycobacterial isolates for drug sensitivity on a routine basis, a number of faster, more sensitive, specific diagnostic procedures are under development for use in hospital laboratories.[77] These procedures take advantage of specific DNA probes, high pressure liquid chromatography, and phages carrying a luminescence reporter gene to provide a reliable detection system for these technically demanding pathogens.[78-80]

Many AIDS patients develop severe intestinal lesions involving large numbers of acid-fast bacilli within the submucosa, giving them a histological appearance similar to that seen in Whipple's disease.[81] Rectal biopsies, as well as feces samples taken from such patients yield copious growth of *M. avium* on appropriate culture media and serve as useful predictors of the disseminated MAC disease that later develops in many of these patients.[82] This intestinal involvement has been taken as evidence of an oral infection route in many of these patients, a

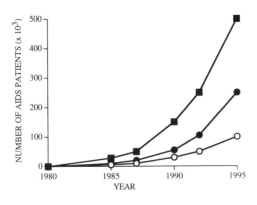

FIGURE 5. Total number of AIDS cases in the United States reported to the Centers for Disease Control from 1980 to 1995 (■). The number of AIDS patients with nontuberculous mycobacterial (●) and disseminated *M. avium* complex disease cases (○) were estimated using reported incidence rates from refs. 8, 11, 13, and 15.

conclusion compatible with the known presence of many *M. avium*-complex serovars in the tap water supplied to patients with DMAC disease.[83] Some of these
mycobacteria have also been detected in feces samples taken from healthy adults,
although their occurrence is usually too sporadic and unpredictable to be a
reliable predictor of a subsequent MAC attack.[84] More efficient recovery of small
numbers of *M. avium* from feces samples was achieved using specific antibody-
coated magnetic beads, followed by PCR expansion and identification of the
DNA with specific probes.[85] As few as 10 viable *M. avium* were detected using this
method, with 18 of 22 samples yielding positive results within 24 h. The presence
of even small numbers of these mycobacteria in the respiratory or gastrointestinal
tracts of HIV-positive individuals has important pathologic implications and the
earliest isolation and identification of these organisms will have crucial importance for these patients.

Once *M. avium* becomes firmly established within the tissues of the HIV-
positive individual, the resulting lesions are more reminiscent of lepromatous
leprosy than tuberculosis. In place of the well-circumscribed lung tubercle, there
will be a diffuse granulomatous response, with loose aggregations of large, foamy
macrophages, many of which are packed with acid-fast bacilli.[86] These tubercles
contain very few lymphocytes, giving them a histological appearance similar to
that described for the lungs of Bacillus Calmette-Guérin (BCG)-infected severe
combined immunogenicity (SCID) and thymectomized, T-cell-deficient mice.[87,88]
When death occurs in these animals, it is the result of a progressive fibrosis and
lung consolidation due to the persistent infection rather than to any toxic effect of
the BCG population within the host tissues. Eventually, this cellular infiltrate
becomes so severe that the functional capacity of the lung is compromised and the
animal dies.

There is no clear consensus regarding the order in which the mycobacterial
and HIV infections develop in the AIDS patient. *M. tuberculosis*-infected AIDS
patients usually develop signs of active disease relatively early in the HIV infection, at a time when the CD4 T-cell population is still relatively high (500 CD4+
cells/mm³ of peripheral blood). Such infections are generally considered to represent reactivation disease rather than newly acquired exogenous infections. However, recent fingerprinting of isolates taken from some AIDS patients indicates
that exogenous infection may occur in some of these highly susceptible patients.
This may be especially important when these patients are housed in confined
environments such as prisons, nursing homes, or homeless shelters where the
incidence of both tuberculosis and HIV infections are likely to be high.[89] On the
other hand, *M. avium* complex infections develop relatively late in the HIV infection when the peripheral CD4 T-cell counts have fallen below 200/mm³ blood.
Because most immunocompetent adults are remarkably resistant to MAC infection, it is assumed that infection with these organisms occurs only after the HIV
infection is well established within the host tissues. However, such an assumption

overlooks the possibility that some of the more "virulent" serovars in the *M. avium* complex may colonize the mucosal surfaces prior to the initiation of the HIV infection. This could explain the presence of a limited number of serotypes in MAC isolates in American AIDS patients if serovars 1, 4, and 8 possess some sort of survival advantage over other members of this group. These three serovars have long been considered to be among the more "virulent" *M. avium* complex strains and this may allow them to establish a temporary residence within the GALTs. The less virulent serovars will be killed by the time they reach the draining lymph node and so will not be recovered from AIDS patients. Such a hypothesis fails to explain the presence of the avirulent, rapid growers *M. gordonae* and *M. fortuitum* in a small number of AIDS patients.[15] It is not possible to determine whether these organisms represent casual bystanders that accidentally gain entry to the tissues of a few immunologically weakened hosts, or are a more virulent variant that can contribute to the developing pathology in the doubly infected patient.[21] Both *M. gordonae* and *M. fortuitum* are known to be widely distributed in nature and are likely to be ingested from time to time. The nature of the host–parasite interactions responsible for their survival in some AIDS patients is unclear and there are no suitable animal models by which to study this problem experimentally. Furthermore, the problem of detecting very small numbers of mycobacteria using the available, technically demanding and notoriously unreliable methods greatly limits any experimental studies of these infections.

Early identification of *M. avium*-complex-infected individuals is an important research goal because these organisms may play a direct role in the development of the deepening immunosuppression characteristic of the terminal phase of AIDS. The heavy bacterial involvement that develops in the periarteriolar regions of the spleen and lymph nodes will deplete the host of its residual T-cell defenses, further increasing the severity of the infection. In addition, the heavy mycobacterial infection will drive these T-cell defenses further into a Th2, nonprotective humoral response, while at the same time providing new T cells to intensify the severity of the viral infection.[90] This chain of events seems consistent with the clinical observation that DMAC markedly enhances the severity of the disease, so that many patients will die weeks or months earlier than the non-MAC-infected patient cohort.[91] Conversely, reduction of the bacterial load within the tissues leads to a substantial improvement to the quality of life for these patients as well as their prolonged survival.[92] It is interesting that DMAC disease can potentiate the severity of the HIV infection compared to patients with *M. tuberculosis* infections. The reason for this difference is unclear but presumably relates to differences in the cytokine profiles produced when macrophages are infected by the different strains.[90,93] These multipathogen–host cell interactions are only now being examined in any detail and are likely to yield important new insights into cellular controls needed to combat this deadly disease combination.

The therapeutic outlook for AIDS patients with disseminated MAC disease was initially extremely bleak.[15] Most members of the *M. avium* complex are innately resistant to streptomycin, isoniazid, and rifampin. Recent studies indicate that some patients will respond to prolonged treatment with a combined regimen of rifabutin, ethambutol, amakasin, cycloserine, and clofazimine.[12] However, this response is bacteriostatic rather than bactericidal and some form of maintenance chemotherapy must be continued for the lifetime of the patient, or the infection recurs whenever therapy is discontinued (usually as a result of toxicity). More recent studies indicated a substantial improvement in the therapy of AIDS patients with DMAC disease using rifabutin, clofazimine, ethambutol, and one of the newer macrolides such as clarithromycin or azithromycin. Dramatic reductions in the size of MAC tissue loads can be produced, provided that the infection is diagnosed early enough.[94–96] This has resulted in prolonged survival times in many of these patients. Despite these encouraging results, a number of pharmacological problems remain to be solved, in particular, interactions between rifabutin and some microlides, and between rifampin and the protease inhibitor needed to control the HIV infection. These interactions are currently under intensive investigation.

Finally, some form of immunotherapy may be required if we are to effectively treat these MAC-infected AIDS patients, especially where no clinical response has been achieved using antituberculous drugs alone.[97] Inclusion of killed *M. vaccae* to the treatment regimen for these patients has been proposed and could be especially useful in the treatment of infections caused by these multidrug-resistant organisms. The results of *M. vaccae* trials currently being carried out in Europe and Africa are being followed with great interest by clinicians and immunologists who are faced with treating these multiply infected patients. More conventional attempts to reconstitute the depleted host defenses of AIDS patients by means of bone marrow transplants, with or without recombinant interleukin-2 (IL-2), IL-12, and IFN-γ, have not been particularly successful to date, although such studies will undoubtedly continue in the future.[12]

5. CONCLUSIONS

The nontuberculous mycobacteria changed from a group of virtually unknown environmental organisms (of little interest to any but a few bacterial taxonomists and environmentalists) into an important group of opportunistic human pathogens with sharply increased public health significance. This shift was largely the result of the AIDS epidemic, which also thrust tuberculosis into the forefront of public health interest, causing the World Health Organization to take the unique step of declaring this disease to be a "global emergency." In addition to the increasing number of tuberculosis patients in this country, there has been a steady increase in the incidence of *M. avium*-complex infections in the AIDS patient population. MAC isolates had been obtained from a number of cancer and transplant patients prior to the advent of the AIDS epidemic. However, it was only after substantial numbers of HIV-infected patients were present in the community that disseminated, life-threatening disease became a significant clinical problem and forced the reevaluation of the pathogenic potential of these highly drug-resistant opportunistic pathogens.

Our understanding of the pathobiology of these *M. avium*-complex infections is greatly limited by the lack of a realistic animal model of the human disease. The host–parasite interactions responsible for establishment of these MAC infections are largely unknown. Most members in this group are nonpathogenic for most immunocompetent adults, being killed by the normal defenses as soon as they enter the tissues without the need for their immunological activation. Some of the more virulent members of this group are able to establish a foothold within the tissues of the immunodepressed host, from which they may be difficult to dislodge. Studies using cytokine-stimulated macrophages harvested from such patients suggest that they are capable of inhibiting the intracellular growth of *M. avium* in tissue culture, but it has been surprisingly difficult to extrapolate these experimental findings into the immunotherapeutic realities of the MAC-infected AIDS patient. As many as 60% of severely immunodepressed AIDS patients may be infected with nontuberculous mycobacteria, many of whom will go on to develop disseminated MAC disease in less than a year. The MAC-infected AIDS patient shows a substantially reduced survival time compared to non-MAC-infected patients. Limiting the extent of MAC involvement can have a substantial effect on the quality of life and survival times for these patients. Epidemiological studies suggest that the MAC infection is the result of ingesting contaminated food or drinking water, although inhalation of infected dust may also be a factor. AIDS patients are highly susceptible to mycobacterial infection, constituting a sentinel population for the presence of these organisms in the community. Fortunately, unlike pulmonary tuberculosis, MAC disease does not constitute a direct person-to-person infectious threat to contacts. This is because the nontuberculous mycobacteria do not induce cavitary disease and aerogenic shedding does not appear to be an important public health problem with these patients.

One of the limiting factors to fuller understanding of the host–parasite interactions responsible for these infections also has been the lack of a suitable animal model of MAC disease. Most members of the *M. avium* complex are virtually avirulent for normal mice and guinea pigs, producing detectable pathology only when injected in very large numbers. *M. avium* can induce progressive lung disease in beige mice and this host has been promoted as a potential model of the human MAC disease. However, the modest increase in susceptibility seen in beige mice, compared to the parent C57BL/6 mouse, hardly justifies the increased costs involved. *M. avium* induces a progressive, fatal infection in intravenously, aerogenically, and intragastrically challenged C57BL/6 mice, although the prolonged incubation periods involved can make these experiments both tedious and costly. *M. avium* infection can be substantially accelerated by its inoculation into T-cell-depleted mice. No such increase occurs when avirulent MAC strains were tested in this system. This suggests that less virulent MAC serovars do not infect AIDS patients because they are inactivated by macrophages as soon as they enter the tissues. This seems to occur even after HIV-induced immunodepression has reached a point where T-cell defenses have been seriously ablated. It seems likely that differences in the size of inoculum and route of infection, as well as the level of immunosuppression, determines the nature of the nontuberculous disease that ultimately develops in these patients. Once established within the tissues, the *M. avium* infection may itself contribute to the deepening immunosuppression characteristic of the terminal AIDS patient by diverting an already limited T-cell response into a nonprotective humoral immunity. For this reason, *M. avium* can no longer be considered to be a casual opportunist but an active contributor to the AIDS infection. It therefore seems prudent to explore the complexities of this viral–mycobacterial–host cell interaction in much greater detail if we are to develop a rational strategy for use against this deadly, dual epidemic.

6. SUMMARY

The *M. avium* complex consists of a group of environmental mycobacteria that are important opportunistic human pathogens for a variety of immunosuppressed cancer, transplant, and HIV-infected patients. Some members of this group are able to colonize the nasopharyngeal and intestinal mucosal membranes of normal individuals who may go on to develop a self-limiting lymphadenitis. The more virulent strains within this group may produce slow, indolent lung disease in some tuberculosis patients as well as in terminally ill renal, diabetic, and cancer patients. More aggressive systemic infections will develop in congenitally and iatrogenically immunosuppressed patients. As much as 60% of AIDS patients have been reported to be infected with nontuberculous mycobacteria, the most common of which are *M. avium*-complex serovars 1, 4, 6, and 8. Half of these patients go on to develop a life-threatening, disseminated form of this disease that can markedly reduce their survival and quality of life. The high level of drug resistance exhibited by these organisms makes effective chemotherapy difficult to achieve and maintain. The response to these drugs is bacteriostatic rather than bactericidal and the disease recurs whenever therapy is discontinued, usually as result of the increasing toxicity of the drug regimen. Development of a suitable immunotherapeutic intervention to help restore cellular immunity to the HIV-infected patient takes on an increasingly urgent priority as the worldwide HIV–MAC epidemic continues its relentless spread.

REFERENCES

1. Collins, F. M., 1982, Immunology of tuberculosis, *Am. Rev. Respir. Dis.* **125:**42–49.
2. Wolinsky, E., 1984, Nontuberculous mycobacteria and associated diseases, in: *The Mycobacteria: A Sourcebook*, Vol. 2 (G. P. Kubica and L. G. Wayne, eds.), Marcel Dekker, New York, pp. 1141–1208.
3. Wayne, L. G., 1984, Mycobacterial speciation, in *The Mycobacteria: A Sourcebook*, Vol. 1 (G. P. Kubica and L. G. Wayne, eds.), Marcel Dekker, New York, pp. 25–65.
4. Wayne, L. G., 1985, The 'atypical' mycobacteria: Recognition and disease association, *Crit. Rev. Microbiol.* **12:**185–222.
5. McClatchy, J. K., 1981, The seroagglutination test in the study of nontuberculous mycobacteria, *Rev. Infect. Dis.* **3:**867–870.
6. Wayne, L. G., Good, R. C., Tsang, A., *et al.*, 1993, Serovar determination and molecular taxonomic correlation in *Mycobacterium avium, M. intracellulare* and *M. scrofulaceum*: A cooperative study of the International Working Group on Mycobacterial Taxonomy, *Int. J. Syst. Bacteriol.* **43:**482–489.
7. Yajko, D. M., Chin, D. P., Gonzalez, P. C., *et al.*, 1995, *M. avium*-complex in water, food and soil samples collected from the environment of HIV-infected individuals, *J. AIDS* **9:**176–182.
8. Young, L. S., Inderlied, C. B., Berlin, O. G., and Gottlieb, M. S., 1986, Mycobacterial infections in AIDS patients with an emphasis on the *Mycobacterium avium* complex, *Rev. Infect. Dis.* **8:**1024–1033.
9. Piot, P., Loga, M., Ryder, R., *et al.*, 1990, The global epidemiology of HIV infection: Continuity, heterogenicity and change, *J. AIDS* **3:**403–412.
10. Dolin, P. J., Raviglione, M. C., and Kochi, A., 1992, Global tuberculosis incidence and mortality during 1990–2000, *Bull. WHO* **72:**213–220.
11. Centers for Disease Control, 1995, First 500,000 AIDS cases—United States, 1995, *Morb. Mort. Wk. Rep.* **44:**849–853.
12. Bermudez, L. E., 1994, Immunobiology of *Mycobacterium avium* infection, *Eur. J. Clin. Microbiol. Infect. Dis.* **13:**1000–1006.
13. O'Brien, R. J., Geiter, L. J., and Snider, D. E., 1987, The epidemiology of nontuberculous mycobacterial diseases in the United States, *Am. Rev. Respir. Dis.* **135:**1007–1014.
14. Hoffner, S. E., Petrini, B., Brennan, P. J., *et al.*, 1989, AIDS and *M. avium* serotypes in Sweden, *Lancet* **ii:**336–337.
15. Kiehn, T. E., Edwards, F. F., Brannon, P., Tsang, A., Maio, M., Gold, J., Whinberg, E., Wang, B., McClatchy, J. K., and Armstrong, D., 1985, Infections caused by *M. avium*-complex in immunocompromised patients: Diagnosis by blood culture and fecal examination, antimicrobial susceptibility test and morphological and serological characteristics, *J. Clin. Microbiol.* **21:**168–173.
16. von Reyn, C. F., Maslow, J. N., Barber, T. W., *et al.*, 1994, Persistent colonization of potable water as a source of *M. avium* infection in AIDS, *Lancet* **343:**1137–1141.
17. duMoulin, G. C., and Stottmeier, K. D., 1986, Waterborne Mycobacteria: An increasing threat to health, *ASM News* **52:**525–529.
18. Gruft, H., Falkinham, J. O., and Parker, B. C., 1981, Recent experience in the epidemiology of disease caused by atypical mycobacteria, *Rev. Infect. Dis.* **3:**990–996.
19. Romanus, V., 1983, Childhood tuberculosis in Sweden, *Tubercle* **64:**101–110.
20. von Reyn, C. F., Waddell, R. D., Eaton, T., *et al.*, 1993, Isolation of *Mycobacterium avium* complex from water in the United States, Finland, Zaire and Kenya, *J. Clin. Microbiol.* **31:**3227–3230.
21. Collins, F. M., 1986, *Mycobacterium avium*-complex infection and the development of acquired immunodeficiency syndrome (AIDS): A casual opportunist or a causal cofactor?, *Int. J. Leprosy* **54:**458–474.

22. von Reyn, C. F., Barber, T. W., Arbeit, R. D., Sox, C. H., *et al.*, 1993, Evidence of previous infection with *Mycobacterium avium-M. intracellulare* complex among healthy subjects: An international study of dominant mycobacterial skin test reactions, *J. Infect. Dis.* **168:**1553–1558.

23. Bates, J. H., 1996, The tuberculin skin test and preventive treatment for tuberculosis, in *Tuberculosis* (W. N. Rom and S. M. Garay, eds.), Little Brown, Boston, pp. 865–871.

24. Chin, D. P., Hopewell, P. C., Yajko, D. M., Vittinghoff, E., *et al.*, 1994, *Mycobacterium avium*-complex in the respiratory or gastrointestinal tract and the risk of *M. avium*-complex bacteremia in patients with human immunodeficiency virus infection, *J. Infect. Dis.* **169:**289–295.

25. Crawford, J. L., 1993, Applications of molecular methods in epidemiology of tuberculosis, *Res. Microbiol.* **144:**111–116.

26. Wolinsky, E., 1981, When is an infection disease?, *Rev. Infect. Dis.* **3:**1025–1027.

27. Schaefer, W. F., Davis, C. L., and Cohn, M. L., 1970, Pathogenicity of translucent, opaque and rough variants of *M. avium* in chickens and mice, *Am. Rev. Respir. Dis.* **123:**343–358.

28. Moulding, T., 1978, The relative drug susceptibility of opaque colony forms of *M. intracellulare-avium*: Does it affect therapeutic results?, *Am. Rev. Respir. Dis.* **117:**1142–1143.

29. Belisle, J. T., and Brennan, P. J., 1994, Molecular basis of colony morphology in *Mycobacterium avium*, *Res. Microbiol.* **145:**237–242.

30. Barrow, W. W., and Brennan, P. J., 1982, Isolation in high frequency of rough variants of *Mycobacterium intracellulare* lacking C-mycoside glycopeptidolipid antigens, *J. Bacteriol.* **150:**381–384.

31. Shiratsuchi, H., Toosi, Z., Mettler, M. A., and Ellner, J. J., 1993, Colonial morphotype as a determinant of cytokine expression by human monocytes infected with *Mycobacterium avium*, *J. Immunol.* **150:**2945–2954.

32. Rastogi, N., Frehl, C., Ryter, A., *et al.*, 1981, Multiple drug-resistance in *M. avium*: Is the wall architecture responsible for the exclusion of antimicrobial agents?, *Antimicrob. Agents Chemother.* **20:**666–667.

33. Runyon, E. H., Karlson, A. G., Kubica, G. P., and Wayne, G. P., 1974, Mycobacterium, in *Manual of Clinical Microbiology* (E. H. Lennette, E. H. Spalding, and J. P. Truant, eds.), ASM, Washington, D.C., pp. 148–174.

34. Iseman, M. D., 1989, *Mycobacterium avium* complex and the normal host: The other side of the coin, *N. Engl. J. Med.* **321:**896–898.

35. Falkinham, J. O., 1996, Epidemiology of infection by nontuberculosis mycobacteria. *Clin. Microbiol. Rev.* **9:**177–215.

36. Good, R. C., and Snider, D. E., 1982, Isolation of nontuberculous mycobacteria in the United States, *J. Infect. Dis.* **146:**829–833.

37. Good, R. C., 1985, Opportunistic pathogens in the genus *Mycobacterium*, *Annu. Rev. Microbiol.* **39:**347–369.

38. Bates, J. H., 1996, The tuberculin skin test and preventive treatment for tuberculosis, in: *Tuberculosis* (W. N. Rom and S. M. Garay, eds.), Little, Brown, Boston, pp. 865–872.

39. Fairchok, M. P., Rouse, J. H., and Morris, S. L., 1995, Age-dependent humoral responses of children to mycobacterial antigens. *Clin. Diagn. Lab. Immunol.* **2:**443–447.

40. Portaels, F., Larsson, L., and Smeets, P., 1988, Isolation of mycobacteria from healthy persons stools. *Int. J. Leprosy* **56:**468–471.

41. Williams, R. C., Hasby, G., and Koster, F. T., 1986, Well defined receptors may be entry points for infectious agents, *Scand. J. Immunol.* **23:**529–533.

42. Malpother, M. E., and Sanger, J. G., 1984, *In vitro* interaction of *Mycobacterium avium* with intestinal epithelial cells, *Infect. Immun.* **45:**67–73.

43. Hubbard, R. D., Flory, C. M., and Collins, F. M., 1992, T-cell immune responses in *Mycobacterium avium*-infected mice. *Infect. Immun.* **60:**150–153.

44. Collins, F. M., and Stokes, R. W., 1987, *Mycobacterium avium*-complex infections in normal and immunodeficient mice, *Tubercle* **68:**127–136.

45. Stokes, R. W., and Collins, F. M., 1990, Passive transfer of immunity to *Mycobacterium avium* in susceptible and resistant strains of mice, *Clin. Exp. Immunol.* **81:**109–115.
46. Lagrange, P. H., 1978, Comparative studies of different strains of BCG vaccine in mice: T-cell dependent immune responses, *Dev. Biol. Stand.* **38:**223–229.
47. Collins, F. M., 1989, Mycobacterial disease, immunosuppression and acquired immunodeficiency syndrome, *Clin. Microbiol. Rev.* **2:**360–377.
48. Collins, F. M., 1991, Pulmonary tuberculosis: The immunology of a chronic infection, in: *Vaccines and Immunotherapy* (S. J. Cryz, ed.), Pergamon Press, New York, pp. 140–155.
49. Collins, F. M., Morrison, N. E., and Montalbine, V., 1978, Immune response to persistent mycobacterial infection in mice, *Infect. Immun.* **19:**430–438.
50. Reddy, V. M., Parikh, K., Luna-Herrera, J., et al., 1994, Comparison of virulence of *Mycobacterium avium* complex (MAC) strains isolated from AIDS and non-AIDS patients, *Microbiol. Pathogen.* **16:**121–130.
51. Goto, Y., Nakamura, R. M., Takahashi, H., and Tokunaga, T., 1984, Genetic control of resistance to *Mycobacterium intracellulare* infections in mice, *Infect. Immun.* **46:**135–140.
52. Barnes, P. F., Modlin, R. L., and Ellner, J. J., 1994, T-cell responses and cytokines, in: *Tuberculosis: Pathogenesis, Protection and Control* (B. R. Bloom, ed.), ASM, Washington, D.C., pp. 417–435.
53. Ellner, J. J., Goldberger, M. J., and Parenti, D. M., 1991, *Mycobacterium avium* infection and AIDS: A therapeutic dilemma in rapid evolution, *J. Infect. Dis.* **163:**1326–1335.
54. Abbott, M. R., and Smith, D. D., 1981, Mycobacterial infections in immunosuppressed patients, *Med. J. Austr.* **1:**351–353.
55. Feld, R., Bodey, G. P., and Groschel, D., 1976, Mycobacteriosis in patients with malignant disease, *Arch. Intern. Med.* **136:**67–70.
56. Watson, S. R., Morrison, N. E., and Collins, F. M., 1979, Delayed hypersensitivity responses in mice and guinea pigs to *Mycobacterium leprae*, *M. vaccae* and *M. nonchromogenicum* cytoplasmic proteins, *Infect. Immun.* **25:**229–236.
57. Gordin, F., and Masur, H., 1994, Prophylaxis of *M. avium* complex bacteremia in patients with AIDS, *Clin. Infect. Dis.* **18:**S223–226.
58. Bermudez, L. E., 1994, Immunobiology of *Mycobacterium avium* infection, *Eur. J. Clin. Microbiol. Infect. Dis.* **13:**1000–1006.
59. Orme, I. M., 1993, Immunity to mycobacteria, *Curr. Opinion Immunol.* **5:**497–502.
60. McCune, R. M., Feldman, F. M., Lambert, H. P., and McDermott, W., 1966, Microbial persistence. I. The capacity of tubercle bacilli to survive sterilization in mouse tissues, *J. Exp. Med.* **123:**455–468.
61. de Wit, D., Wooton, M., Dhillon, J., and Mitchison, D. A., 1995, The bacterial DNA content of mouse organs in the Cornell model of dormant tuberculosis, *Tubercle Lung Dis.* **76:**555–562.
62. Grange, J. M., 1992, The mystery of the mycobacterial 'persistor,' *Tubercle Lung Dis.* **73:**249–251.
63. Khansari, D. N., Murgo, A. J., and Faith, R. E., 1990, Effects of stress on the immune system, *Immunol. Today* **10:**170–175.
64. Stead, W. W., 1989, Special problems in tuberculosis. Tuberculosis in the elderly and in residents of nursing homes, correctional facilities, long-term hospitals, mental hospitals, shelters for the homeless and jails, *Clin. Chest Med.* **10:**397–405.
65. Orme, I. M., 1989, Aging and immunity to tuberculosis: Prolonged survival of old mice infected with *Mycobacterium tuberculosis* by adoptive immunization with memory-immune T lymphocytes, *Cell. Immunol.* **118:**229–233.
66. North, R. J., 1993, Minimal effect of advancing age on susceptibility of mice to infection by *Mycobacterium tuberculosis*, *J. Infect. Dis.* **168:**1059–1062.
67. Fauci, A. S., 1984, Acquired immunodeficiency syndrome: Epidemiologic, immunologic and therapeutic considerations, *Ann. Intern. Med.* **100:**92–106.

68. Collins, F. M., 1990, Bacterial cofactors in AIDS, in: *Cofactors in HIV-1 infection and AIDS* (R. R. Watson, ed.), CRC Press, Boca Raton, FL, pp. 61–78.
69. Morrissey, A. B., Aisa, T. O., Falkinham, J. O., *et al.*, 1992, Absence of *M. avium* complex disease in patients with AIDS in Uganda, *J. AIDS* **5:**477–478.
70. Horsburgh, C. R., Hanson, D. L., Jones, J. L., and Thompson, S. E., 1996, Protection from *Mycobacterium avium* complex disease in human immunodeficiency virus-infected persons with a history of tuberculosis, *J. Infect. Dis.* **174:**1212–1217.
71. Gilks, C. F., Brindle, R. J., Mwachari, C., *et al.*, 1995, Disseminated *M. avium* infection among HIV-infected patients in Kenya, *J. AIDS* **8:**195–198.
72. Pitchenik, A. E., Cole, C., Russell, B. W., *et al.*, 1984, Tuberculosis, atypical mycobacteriosis and the acquired immunodeficiency syndrome among Haitian and non-Haitian patients in South Florida, *Ann. Intern. Med.* **101:**641–645.
73. Horsburg, C. R., Chin, D. P., Yajko, D. M., *et al.*, 1994, Environmental risk factors for acquisition of *Mycobacterium avium* complex in persons with human immunodeficiency virus infection, *J. Infect. Dis.* **170:**362–367.
74. von Reyn, C. F., Jacobs, N. J., Arbeit, R. D., *et al.*, 1995, Polyclonal *Mycobacterium avium* infection in patients with AIDS: Variations in antimicrobial susceptibilities of different strains of *M. avium* isolated from the same patient, *J. Clin. Microbiol* **33:**1008–1010.
75. von Reyn, C. F., Green, P. A., McCormick, D., *et al.*, 1994, Dual skin testing with *M. avium* sensitin and purified protein derivative: An open study of patients with *M. avium*-complex infection or tuberculosis, *Clin. Infect. Dis.* **19:**15–20.
76. Lucas, S. B., Hounnou, A., Peacock, C. S., *et al.*, 1993, The mortality and pathology of HIV disease in a West African city, *AIDS* **7:**1569–1579.
77. Welch, K., Finkbeiner, W., Alpers, C. E., *et al.*, 1984, Autopsy findings in the acquired immune deficiency syndrome, *JAMA* **252:**1152–1159.
78. Crawford, J. L., 1994, Development of rapid techniques for identification of *Mycobacterium avium* infections, *Res. Microbiol.* **145:**171–178.
79. Woods, G. L., 1994, Disease due to *Mycobacterium avium* complex in patients infected with human immunodeficiency virus: Diagnosis and susceptibility testing, *Clin. Infect. Dis.* **18:**S227–232.
80. Jost, K. C., Dunbar, D. F., Barth, S. S., *et al.*, 1995, Identification of *M. tuberculosis* and *M. avium* complex directly from smear-positive sputum specimens and BACTEC 12B cultures by high performance liquid chromatography with fluorescence detection and computer-driven pattern recognition models, *J. Clin. Microbiol.* **33:**1270–1277.
81. Jacobs, W. R., Barletta, R. G., Udani, R., *et al.*, 1993, Rapid assessment of drug susceptibilities of *M. tuberculosis* by means of luciferase reporter genes, *Science* **260:**819–822.
82. Roth, R. J., Owen, R. L., and Keren, D. F., 1983, AIDS with *M. avium-intracellulare* lesions resembling those of Whipple's disease, *N. Engl. J. Med.* **309:**1324–1325.
83. Hellyer, T. J., Brown, I. N., Taylor, M. B., *et al.*, 1993, Gastrointestinal involvement in *M. avium-intracellulare* infection in patients with HIV, *J. Infect.* **26:**55–66.
84. Montecalvo, M. A., Forester, G., Tsang, A. Y., *et al.*, 1994, Colonization of potable water with *Mycobacterium avium* complex in homes of HIV-infected patients, *Lancet* **343:**1639.
85. Morris, A., Reller, L. B., Salfinger, M., *et al.*, 1993, Mycobacteria in stool samples: The non-value of smears for predicting culture results, *J. Clin. Microbiol.* **31:**1385–1387.
86. Li, Z., Bai, G. H., von Reyn, C. F., *et al.*, 1996, Rapid detection of *M. avium* in stool samples from AIDS patients by immunomagnetic PCR, *J. Clin. Microbiol.* **34:**1903–1907.
87. Nash, G., and Fliegel, S., 1984, Pathological features of the lung in acquired immune deficiency syndrome (AIDS): An autopsy study of seventeen homosexual males, *Am. J. Clin. Pathol.* **81:**6–12.
88. Morrison, N. E., and Collins, F. M., 1975, Immunogenicity of an aerogenic BCG vaccine in T-cell depleted and normal mice, *Infect. Immun.* **11:**1110–1121.

89. North, R. J., and Izzo, A. A., 1993, Granuloma formation in severe combined immunodeficient (SCID) mice in response to progressive BCG infection, *Am. J. Pathol.* **142:**1959–1966.

90. Centers for Disease Control, 1992, Transmission of multidrug-resistant tuberculosis among immunocompromised persons in a correctional system—New York, *Morb. Mort. Wk. Rep.* **41:**507–509.

91. Goletti, D., Weissman, D., Jackson, R. W., *et al.*, 1996, Effect of *Mycobacterium tuberculosis* in HIV replication: Role of immune activation, *J. Immunol.* **157:**1271–1278.

92. Horsburg, C. R., and Selik, R. M., 1989, The epidemiology of disseminated tuberculous mycobacterial infection in the acquired immunodeficiency syndrome (AIDS), *Am. Rev. Respir. Dis.* **139:**4–7.

93. Olliaro, P., and Dautzenberg, B., 1994, Control of the body burden of *M. avium* complex is associated with improved quality of life and prolonged survival of patients with AIDS: A prospective trial with rifabutin combined with isoniazid, clofazimine and ethambutol, *J. Chemother.* **6:**189–196.

94. Gordin, F., and Masur, H., 1994, Prophylaxis of *M. avium*-complex bacteremia in patients with AIDS, *Clin. Infect. Dis.* **18:**S223–226.

95. Young, L. S., 1996, Mycobacterial infections in immunocompromised patients. *Curr. Opinion Infect. Dis.* **9:**240–245.

96. Chin, D. P., Reingold, A. L., Stone, E. N., *et al.*, 1994, The impact of *Mycobacterium avium* complex bacteremia and its treatment or survival of AIDS patients—a prospective study. *J. Infect. Dis.* **170:**578–584.

97. Stanford, J. L., and Grange, J. M., 1994, The promise of immunotherapy for tuberculosis, *Respir. Med.* **88:**3–7.

8

Pathogenesis of *Legionella pneumophila* Infection

PAUL S. HOFFMAN and RAFAEL GARDUNO

1. INTRODUCTION

Legionella pneumophila is an opportunistic Gram-negative, facultative-intracellular pathogen that gained notoriety in 1976 as the etiologic agent of Legionnaires' disease, an atypical pneumonia.[1] Inhalation of *Legionella*-laden aerosols is the most common route of infection and once in the lungs, the bacteria invade and multiply within alveolar macrophages.[2] Like *Mycobacterium tuberculosis*, *Chlamydia psittaci*, *Toxoplasma gondii*, and *Brucella abortus*, *L. pneumophila* resides in a specialized phagosome which does not fuse with secondary lysosomes.[2-5] Of the ~40 named species of *Legionella*, *L. pneumophila* is considered the most virulent, accounting for nearly 90% of cases.[6,7] Legionnaires' disease is still problematic, accounting for nearly 4% of all community- and nosocomial-acquired pneumonia, with an estimated annual incidence in the United States of more than 20,000 cases.[7] Explosive outbreaks can still be traced to improperly maintained cooling towers, hot tubs and dehumidifiers which have the common property of producing aerosols. The legionellae are ubiquitous in aquatic environments, including moist soils, where they live in biofilms or intracellularly in a variety of protozoa.[8] Our technology has brought the legionellae into proximity with an ever increasing

PAUL S. HOFFMAN • Departments of Microbiology, Immunology, and Medicine, Division of Infectious Diseases, Dalhousie University, Halifax, Nova Scotia B3H 4H7, Canada. RAFAEL GARDUNO • Departments of Microbiology and Immunology, Dalhousie University, Halifax, Nova Scotia B3H 4H7, Canada.

Opportunistic Intracellular Bacteria and Immunity, edited by Lois J. Paradise *et al.* Plenum Press, New York, 1999.

population of immunocompromised individuals. Therefore, environmental control of the disease is largely limited to continuous monitoring and treatment of man made devices and to distancing susceptible individuals from known sources of infection.[9]

Legionnaires' disease is recognized as primarily a disease of the immunocompromised and elderly, two of the fastest growing segments of the population.[7] Immunity as well as recovery from legionellosis is largely dependent on the cellular immune status of the individual. In particular, an individual's ability to initiate a Type-1 interferon-γ (IFN-γ) producing response is believed to be crucial because *L. pneumophila* is unable to replicate in interferon-activated macrophages.[10] One of the emerging themes of recent studies is that *Legionella* proteins associated with pathogenesis also specifically induce the production of inflammatory cytokines [interleukin-1 (IL-1) and IL-12] by the infected macrophages, leading to development of the Th1 response.[11,12] Thus, macrophages of immunocompromised individuals, who are unable to mount a cellular immune response, remain permissive to the growth of *L. pneumophila* and even with antimicrobial intervention, the mortality rate for immunocompromised individuals is very high.

Although the legionellae are not the only environmental microorganisms with a capacity to produce disease in humans, like *Listeria monocytogenes* and *Mycobacterium* spp., they are proving extremely useful as tools for dissecting the cell biology of eukaryotic cells, including host immune recognition and response to intracellular parasites. Most of our understanding of the biology of Legionnaires' disease has come from studies with macrophages or macrophage-like cell lines. However, because Legionnaires' disease is not a communicable disease and therefore provides no survival advantage for the pathogen, more recent attention has been given to the interactions of *L. pneumophila* with natural hosts including *Hartmannella* and *Acanthamoeba*.[6,8,13] These studies have contributed substantially to our understanding of common pathogenesis mechanisms plied by *L. pneumophila* on eukaryotic cells. These mechanisms of pathogenesis are emphasized throughout this chapter. Readers are referred to other reviews for additional information and citations on the history of Legionnaires' disease,[14] discussions of virulence determinants,[15] genetics,[16,17] and to the following chapter on the Immunology of Legionnaires' disease (Chapter 9).

2. NATURAL AND MAMMALIAN HOSTS

The genus *Legionella* is one of the largest genera of aquatic microorganisms that survive as intracellular parasites of freshwater protozoa. The genus will become even larger with the eventual inclusion of a group of recently described obligate intracellular parasites of amoebae referred to as *Legionella*-like amebal parasites, or LLAPs.[18] *L. pneumophila*, the most virulent of the legionellae, is capable of multiplying in the intracellular compartment of more than 10 species of amoebae, and in at least three species of ciliated protozoa.[6] The bacteria also replicate in human macrophages, monocytes, and in at least 14 mammalian cell lines.[6] Therefore, *L. pneumophila* exhibits a wide host range. In contrast, other species of *Legionella*, including the LLAPs, exhibit a very limited host range, and in the case of the X-bacteria, a group of *Legionella*-like obligate parasites of *Amoeba proteus*, infection is required for survival of the amoeba.[19] Although all of the legionellae are considered potentially pathogenic for humans, those species displaying the widest host range (e.g., *L. pneumophila*) are more frequently associated with human infection.

Morphological, biochemical, and molecular studies with natural and mammalian hosts suggest that *L. pneumophila* employs a common strategy for infection.[20] Table I lists some of the similarities and differences noted among these model systems. Both natural and mammalian hosts phagocytize *L. pneumophila* via coiling phagocytosis, first described by Horwitz.[21] The second common feature observed in these models is the recruitment of organelles that surround the bacterium-laden phagosome or endosome (see Fig. 1A, B, C).[3,22] This is a virulence related feature, as endosomes harboring laboratory-generated avirulent variants do not recruit these organelles and eventually fuse with secondary lysosomes. An essential feature for intracellular growth is the association of the *Legionelle*-laden endosomes with the endoplasmic reticulum (ER).[3] The ER completely surrounds the bacteria-laden endosomes and presumably facilitates the

TABLE I
Similarities and Differences Noted between the Infection of Mammalian Host Cells and Protozoa by *L. pneumophila*

	Host		
Trait	Mammalian	Protozoan	References
Internalization via coiling phagocytosis	+	+	21, 48, 62
Inhibition of phagosome–lysosome fusion	+	+	62, 63
Organelle recruitment	+	+	6, 53, 63
Formation of large, bacteria-laden vacuoles	+	+	64, 65
Internalization driven by actin polymerization	+	−	6, 21, 39
Growth dependent on host protein synthesis	−	+	8, 24
Induction of apoptosis	+	−	50

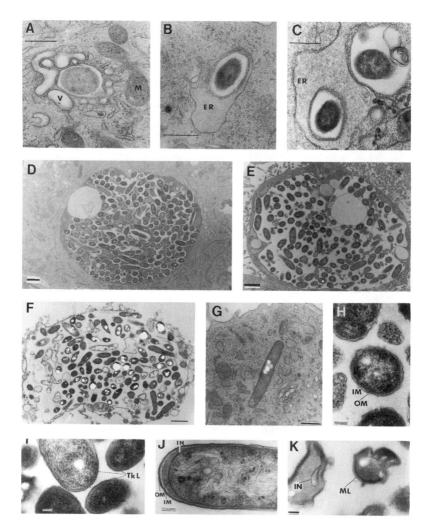

FIGURE 1. Intracellular replication and maturation of *L. pneumophila* in HeLa cells. Shortly after entry, bacterium-containing endosomes become associated with smooth vesicles (V) and mitochondria (M) (A). Later, the endoplasmic reticulum (ER) is recruited and it surrounds the legionellae-containing endosome (B). It is important to notice that where the endosome and the ER meet, there is a double membrane studded with ribosomes, as clearly seen in C. Recruitment of the ER is very important for replication of *L. pneumophila*. The replicative endosome supports growth of many bacterial cells (D) that mature inside the replicative endosome (E) and transform it into a legionellae-laden vesicle lined by a single smooth membrane with no associated organelles (F). The few non-virulent legionellae that are taken up by HeLa cells remain in unchanged, smooth endosomes (G) and do not replicate. The mature intracellular bacteria observed in F are morphologically different from the replicating bacteria shown in D. The latter have a typical Gram-negative morphology (H) with a cell envelope clearly defined by an inner membrane (IM) and an outer membrane (OM), separated by the periplasmic space. Mature intracellular forms would have a defined thick layer (TkL) associated with the inner leaflet of the outer membrane (I), or extra lipid bilayers running internally within the cytoplasm (IN in J and K), or a series of multiple layers (ML) enveloping the bacterial cell. Bars represent 1 μm in D, E, and F; 0.5 μm in A, B, C, and D; and 0.1 μm in H, I, J, and K.

entry of nutrients into the endosomal lumen (see Fig. 1C). Interestingly, disruption of the endoplasmic reticulum with brefeldn A leads to cessation of growth of the bacteria.[3] The growth kinetics of *L. pneumophila* in natural and mammalian hosts are also very similar, as is the observation of increased motility of intracellular bacteria late in infection. The increased motility of released bacteria enhances the likelihood of finding another susceptible host.

There are several differences between infection of natural and mammalian hosts. Fields *et al.* demonstrated that the microfilament inhibitor cytochalasin D prevents uptake of *L. pneumophila* by monocytes and various cell lines, but has no effect on entry of the bacteria into *Hartmannella*.[6] A second major difference relates to a requirement for host protein synthesis for intracellular growth of *L. pneumophila*. Several studies have indicated that *L. pneumophila* grows in mammalian cell lines and macrophage systems in the presence of cycloheximide, an inhibitor of eukaryotic protein synthesis.[20] In contrast, studies by King *et al.*[23] demonstrate a requirement for host protein synthesis to facilitate intracellular growth of *L. pneumophila* in *Hartmannella*. In fact, 33 host proteins are specifically synthesized in response to interaction with *L. pneumophila*.[24] The response of natural hosts to *L. pneumophila* infection may be related to establishment of a symbiotic relationship rather than an effort to eradicate the invading microbe. From a survival perspective, quick destruction of either partner would not be beneficial. One could argue that the uncompromising nature of the macrophage leads to its early demise by *L. pneumophila*. Finally, recent studies show that mammalian cells, including macrophages, undergo apoptosis as a consequence of *L. pneumophila* infection.[25] Apoptosis does not occur in natural hosts.

3. ANTIGENS

The major antigenic determinants of *L. pneumophila* were characterized shortly after the original epidemic because of the urgent need for diagnostic reagents. The serogrouping antigen as well as the dominant humoral antigen is lipopolysaccharide (LPS). Diagnosis of legionellosis is frequently retrospective and based on a four-fold rise in antibody titer to LPS in convalescing patients. The *O*-chain of this LPS constitutes a homopolymer of an unusual sugar, 5-acetamidino-7-acetamido-8-*O*-acetyl-3,5,7,9-tetradeoxy-*D*-glycero-*L*-galactononulosonic   acid (legionaminic acid).[26] It is believed that this polymer confers hydrophobicity on the outer membrane, a property that might enhance nonspecific binding of bacteria to host cells. The LPS exhibits low endotoxicity that is attributed to long-chain fatty acid [28:0(27-oxo) and 27:0-dioic] side chains of lipid A. In contrast, humoral responses against protein antigens are generally weak and often are obscured by the overwhelming antibody response against LPS.[27] Major protein antigens for which human or guinea pig humoral responses have been identified by immunoblot include OmpS, the major outer membrane protein;[28] 60-kDa heat-shock protein (Hsp60) or common antigen;[28] proteins of 14 and 18 kDa;[27] and a secreted metalloprotease.[29] It should be noted that many of these antigens are detected only in sera exhibiting very high antibody titers to LPS. Only a few antigens associated with development of cellular immunity have been described. Horwitz demonstrated that vaccination of guinea pigs with purified metalloprotease led to protection of immunized animals against lethal challenge.[30] The protease is secreted by intracellular bacteria, but is not essential for virulence. In this regard, immunization of animals with *L. pneumophila* mutants defective in expression of the metalloprotease also conferred protection from lethal challenge, indicating that additional factors were involved with cellular immunity. Hsp60, which was identified initially as the major cytoplasmic membrane protein of *L. pneumophila*, was found to stimulate a cellular immune response and to protect guinea pigs against lethal challenge.[31] However, another study demonstrated that Hsp60 did not confer protection against lethal challenge in guinea pigs,[28] which is more consistent with results obtained with heat-shock proteins from other microbial pathogens. Interestingly, peripheral blood lymphocytes from patients with acute legionellosis proliferate in response to Hsp60, suggesting that Hsp60 may be one of the early proteins recognized by host defenses.[28] Consistent with this conclusion is the knowledge that Hsp60 is the dominant protein synthesized by *L. pneumophila* throughout the course of intracellular infection.[32–34] The next chapter deals specifically with the role of Hsp60 in induction of cytokines and recruitment of immune effector cells by infected macrophages. Immunization with *L. pneumophila* major outer membrane protein (MOMP; OmpS) was found to protect guinea pigs from lethal challenge and by lymphocyte proliferation assays, it was demonstrated that humans who have recovered from legionellosis exhibit a proliferative response against OmpS for years after infection.[28] It should be emphasized that cellular immune responses have been determined only for a small number of protein antigens, which might reflect the current low priority given to development of a *Legionella* vaccine.

4. INTRACELLULAR LIFE CYCLE OF *L. PNEUMOPHILA*

4.1. Attachment and Invasion

Legionella pneumophila, like *Leishmania donovani* and *Borrelia burgdorferi*, enters host cells by coiling phagocytosis.[21] In this form of phagocytosis, the pseudopodia enveloping the bacterium proceed asymmetrically, resulting in one of the pseudopods winding around the bacterium. Once the bacterium becomes internalized, the pseudopodial membranes appear to fuse and the multilamellar appearance of the phagosome is lost. Coiling phagocytosis is inhibited by anti-*L.*

pneumophila antibodies, suggesting that a specific component of the *L pneumophila* surface induces this uncommon internalization mechanism. Despite the wide host range observed for *L. pneumophila*, relatively few studies, with the exception of macrophage studies, have addressed mechanisms of invasion. The Horwitz group demonstrated that complement components C3b and C3bi bound specifically to the MOMP (OmpS) of *L. pneumophila* and mediated phagocytosis by macrophages via complement receptors CR1 and CR3.[35] In contrast, Husmann and Johnson demonstrated that complement receptors facilitated phagocytosis of bacteria treated with complement only in the presence of a specific antibody.[36] They further demonstrated that specific antibodies mediated endocytosis of *L. pneumophila* by macrophages via Fc receptors. Several studies provide evidence for the participation of both the alternate and classic complement fixation pathways in endocytosis. However, both the lack of complement in bronchial washings and the likely absence of anti-*L. pneumophila* antibodies during the initial infection suggest that *L. pneumophila* enters alveolar marcrophages by other means.[20] This conclusion is also supported by the knowledge that *L. pneumophila* can invade and replicate in some mammalian cell lines that are nonphagocytic and lack both complement and Fc receptors.[20] Finally, there are no functional equivalents of complement or antibody in aquatic systems. Therefore, it is likely that *L. pneumophila* enters host cells by parasite-directed endocytosis, a mechanism common to many other intracellular parasites. According to Gibson *et al.*,[37] the opsonin-independent interaction of *L. pneumophila* with human phagocytes and other mammalian cells is mediated by a bacterial surface protein with lectin-like properties, intimately associated with carbohydrates or lipids on the outer membrane of *L. pneumophila*. This putative component must be constitutively expressed on the surface of virulent *L. pneumophila* (i.e., it is not induced upon contact with the host cell) because formalin-killed or antibiotic-treated bacteria still induce coiling phagocytosis in human phagocytes,[38] and enter nonphagocytic HeLa cells.[39-43]

The bacterial mediators of attachment may include OmpS, which is the most abundant protein associated with the outer membrane. In this regard, antibodies raised against OmpS were found to effectively block attachment of *L. pneumophila* to mammalian cells.[39-40] More recent studies in this laboratory clarify these findings and suggest that OmpS, present on both virulent and isogenic avirulent strains, is one of several mediators of attachment.[66] However, OmpS does not appear to mediate invasion. Other proteins found in the outer membrane that may be involved in invasion include Mip (macrophage invasion potentiator),[41] which has been demonstrated to be a prolyl-isomerase.[42] The role of Mip in invasion is not clear because Mip is also expressed by avirulent mutants that do not invade nonphagocytic cells.[41] However, the fact that mutations in Mip reduce the efficiency of infection of macrophage cell lines, without affecting subsequent intracellular replication, suggests that Mip may have an indirect influence on invasion.[42] For example, defects in Mip might affect the topography of the bacterial cell surface or the efficiency at which surface-expressed molecules mediate attachment and invasion.

We have been using HeLa cells as a model system for studies of invasion because only virulent strains of *L. pneumophila* efficiently enter these cells.[39,43] These investigations revealed a rather novel use of the bacterial chaperone protein Hsp60 by virulent strains of *L. pneumophila* as both an adhesin and an invasin.[39,66,67] In general, the Hsp60 class of heat-shock proteins are located in the cytosol, as exemplified with *Escherichia coli*, where they function in assembly and secretion of proteins.[44,67] However, recent studies indicate heat-shock proteins may exhibit much more varied roles in the biology of Gram-negative bacteria, and localization studies reveal both periplasmic and surface locations where they mediate adhesion. In the case of *L. pneumophila*, four lines of evidence suggest that Hsp60 participates in attachment: (1) attachment-invasion by virulent strains of *L. pneumophila* is effectively inhibited by anti-Hsp60 antibodies, as well as by the preincubation of host HeLa cells with purified Hsp60; these treatments have little or no effect on avirulent strains; (2) latex beads coated with purified Hsp60 adhere to HeLa cells rapidly and tightly, and are subsequently internalized 10- to 20-foled more efficiently than bovine serum albumin (BSA)-coated beads; (3) purified Hsp60 binds to HeLa cell membrane preparations, as detected in ELISA assays; and (4) the Hsp60-coated beads, but not BSA-coated beads, readily agglutinate cell suspensions of HeLa cells. Members of the Hsp60 family have been involved in the attachment of other bacterial pathogens to host cells. *Helicobacter pylori* displays Hsp60 on its surface and this protein mediates specific attachment to host membrane sulfatides.[45] Further experimentation is required to unequivocally demonstrate that the interaction of Hsp60 with host cell receptors triggers the cytoskeletal changes required to drive the internalization of *L. pneumophila*. Finally, the nature of the host cell receptor(s) for nonopsonized *L. pneumophila* remains to be determined as does the possibility that *L. pneumophila* targets a conserved class of receptor common to natural as well as mammalian hosts.

4.2. Subversion of Organelle Trafficking

Once intracellular, *L. pneumophila* resides in modified phagosomes that do not become acidified or fuse with lysosomes. The observation that blockage of *de novo* protein synthesis does not affect the ability of *L. pneumophila* to inhibit phagosome–lysosome fusion[38] indicates that a constitutively expressed bacterial factor must be involved in the process. It is generally accepted that *L. pneumophila* modifies the bacteria-laden phagosome through unknown mechanisms, leading to the sequential recruitment of smooth vesicles, mitochondria, endoplasmic reticulum, and numerous ribosomes. Because the events associated with phagosome–lysosome fusion begin with the initiation of phagocytosis,[46] it is very likely that *L. pneumophila* modifies the developing phagosome early in the invasion process. The fact that avirulent mutants are unable to replicate intracellularly and cannot recruit organelles supports the idea that they are defective for phagosome modification and implies that organelle recruitment is essential for *L. pneumophila* replication, and therefore should be considered a virulence trait. It also implies that the constitutive bacterial factor is either absent or nonfunctional in avirulent strains.[20] Interestingly, Hsp60 was found to be the most dominant protein synthesized and secreted by intracellular bacteria throughout intracellular infection[32–34] (see below). Electron microscopic studies with specific anti-Hsp60 antibodies demonstrated that Hsp60 was both suface exposed and secreted into the phagosome of infected monocytes and L929 cells.[33] The inability of avirulent mutants to block phagosome–lysosome fusion correlated with an inability to synthesize or secrete appreciable levels of Hsp60 upon interaction with host cells. Although no mechanism has been ascribed for how molecular chaperones, such as Hsp60, might disrupt organelle trafficking, it is known that the Hsp60 class of proteins possess both autophosphorylase and phosphotransferase activities.[47] One can envision Hsp60 disrupting cellular events that are dependent, for example, on GTP/GDP ratios by indiscriminately phosphorylating GDP. Whether Hsp60 affects signal transduction mechanisms directly or does so indirectly through assembly or secretion of other factors that disrupt organelle trafficking remains to be determined. Although inhibition of phagosome–lysosome fusion appears to be a trait restricted to some strains of *L. pneumophila*,[48] organelle recruitment is a generalized feature of all legionellae that is displayed in all their hosts.

Two adjacent loci have been identified through complementation studies of mutants defective in intracellular replication. One locus is known as *dot* (for *defect in organelle trafficking*),[49] and the other as *icm* (for *intracellular multiplication*).[50] Both loci contain several genes, apparently organized in operons, with no known function or sequence similarity to other known proteins. The DotA protein, however, is a high molecular weight cytoplasmic membrane protein with eight membrane-spanning domains and one large, cysteine-rich periplasmic domain.[51] There are similarities with ABC-type transporter proteins that are further supported by the recent cloning of an additional *dot* gene exhibiting similarity with nucleotide binding proteins known to transduce energy to ABC-type transporters. Besides *dot* and *icm* loci, other loci may be involved in the subversion of organelle trafficking, since several chemically-induced mutants, none with defects in the *dot* locus, displayed defects in organelle recruitment and impaired ability to establish a replicative endosome.[53] Also, a genetic characterization of transposon insertion mutants, defective for intracellular replication (but not related to the *dot/icm* region), could be grouped into 15 distinct DNA hybridization groups.[54] Recent studies have demonstrated that some of these mutations map to a 22 kbp locus whose genes exhibit some homology to *tra* genes which are involved in conjugation.[68,69] Mutational analysis of this locus further demonstrated a requirement for several of these genes in both conjugation of plasmids as well as for virulence. It has been suggested that the protein products from the 22 kbp locus together with proteins from the *dot/icm* locus assemble into a protein complex that facilitates DNA transfer as well as possibly delivering protein(s) to eukaryotic hosts.[69] DotA, a protein that might anchor this conjugation complex into the cytoplasmic membrane, is functionally required for early phagosome trafficking decisions, but whose activity, when turned off is not required for intracellular multiplication.[70] It will likely be demonstrated that the conjugation complex, which appears to be essential for virulence of *L. pneumophila*, is required for the proper targeting of Hsp60 to the bacterial surface. Another group of membrane proteins believed to be associated with ion transport and resistance to heavy metals in *L. pneumophila* have recently been identified following transposon mutagenesis. The locus named *hel* is involved in cytopathicity, though the specific mechanisms remain unresolved.[52] The number of mutants displaying defects in transport functions underscores the complexity of studying virulence in an intracellular pathogen, in which communication and nutrient acquisition are essential to survival.

4.3. Stage-Specific Gene Expression

Several investigators have surmised that the complex intracellular cycle of *L. pneumophila* involves the coordinated expression of many genes, as has been demonstrated for other intracellular parasites.[20,34] However, only a few studies have attempted to catalogue specific *L. pneumophila* proteins selectively synthesized during the distinct stages of intracellular residence and(or) replication.

During the first 2 h postinfection, synthesis of Hsp60 is increased, coordinate with a decrease in the synthesis of many proteins including OmpS.[33] Elevated synthesis of Hsp60 in response to the intracellular milieu is a common theme for many intracellular parasites and it is generally believed to result from the stresses associated with phagocytosis. An alternative view is that the response is a parasite-directed virulence trait required to suppress host cellular defense mechanisms. This view is supported by the observation that Hsp60 levels remain high throughout the course of intracellular infection as opposed to transient expression, as noted for a typical heat shock response.[33] Apparently Hsp60 plays a major role in the establishment of endosymbiotic relationships as exemplified by the endosymbionts of aphids. Symbionin, the major 60-kDa protein thought to be essential for the endosymbiotic relationship between bacteria and insect cells, is a homologue of Hsp60 or GroEL.[47,55] The overwhelming synthesis of Hsp60 early in the course of *L. pneumophila* infection may mask the synthesis of additional proteins whose functions may also be necessary for establishment of the replicative phagosome. Abu Kwaik has employed differential display polymerase chain reaction (PCR) techniques to identify genes expressed early in infection. In addition to Hsp60, another locus, *eml* (for early-stage macrophage-incuded), has been identified.[56] It is reasonable to expect that additional early genes will be discovered by this technique, as bacterial replication postinfection is delayed several hours, presumably a time during which genes required for intracellular growth are expressed. Several proteins exclusively synthesized around the fourth hour postinfection have also been identified by Susa *et al.*[57] Among these, there is a 44-kDa protein that follows different kinetics of expression in different hosts. Interestingly, whereas expression of this protein peaks 2 to 4 h after infection of mammalian phagocytes, it peaked at 2 days after infection of mammalian nonphagocytic cells. Studies are currently in progress to determine if the gene encoding the 44-kDa protein is part of the *eml* locus and if it is identical to an ~40-kDa protein exclusively expressed in the intracellular environment, as previously found by Abu Kwaik *et al.*[34] The function of the 44-kDa antigen and the gene products of the *eml* locus has not yet been elucidated.

The most complete record of protein changes that occur in the replicative phase of the intracellular cycle has been reported by Abu Kwaik *et al.*[34] Using two-dimensional gel electrophoresis of selectively radiolabeled bacterial proteins, it was determined that at least 35 proteins were selectively induced and at least 32 proteins were selectively repressed at 10 to 20 h postinfection, when *L. pneumophila* is actively replicating in modified endosomes. Because 13 of the induced proteins were identified as stress proteins, it was assumed that the phenotypic modulation in intracellular *L. pneumophila* primarily reflects a stress response to the intracellular environment. However, we believe that *L. pneumophila* is well adapted to the intracellular environment and that these changes reflect more a developmental program (see below) than a generalized stress response. Therefore, the participation of stress proteins in this process may follow rules still unknown to us, but essential in the evolution of intracellular parasites. Prominent among the induced stress proteins are the global stress protein GspA and, as mentioned previously, the heat-shock protein Hsp60. The gene *gspA* has been cloned, sequenced, and characterized; it forms part of an operon regulated by a σ-70 promoter, and a σ-32 heat-shock promoter.[58] GspA has strong homology to the heat-shock proteins LbpA and LbpB or *E. coli*, but no specific function has yet been ascribed to it.[58]

Finally, other gene products known to be expressed or required during intracellular growth are involved in iron uptake.[59,60] Cianciotto and coworkers identified and characterized the iron regulatory protein Fur in *L. pneumophila*. They have further used several selection procedures to identify genes associated with iron acquisition including sensitivity to iron chelators and resistance to streptonigrin, as well as screening *L. pneumophila* mutants containing Tn10*lacZ* insertions for genes demonstrating elevated expression under iron-limiting conditions.[60] One of these genes (*frg*) exhibits homology with genes of the aerobactin biosynthetic pathway, raising the possibility for an intracellularly induced iron acquisition system. These are novel areas of study because few studies have rigorously addressed how intracellular parasites acquire nutrients and essential elements from their host. These studies suggest that iron-regulated genes may also be activated during intracellular growth, suggesting that iron may not be readily available within host phagosomes.[60]

4.4. Late Intracellular Events and Development of Infectious Forms

We have studied the intracellular cycle of *L. pneumophila* in HeLa cells[39] (see Fig.1). In the late stages of the infection we noticed the presence of large, free vacuoles containing large numbers of *L. pneumophila* (Fig. 1F). These vacuoles excluded trypan blue dye, suggesting that the vacuolar membrane was energized. Interestingly, Cirillo *et al.* also noted that amoeba-grown legionellae were morphologically different from agar-grown bacteria and could be distinguished by their retention of the Gimenez stain.[13] Moreover, the amoeba-grown bacteria were more infectious than agar-grown bacteria. Similarly, we found that the HeLa cell-grown bacteria contained in the free vacuoles were ultrastructurally different and were ~100-fold more infective to HeLa cells than agar-grown *L. pneumophila*.[39,66] We named these bacteria the mature intracellular forms or MIFs.[39] The ultrastructural differences as noted by electron microscopy included the presence of a thick, electron-dense layer closely associated with the inner leaflet of the outer membrane (also observed in intracellular *L. micdadei*[61]), as well as the presence of complex intracytoplasmic membrane inclusions (Fig. 1F to K). Furthermore, the MIFs stained bright red after the Gimenez stain (Gimenez-positive), which uses carbol fuchsin as the primary stain and malachite green as counterstain. In contrast, agar-grown legionellae stained green or bluish red (Gimenez-negative) after the Gimenez stain. We have followed the Gimenez stain phenotype of agar-grown legionellae and MIFs at different times during growth, and have established the existence of a developmental cycle in which green bacteria give rise to red bacteria upon intracellular growth, and the red bacteria give rise to green bacteria upon reinfection of new HeLa cells or upon subculture on artificial media. Because the MIFs are highly infectious and were never observed in division by electron microscopy, we have assumed that they represent a resting form, perhaps similar to the nonreplicative, infectious elementary body of *Chlamydia* spp. The green bacterial form, which has a typical Gram-negative envelope, is frequently seen in division by electron microscopy (Fig. 1D, E, and H) and is referred to as the replicative form or RF. Interestingly, when agar-grown *L. pneumophila* is suspended in distilled water, over time, bacteria become completely red, a process that can be inhibited by added chloramphenicol (unpublished observations). This observation raises the possibility that MIFs may be present in environmental sources, particularly because the legionellae can still be recovered from distilled water a year after inoculation. The existence of such a developmental cycle may explain the complex stage-specific gene expression pattern discussed earlier, as well as provide additional understanding of the biology of the legionellae.

Interestingly, intracellular growth of *L. pneumophila* in cultured macrophages does not seem to lead to the formation of mature intracellular forms and no bacteria-laden vacuoles have been reported to be present in infected macrophage cultures. However, MIFs were observed in lung biopsy material from several of the original cases of Legionnaires' disease which had led to the notion that *L. pneumophila* may be weakly acid-fast. Fernandez *et al.* have suggested that *L. pneumophila* is more aggressive to macrophages than to nonphagocytic cell lines or natural hosts.[33] High multiplicities of infection (MOIs) result in immediate destruction of macrophage monolayers in culture, whereas high MOIs do not destroy L929 or HeLa cell monolayers, an effect perhaps related to differential expression of virulence traits in the two host cell populations. As noted earlier, a 44-kDa antigen of *L. pneumophila* is expressed early in macrophage-like cells and late in nonphagocytic cells.[57] In addition, *L. pneumophila* appears to synthesize much higher levels of Hsp60 in response to macrophage infection than to infection of either L929 or HeLa cells.[33] The association between levels of Hsp60 or other *L. pneumophila* proteins, formation of bacteria-laden vesicles, and differentiation of *L. pneumophila* into MIFs has yet to be established.

5. CONCLUSIONS

We have attempted to present new information on the biology of the legionellae. Most new developments have focused on the events that follow host cell entry and lead to intracellular replication in macrophages or macrophage-like cell lines. However, we have also presented recent findings addressing the early events of invasion of nonphagocytic cells by *L. pneumophila* and the unusual role that the heat-shock protein Hsp60 may play in these early events. Readers may have grasped the wealth of potential knowledge that could be extracted from using the legionellae to model the pathogenesis and evolution of intracellular bacterial pathogens. In particular, the study of the recently discovered developmental cycle of *L. pneumophila* offers unique opportunities, as developmental cycles have been basically described only for obligate intracellular pathogens.

REFERENCES

1. Fraser, D. W., Tsai, T. R., Orenstein, W., Parkin, W. E., Beecham, H. J., Sharrar, R. G., Harris, J., Mallison, G. F., Martin, S. M., McDade, J. E., Shepard, C. C., and Brachman, P. S., 1977, Legionnaires' disease: Description of an epidemic of pneumonia, *N. Engl. J. Med.* **297:**1189–1197.

2. Horwitz, M. A., and Silverstein, S. C., 1980, Interaction of the Legionnaires' disease bacterium *(Legionella pneumophila)* multiplies intracellularly in human monocytes, *J. Clin. Invest.* **66:**441–450.

3. Swanson, M. S., and Isberg, R. R., 1995, Association of *Legionella pneumophila* with the macrophage endoplasmic reticulum, *Infect. Immun.* **63:**3609–3620.

4. Horwitz, M. A., 1983, The Legionnaires' disease bacterium *(Legionella pneumophila)* inhibits phagosome-lysosome fusion in human monocytes, *J. Exp. Med.* **158:**2108.

5. Moulder, J. W., 1985, Comparative biology of intracellular parasitism, *Microbiol. Rev.* **49:**298–337.

6. Fields, B. S., 1996, The molecular ecology of legionellae, *Trends Microbiol.* **4:**286–290.

7. Marston, B. J., Lipman, H. B., and Breiman, R. F., 1994, Surveillance for Legionnaires' disease: Risk factors for morbidity and mortality, *Arch. Intern. Med.* **154:**2417–2422.

8. Fields, B. S., 1993, *Legionella* and protozoa: Interaction of a pathogen and its natural host, in: *Legionella: Current Status and Emerging Perspectives* (J. M. Barbaree, R. F. Breiman, and A. P. Dufour, eds.), American Society for Microbiology Press, Washington, D. C., pp. 129–136.

9. Joly, J. R., 1993, Monitoring for the presence of *Legionella:* Where, when and how? In: *Legionella: Current Status and Emerging Perspectives* (J. M. Barbaree, R. F. Breiman, and A. P. Dufour, eds.) American Society for Microbiology Press, Washington, D. C., pp. 211–216.

10. Bhardwaj, N., Nash, T. W., and Horwitz, M. A., 1986, Interferon-gamma activated human monocytes inhibit the intracellular multiplication of *Legionella pneumophila, J. Immunol.* **17:**2662–2669.

11. Skeen, M. J., Miller, M. A., Shinnick, T. M., and Ziegler, H. K., 1996, Regulation of murine macrophage IL-12 production: Activation of macrophages *in vivo,* restimulation *in vitro,* and modulation by other cytokines, *J. Immunol.* **156:**1196–1206.

12. Retzlaff, C., Yamamoto, Y., Hoffman, P. S., Friedman, H., and Klein, T. W., 1996, *Legionella pneumophila* heat-shock protein-induced increase of interleukin-1β mRNA involves protein kinase C signalling in macrophages, *Immunology* **89:**281–288.

13. Cirillo, J. D., Falkow, S., and Tompkins, L. S., 1994, Growth of *Legionella pneumophila* in *Acanthamoeba castellanii, Infect. Immun.* **62:**3254–3261.

14. Winn, W. C., Jr, 1988, Legionnaires' disease: Historical perspective, *Clin. Microbiol. Rev.* **1:**60–81.

15. Dowling, J. N., Saha, A. K., and Glew, R. H., 1992, Virulence factors of the family *Legionellaceae, Microbiol. Rev.* **56:**32–60.

16. Cianciotto, N. Eisenstein, B. I., Engleberg, N. C., and Shuman, H., 1989, Genetics and molecular pathogenesis of *Legionella pneumophila,* an intracellular parasite of macrophages, *Mol. Biol. Med.* **6:**409–424.

17. Marra, A., and Shuman, H. A., 1992, Genetics of *Legionella pneumophila* virulence, *Annu. Rev. Genet.* **26:**51–69.

18. Adeleke, A., Pruckler, J., Benson, R., Rowbotham, T., Halablab, M., and Fields, B., 1996, *Legionella*-like amebal pathogens—phylogenetic status and possible role in respiratory disease, *Emerg. Infect. Dis.* **2:**225–230.

19. Ahn, T. I., Lim, L. T., Leeu, H. K., Lee, J. E., and Jeon, K. W., 1994, A novel strong promoter of the groEx operon of symbiotic bacteria in *Amoeba proteus, Gene* **128:**43–49.

20. Hoffman, P. S., 1998, Invasion of eukaryotic cells by *L. pneumophila:* A common strategy for all hosts?, *Can. J. Infect. Dis.* **8:**139–146.

21. Horwitz, M. A., 1984, Phagocytosis of the Legionnaires' disease bacterium *(Legionella pneumophila)* occurs by a novel mechanism: Engulfment within a pseudopod coil, *Cell* **36:**27–33.

22. Horwitz, M. A., 1983, Formation of a novel phagosome by the Legionnaires' disease bacterium *(Legionella pneumophila)* in human monocytes, *J. Exp. Med.* **158:**13–31.

23. King, C. H., Fields, B. S., Shotts, E. B., Jr., and White, E. H., 1991, Effects of cytochalasin D and methylamine on intracellular growth of *Legionella pneumophila* in amoebae and human monocyte-like cells, *Infect. Immun.* **59:**758–763.

24. Abu Kwaik, Y., Fields, B. S., and Engleberg, N. C., 1994, Protein expression by the protozoan *Hartmannella vermiformis* upon contact with its bacterial parasite *Legionella pneumophila, Infect. Immun.* **62:**1860–1866.

25. Muller, A., Hacker, J., and Brand, B. C., 1996, Evidence for apoptosis of human macrophage-like HL-60 cells by *Legionella pneumophila* infection, *Infect. Immun.* **64:**4900–4906.

26. Zahringer, U., Knirel, Y. A., Lindner, B., Helbig, J. H., Sonesson, A., Marre, R., and T. Rietschel, E. T., 1995, The lipopolysaccharide of *Legionella pneumophila* serogroup 1 (strain Philadelphia 1): Chemical structure and biological significance, *Prog. Clin. Biol. Res.* **392:**113–119.

27. Sampson, J. S., Plikaytis, B. B., and Wilkinson, H. W., 1986, Immunologic response of patients with legionellosis against major protein-containing antigens of *Legionella pneumophila* serogroup 1 as shown by immunoblot analysis, *J. Clin. Microbiol.* **23:**92–99.

28. Weeratna, R., Stamler, D. A., Edelstein, P. H., Ripley, M., Marrie, T. J., Hoskin, D., and Hoffman, P. S., 1994, Human and guinea pig immune responses to *Legionella pneumophila* protein antigens: Vaccination of guinea pigs with OmpS, but not Hsp60, induces cell-mediated and protective immunity, *Infect. Immun.* **62:**3454–3462.

29. Keen, M. G., and Hoffman, P. S., 1989, Characterization of a *Legionella pneumophila* extracellular protease exhibiting hemolytic and cytotoxic activities, *Infect. Immun.* **57:**732–738.

30. Blander, S. J., and Horwitz, M. A., 1991, Vaccination with the major secretory protein of *Legionella* induces humoral and cell-mediated immune responses and protective immunity across different serogroups of *L. pneumophila* and different species of *Legionella, J. Immunol.* **147:**285–291.

31. Blander, S. J., and Horwitz, M. A., 1993, Major cytoplasmic membrane protein of *Legionella pneumophila*, a genus common antigen and member of the hsp60 family of heat shock proteins, induces protective immunity in a guinea pig model of Legionnaires' disease, *J. Clin. Invest.* **91:**717–723.

32. Hoffman, P. S., Houston, L., and Butler, C. A., 1990, *Legionella pneumophila htpAB* heat shock operon: Nucleotide sequence and expression of the 60-kilodalton antigen in *L. pneumophila*-infected HeLa cells, *Infect. Immun.* **58:**3380–3387.

33. Fernandez, R. C., Logan, S. M., Lee, S. H. S., and Hoffman, P. S., 1996, Elevated levels of *Legionella pneumophila* stress protein Hsp60 early in infection of human monocytes and L929 cells correlate with virulence, *Infect. Immun.* **64:**1968–1976.

34. Abu Kwaik, Y., Eisenstein, B. I., and Engleberg, N. C., 1993, Phenotypic modulation by *Legionella pneumophila* upon infection of macrophages, *Infect. Immun.* **61:**1320–1329.

35. Bellinger-Kawahara, C. G., and Horwitz, M. A., 1990, Complement component C3 fixes selectively to the major outer membrane protein (MOMP) of *Legionella pneumophila* and mediates phagocytosis of liposome–MOMP complexes by human monocytes, *J. Exp. Med.* **172:**1201–1210.

36. Husmann, L. K., and Johnson, W., 1992, Adherence of *Legionella pneumophila* to guinea pig peritoneal macrophages, J774 mouse macrophages, and undifferentiated U937 human monocytes: Role of Fc and complement receptors, *Infect. Immun.* **60:**5212–5218.

37. Gibson, F. C., Tzianabos, A. O., and Rodgers, F. G., 1994, Adherence of *Legionella pneumophila* to U-937 cells, guinea pig alveolar macrophages, and MRC-5 cells by a novel, complement-independent binding mechanism, *Can. J. Microbiol.* **40:**865–872.

38. Horwitz, M. A., and Silverstein, S. C., 1983, Intracellular multiplication of Legionnaires' disease bacterium *(Legionella pneumophila)* in human monocytes is reversibly inhibited by erythromycin and rifampin, *J. Clin. Invest.* **71:**15–26.

39. Garduno, R. A., Quinn, F. D., and Hoffman, P. S., 1998, HeLa cells as a model to study the invasiveness and biology of *Legionella pneumophila, Can. J. Microbiol.* **44:**430–440.

40. Quinn, F. D., Butler, C. A., and Hoffman, P. S., 1987, Characterization and cloning of the disulfide-cross-linked major outer membrane protein of *Legionella pneumophila, J. Cell. Biochem.* **115:**116.

41. Cianciotto, N. P., Eisenstein, B. I., Mody, C., and Engleberg, N. C., 1990, A mutation in the *mip* gene results in attenuation of *Legionella pneumophila* virulence, *J. Infect. Dis.* **162:**121–126.

42. Wintermeyer, E., Ludwig, B., Schmidt, B., Fischer, G., and Hacker, J., 1995, Influence of site specifically altered Mip proteins on intracellular survival of *Legionella pneumophila* in eukaryotic cells, *Infect. Immun.* **63:**4576–4583.

43. Dreyfus, L. A., 1987, Virulence associated ingestion of *Legionella pneumophila* by HeLa cells, *Microb. Pathog.* **3:**45–52.

44. Gaitanaris, G. A., Vysokanov, A., Hung, S. C., Gottesman, M. E., and Gragerov, A., 1994, Successive action of *Escherichia coli* chaperones *in vivo, Mol. Microbiol.* **14:**861–869.

45. Huesca, M., Borgia, S., Hoffman, P. S., and Lingwood, C. A., 1996. Acidic pH changes receptor binding specificity of *Helicobacter pylori:* A binary adhesion model in which surface heat shock (stress) proteins mediate sulfatide recognition in gastric colonization, *Infect. Immun.* **64:**2643–2648.

46. Hall, B. F., and Joiner, K. A., 1991, Strategies of obligate intracellular parasites for evading host defenses, *Immunol. Today* **12:**A22–A27.

47. Morioka, M., Muraoda, H., and Ishikawa, H., 1993, Chaperonin produced by an intracellular symbiont is an energy-coupling protein with phosphotransferase activity, *J. Biochem.* **114:**246–250.

48. Rechnitzer, C., and Blom, J., 1989, Engulfment of the Philadelphia-1 strain of *Legionella pneumophila* within pseudopod coils in human phagocytes. Comparison with other *Legionella* strains and species, *APMIS* **97:**105–114.

49. Berger, K. H., Merriam, J. J., and Isberg, R. R., 1994, Altered intracellular targeting properties associated with mutations in the *Legionella pneumophila dotA* gene, *Mol. Microbiol.* **14:**809–822.

50. Brand, B. C., Sadosky, A. B., and Shuman, H. A., 1994, The *Legionella pneumophila icm* locus; a set of genes required for intracellular multiplication in human macrophages, *Mol. Microbiol.* **14:**797–808.

51. Roy, C., and Isberg, R. R., 1997. Topology of *Legionella pneumophila* DotA: An inner membrane protein required for replication in macrophages, *Infect. Immun.* **65:**571–578.

52. McClain, M. S., Hurley, M. C., Brieland, J. K., and Engleberg, N. C., 1996, The *Legionella pneumophila hel* locus encodes intracellularly induced homologs of heavy-metal ion transporters of *Alcaligenes* spp., *Infect. Immun.* **64:**1532–1520.

53. Swanson, M. S., and Isberg, R. R., 1996, Identification of *L. pneumophila* mutants that have aberrant intracellular fates, *Infect. Immun.* **64:**2585–2594.

54. Sadosky, A. B., Wiater, L. A., and Shuman, H. A., 1993, Identification of *Legionella pneumophila* genes required for growth within and killing of human macrophages, *Infect. Immun.* **61:**5361–5373.

55. Morioka, M., and Ishikawa, H., 1992, Mutualism based on stress: Selective synthesis and phosphorylation of a stress protein by an intracellular symbiont, *J. Biochem.* **111:**431–435.

56. Abu Kwaik, Y., and Pederson, L. L., 1996, The use of differential display-PCR to isolate and characterize a *Legionella pneumophila* locus induced during the intracellular infection of macrophages, *Mol. Microbiol.* **21:**543–556.

57. Susa, M., Hacker, J., and Marre, R., 1996, De novo synthesis of *Legionella pneumophila* antigens during intracellular growth in phagocytic cells, *Infect. Immun.* **64:**1679–1684.

58. Abu Kwaik, Y., and Engleberg, N. C., 1994, Cloning and molecular characterization of a *Legionella pneumophila* gene induced by intracellular infection and by various *in vitro* stress stimuli, *Mol. Microbiol.* **13:**243–251.

59. Pope, C. D., O'Connell, W. A., and Cianciotto, N. P., 1996, *Legionella pneumophila* mutants that are defective for iron acquisition and assimilation and intracellular infection, *Infect. Immun.* **64:**629–636.

60. Hickey, E. K., and Cianciotto, N. P., 1997, An iron- and Fur-repressed *Legionella pneumophila* gene

that promotes intracellular infection and encodes a protein with similarity to the *Escherichia coli* aerobactin synthetases, *Infect. Immun.* **65:**133–143.

61. Gress, F. M., Myerowitz, R. L., Pasculle, A. W., Rinaldo, C. R., and Dowling, J. N., 1980, The ultrastructural morphologic features of Pittsburgh pneumonia agent, *Am. J. Pathol.* **101:**63–77.

62. Bozue, J. A., and Johnson, W., 1996, Interaction of *Legionella pneumophila* with *Acanthamoeba castellanii:* Uptake by coiling phagocytosis and inhibition of phagosome–lysosome fusion, *Infect. Immun.* **64:**668–673.

63. Horwitz, M. A., 1988, Phagocytosis and intracellular biology of *Legionella pneumophila*, in: *Bacteria–Host Cell Interaction* (M. A. Horwitz, ed.) Alan R. Liss, New York, pp. 283–302.

64. Oldham, L. J., and Rodgers, F. G., 1985, Adhesion, penetration and intracellular replication of *Legionella pneumophila:* An *in vitro* model of pathogenesis, *J. Gen. Microbiol.* **131:**697–706.

65. Rowbotham, T. J., 1980, Preliminary report of the pathogenicity of *Legionella pneumophila* for fresh water and soil amoebae, *J. Clin. Pathol.* **33:**1179–1183.

66. Garduno, R. A., Garduno, E., and Hoffman, P. S., 1998, Surface-associated Hsp60 chaperonin of *Legionella pneumophila*, mediates invasion in a HeLa cell model, *Infect. Immun.* **66:**4602–4610.

67. Garduno, R. A., Faulkner, G., Trevors, M. A., Vats, N., and Hoffman, P. S., 1998, Immunolocalization of Hsp60 in *Legionella pneumophila*, *J. Bacteriol.* **180:**505–513.

68. Segal, G., Purcell, M., and Shuman, H. A., 1998, Host cell killing and bacterial conjugation require overlapping sets of genes within a 22-kb region of the *Legionella pneumophila* genome, *Proc. Natl. Acad. Sci.* **95:**1669–1674.

69. Vogel, J. P., Andrews, H. L., Wong, S. K., and Isberg, R. R., 1998, Conjugative transfer by the virulence system of *Legionella pneumophila*, *Science (Washington, D.C.)* **279:**873–876.

70. Roy, C. R., Berger, K. H., and Isberg, R. R., 1998, *Legionella pneumophila* DotA protein is required for early phagosome trafficking decisions that occur within minutes of bacterial uptake, *Mol. Microbiol.* **28:**663–674.

9

Immune Responses to *Legionella*

THOMAS W. KLEIN, CATHERINE NEWTON,
YOSHIMASA YAMAMOTO, and HERMAN FREIDMAN

1. INTRODUCTION

Legionella pneumophila is a Gram-negative, facultative, intracellular pathogen first reported in 1977 as the causative agent of the fatal pneumonia termed Legionnaires' disease[1,2] and later reported to cause a nonpneumonic illness termed Pontiac fever.[3,4] Since then, approximately 40 more species of *Legionella* have been described[5] and sporadic outbreaks of human illness are still reported,[6,7] with the annual number of cases reported to the CDC running between 1000 and 1500. The severe pneumonic form of the disease occurs most frequently in immunocompromised patients with lowered innate and acquired immunity and is a concern in the etiology of nosocomial infections.[8-10] Relatively healthy individuals can also become infected if exposure to virulent organisms is significant.[7] *Legionella* organisms occur naturally in fresh water ponds and lakes where they multiply in free-living protozoa.[11] The intracellular life cycle in the protozoa appears to be very similar to that reported for mammalian phagocytes[12] and infected protozoa in air conditioning cooling towers and potable water systems such as hot tubs and institutional hot water tanks serve as a major source of human infection.[13,14] The molecular mechanisms involved in the attachment,

THOMAS W. KLEIN, CATHERINE NEWTON, YOSHIMASA YAMAMOTO, and HERMAN FRIEDMAN • Department of Medical Microbiology and Immunology, University of South Florida, College of Medicine, Tampa, Florida 33612.

Opportunistic Intracellular Bacteria and Immunity, edited by Lois J. Paradise *et al.* Plenum Press, New York, 1999.

uptake, and replication of *Legionella* in protozoan and mammalian host cells are poorly understood at this time; however, progress is being made in our understanding, and these mechanisms are reviewed elsewhere in this volume (Chapter 8).

Legionella organisms are very immunostimulatory as evidenced by the fact that (1) the severe symptoms of Legionnaires' disease begin abruptly and parallel those of a severe acute phase response, (2) humans readily develop humoral and cellular immune responses to *Legionella* antigens, and (3) *Legionella* antigens are immunostimulatory in immune cell cultures and animal models. However, as with the mechanisms responsible for intracellular multiplication, those controlling immunostimulation are also incompletely understood. In the following, we review the types of immune responses observed in humans and animals following infection with *Legionella* and where possible identify the *Legionella* antigens involved in immune stimulation. In addition, we focus on the impact of *Legionella* infection on the cytokine network of the host and the role this might have in pathogenesis as well as host resistance to and recovery from infection. It is now apparent that the overall host response to *Legionella* infection involves aspects of both innate immunity encompassing phagocytic cells and acute phase cytokines as well as aspects of acquired immunity involving T and B lymphocytes mechanisms. This is generally true for all intracellular, bacterial pathogens and therefore *Legionella* represents a good model to study host immune mechanisms for this class of pathogens.

2. IMMUNE RESPONSES IN HUMANS

2.1. Antibodies

The first report describing the pathogen, *Legionella pneumophila*, and the index outbreak of 1976 in Philadelphia, also reported extensive information on antibody titers of the Legionnaires' disease patients.[2] Indirect fluorescent antibody tests were carried out using smears of hen's egg yolk sac preparations containing *Legionella* antigens and the results showed that 75% of 136 patients with serum samples available for study were antibody positive for *Legionella* antigens with some convalescent serum titers higher than 1000. Serum samples from previous outbreaks of Legionnaires'-like disease in Washington, D. C. and Pontiac, MI were also reported and averaged around 90% positive for anti-*Legionella* antibodies.[2] Thus, from the beginning, it was noted that humans readily produced antibodies following exposure to *Legionella*. Subsequent serum surveillance studies in the general population have shown the low prevalence (10% to 25%) of significant serum titers to various *Legionella pneumophila* serogroups, suggesting a low level of community exposure to *L. pneumophila* and confirming antibody responsiveness by a wide sampling of human subjects.[15,16]

The antigens responsible for stimulating this antibody response include li-popolysaccharide (LPS) endotoxin as well as protein antigens (Fig. 1). Antibodies to distinct serogroup antigens were first described in very high titers in convales-cent sera from Legionnaires' patients[17,18] and these antigens were identified as lipid–protein–carbohydrate complexes.[18] Later studies showed that *Legionella* contained LPS[19,20] and that the serogroup antigens were of high molecular weight, heat stable, and located on the outer surface of the organism,[21,22] suggest-ing a relationship to LPS. Sera from legionellosis patients also contain antibodies to protein antigens such as the 58-kDa genus-specific antigen and the 11- and 25-kDa species-specific antigens described by Sampson *et al.*[23] These antigens could be related to heat-shock protein 60 (hsp60) and the 28-kDa major outer mem-brane protein antigens also shown to be immunogenic,[24] but this is unclear at this time. Patient serum also contains limited reactivity to the *Legionella* extracellular protease[25] but the overall extent and significance of these antibodies is unclear. Finally, flagella antigens have been described for *Legionella* and these appear to be immunogenic in animals ([26,27]; also see below). However, the immunogenicity of these antigens in humans is unknown and therefore their importance in host immunity is unclear. In addition to these antigens, a variety of *Legionella* virulence factors and other antigens have been described over the last decade. The impor-tance of these proteins as antigens for humoral immunity in humans has not been defined and therefore the role of these various immune complexes and immune reactivites in the immunopathogenesis of legionellosis has yet to be determined. Furthermore, the role of antibodies in resistance to and recovery from le-gionellosis is believed to be minimal and in fact antibodies have been implicated in promoting uptake and replication in host phagocytes rather than promoting elimination of the microbe.[21,28]

2.2. Cellular Immunity

From the very beginning, it was recognized that *Legionella* infected and colonized host cells in the lung. Initial electron micrographs of lung tissues of Legionnaires' patients documented that only a few bacterial cells were seen

FIGURE 1. *Legionella* antigens stimulate various levels of immunity. Antigens reported to directly stimulate cytokine production are flagella proteins, lipopolysaccharide (LPS), heat-shock protein 60 (hsp60), and poorly defined microbial surface antigens or moieties. Antigens reported to stimulate cellular immunity are LPS, hsp60, outer membrane protein (OmpS), and major secretory protein (MSP). These same antigens along with flagella antigens have been shown to also stimulate humoral immunity.

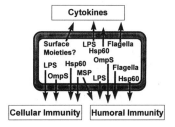

extracellularly while most of the bacteria were intracellular.[29] The type of cell harboring *Legionella* was not clear but the intracellular location was within endosomes and in membrane-bound structures resembling dilated endoplasmic reticulum. This observation had special relevance because it was eventually established that *Legionella* grew and replicated in endosomes in close association with the rough endoplasmic reticulum—the meaning of this is still unclear.[30] In addition to lung cells, human blood monocytes in culture were also shown to harbor and support the growth of *Legionella*.[31] This seminal finding suggested that *Legionella* was a facultative, intracellular microbe (similar to *Listeria monocytogenes* and *Mycobacterium tuberculosis*) and therefore might be controlled by cell-mediated immunity (CMI). CMI involvement was subsequently shown by a number of human and animal studies, among the first of which showed that human peripheral blood mononuclear cell cultures could be activated by mitogen to restrict the intracellular growth of *Legionella* and that this was due to the generation of cytokines.[32] In addition, blood cells from Legionnaires' disease patients were shown to be sensitive to *Legionella* antigens in lymphocyte blast transformation assays.[33] Blood lymphocytes from 17 subjects recovered from legionellosis and 63 control subjects were culture with sonicated extracts of *Legionella* and the proliferation responses (i.e., stimulation indices) were significantly different between the two groups. Samples from legionellosis patients averaged an index of 48 whereas control samples averaged only 18. This increase in antigen-specific lymphocyte proliferation was extended to samples from patients with acute legionellosis, reinforcing the hypothesis that humans exposed to *Legionella* harbored lymphocytes sensitized to *Legionella* antigens.[34] Such sensitized lymphocytes were subsequently shown, in response to *Legionella* antigens, to secrete cytokines capable of activating normal blood monocyte cultures to restrict the growth of *Legionella*.[35] This was strong evidence that the classic mechanisms of CMI were operating in humans and eventually it was shown that the T helper 1 (Th1) cytokine, interferon-γ (IFN-γ), could activate monocytes to inhibit *Legionella* growth.[36] Th1 cells are essential in the development of CMI to intracellular pathogens.[37]

    The identity of *Legionella* antigens capable of inducing CMI in humans has not been elucidated. Indeed, only one study has addressed this issue in a systematic way.[24] Working with OmpS (28-kDa major outer membrane protein) and hsp60 it was shown that peripheral blood lymphocytes from culture confirmed legionellosis patients proliferated in culture in response to *Legionella* antigens to a greater extent that lymphocytes from volunteers with no history of *Legionella* infection. The OmpS antigen (Fig. 1) appeared to have a greater effect on proliferation, suggesting it to be a better immunogen for CMI but other studies are needed to confirm this idea. OmpS also appeared to be a better immunogen in a guinea pig infection model (see below), emphasizing its importance as a possible Th1-selective immunogen in animals. Many *Legionella* antigens have been cloned (see Chapter 8, *this volume*) and are now available for studying the specific immune response in humans. Using peripheral blood cells as a source of tissue, a variety of studies are possible designed to examine which antigens and epitopes are important in stimulating in humans the Th1 axis as opposed to those that stimulate Th2 or other immune responses.

3. ANIMAL STUDIES

3.1. Antibodies

Early animal studies employed infection paradigms with guinea pigs to examine the possibility of airborne transmission of *Legionella* as well as to examine the relative susceptibility and pathophysiology of experimental animals following *Legionella* exposure. It was observed that guinea pigs were more susceptible to *Legionella* administered by aerosols wherein the LD_{50} was 140,000 bacteria,[38] as opposed to the intraperitoneal route wherein the LD_{50} was 3×10^6. Signs of infection included fever, weight loss, dyspnea, and bacteremia as well as a rise in the titer of serum agglutinating antibodies. The antibody titer was highest in animals infected by the aerosol route and reached a peak at 14 days following infection. Rats were also shown to be susceptible and to produce antibodies to *Legionella* infection.[39] However, these animals were several orders of magnitude less sensitive than guinea pigs and they died much more rapidly, that is, within 24 h. The agglutinating antibody response in serum reached a peak between 1 and 2 weeks following infection and interestingly, rats could be protected from *Legionella* infection in a serotype-specific way by pretreatment with immune serum. Protection by antibodies was not seen in a guinea pig model[40] wherein animals were immunized with a large molecular weight, serotype-specific antigen in Freund's complete adjuvant and challenged 30 days later when antibody titers were quite high. None of the animals survived the aerosol challenge infection in fact, the immunized animals died at an accelerated rate compared to controls and the lung histopathology was greater in the immunized group. The increased sensitivity to infection in immunized animals was suggested to be due to antibody-mediated increase in *Legionella* uptake, antibody activation of the complement pathway, or perhaps activation of humoral hypersensitivity pathways.[40]

Vaccination and antibody titers had a mixed efficacy in the studies by Eisenstein *et al.*[41] Guinea pigs were immunized with an intraperitoneal injection of heat- or acetone-killed serogroup 1 cells and 2 weeks later were bled for antibody titers and challenged with virulent *Legionella*. The route of challenge infection was either intraperitoneal or pulmonary. It was observed that titers of antibodies to outer membrane antigens increased following injection of both vaccine preparations and animals challenged by the intraperitoneal route were completely protected by either vaccine preparation. Interestingly, however, guinea pigs challenged by the pulmonary route were not protected by prior vaccination in spite of the rise in specific antibodies. The authors discussed several possibilities to account for the variation in effect with route of infection including hypersensitivity mechanisms and failure to induce cell-mediated immunity.[41] However, the overriding conclusion from this study confirmed that high titers of circulating antibodies did not correlate with resistance to infection with *Legionella*.

The above studies documented that *Legionella* antigens induced a strong antibody response however, they provided little information regarding the cellular and molecular mechanisms involved. In this regard, *Legionella* antigens were shown to induce the proliferation of mouse splenocytes[42] as well as augment the splenocyte antibody-forming response to sheep red blood cell antigens.[43] B cells appeared to be more sensitive than T cells to the immunostimulatory effects of *Legionella* antigens[42] and the antigens involved included LPS as well as protein antigens such as those associated with flagella.[43] A portion of this immunostimulatory effect is now known to be due to the potent cytokine-inducing potential of *Legionella* antigens such as hsp60 which has been shown to selectively induce a humoral response in guinea pigs[24] and to induce macrophages to increase the production of cytokines such as interleukin-1 (IL-1), IL-6, tumor necrosis factor (TNF), and granulocyte/macrophage-colony-stimulating factor (GM-CSF) (see below).

3.2. Cellular Immunity

As it became apparent from human studies that CMI was involved in immunity to Legionnaires' disease, animal models were sought to examine the putative CMI response in greater detail. Delayed-type hypersensitivity (DTH) skin reactions were first reported in guinea pigs sensitized to *Legionella* antigens.[44] Skin responses could be elicited with both "serotypic" and "cross-reacting" antigens. Similar skin responses as well as other manifestations of CMI such as antigen-specific lymphocyte proliferation and migration inhibition were subsequently demonstrated in guinea pigs sensitized to *Legionella* antigens.[45,46] Furthermore, CMI responses were quite pronounced in animals infected with small numbers of virulent organisms, suggesting that moderate exposure to *Legionella* antigens could prime the animal for specific cell-medited immunity.[46] Such priming of guinea pigs by sublethal infection was subsequently demonstrated to increase CMI and resistance to a pulmonary challenge infection.[47]

Several reports have helped to define the *Legionella* antigens responsible for CMI in guinea pigs. One of these antigens is the extracellular protease also referred to as the major secretory protein (MSP).[25] This protein is a metalloprotease with a molecular mass of 38 to 40 kDa. Blander and Horwitz[48] reported that this protein, when injected into guinea pigs subcutaneously in adjuvant, induced anti-*Legionella* CMI responses such as DTH (Fig. 1) and lymphocyte proliferation and also cross-protected animals to challenge infections with three different serotypes of *L. pneumophila*. These investigators subsequently reported that the genus common antigen, hsp60, immunized guinea pigs to a lethal, aerosol challenge infection with *Legionella*.[49] This 60-kDa, heat-shock protein (hsp), which is a member of the GroEL family,[50,51] was also shown to sensitize guinea pigs for stong DTH responses (Fig. 1).[49] More recently, Weeratna *et al.*[24] have examined the sensitizing effect in guinea pigs (and humans) of *Legionella* antigens including MSP, hsp60, and the 28-kDa subunit (OmpS) of the major outer membrane protein of *Legionella*.[52,53] Animals recovering from *Legionella* infection were shown to exhibit strong DTH responses to OmpS and hsp60 while weaker responses were noted to MSP. Lymphocyte proliferation in response to OmpS and hsp60 were also strong in cells from sensitized animals. Of particular interest was the divergence in immune response potential in animals immunized with the various antigens. Vaccination with OmpS induced a relatively low antibody response but strong DTH and lymphocyte proliferation responses while hsp60 induced the reversed balance between humoral and CMI, that is, high antibody with low CMI (Fig. 1). Of further interest was the finding that OmpS-vaccinated animals (high CMI) were more resistant to challenge infection than hsp60-vaccinated (high antibody) animals. These findings suggest that *Legionella* OmpS in guinea pigs preferentially induces CMI or Th1 type of immunity whereas the hsp60 antigen induces humoral or Th2 responses (Fig. 2).This selection of Th responses has been observed in other systems[54,55] and in the case of *Legionella* antigens warrants further study to determine the relative immune potential of these immunodominant antigens.

Besides the use of guinea pigs for studying immunity to *Legionella*, other animal models such as hamster and rat have been examined. Hamsters were shown to be susceptible to intraperitoneal infection with large doses of *Legionella* and displayed mortality and culture-positive evidence of systemic infection within days of infection.[56] Rats infected by aerosol challenge mobilized and activated alveolar macrophages, thus showing evidence of an augmented CMI response.[57] Mice were also examined and, although generally more resistant to *Legionella*, the A/J strain was shown to be more susceptible to infection and to contain peritoneal macrophages permissive for the growth of *Legionella*.[58,59] The interaction of *Legionella* with A/J, exudate macrophages is very similar to that of macrophages from guinea pigs[59,60] and the permissive nature of the strain appears to be genetically determined and related to a single genetic locus termed *Lgn1*.[61-63] Recently, this strain has been suggested to be a good murine model of Legionnaires' disease.[64,65] Regarding the CMI response of these animals, they have been shown to possess *Legionella* responsive lymphocytes that can produce Th1 cytokines such as IFN-γ that protect the animal from *Legionella* infection.[66-69]

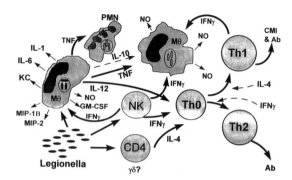

FIGURE 2. *Legionella* antigens stimulate cells and cytokines of both the innate and acquired immune response. Regarding innate immunity, *Legionella* induces macrophages (MΘs) to secrete interleukins 1, 6, 10, and 12, TNF-α, GM-CSF, nitric oxide (NO), and the chemokines KC (platelet-derived growth factor inducible), MIP-1B (macrophage inflammatory peptide), and MIP-2. The TNF-α activates PMNs and MΘs to kill ingested *Legionella*, the IL-10 inhibits MΘ function, and the IL-12 probably augments the development of Th0 cells to Th1 cells. The function of IL-1, IL-6, GM-CSF, NO, and the chemokines is unclear at this time. *Legionella* also stimulates NK cells to produce IFN-γ that activates MΘs to kill *Legionella*, induces the maturation of Th1 immunity, and costimulates MΘs to produce cytokines. IL-4 is also induced by *Legionella* antigens, possibly by cells such as γδ T cells. The IL-4 as well as IFN-γ regulates the maturation of Th1 and Th2 cells. Th1 cells promote cell-mediated immunity (CMI) and certain types of antibody production (Ab) while Th2 cells promote Ab production. Dashed lines indicate inhibition of the response.

4. IMMUNITY AND CYTOKINES

4.1. Acute Phase Cytokines

Patients presenting with Legionnaires' disease or Pontiac fever show abrupt onset of high fever, headache, myalgia, cough, and changes in mental status.[9] This symptom complex is suggestive of an explosive release of acute phase cytokines such as IL-1, TNF-α, and IL-6 by cells of the innate immune response. The first evidence that *Legionella* antigens induce acute phase cytokines in nonimmune hosts came from studies showing that *Legionella* antigen preparations added to normal mouse spleen cell cultures nonspecifically augmented the antibody response to the unrelated antigens on sheep red blood cells (SRBCs).[43] The immunostimulating activity was induced by a semipurified antigen similar to endotoxin as well as flagella protein from *Legionella*. In addition, at least a portion of the immunoenhancing activity came from the splenic macrophages as determined by cell purification studies. This study was followed by several others showing that *Legionella* antigens directly induce TNF and IL-1 (Fig. 2). TNF was detected in lung lavage fluid from *Legionella*-infected mice and in addition adherent lung cells and PU 5-1.8 macrophages were induced in culture to produce TNF and this effect was augmented by the addition of IFN-γ.[70] IL-1 was also shown to be induced by *Legionella* antigens in mouse splenocyte, peritoneal macrophage, and human monocyte cultures.[71] Supernatants rich in IL-1 augmented the antibody response to SRBCs and the IL-1 was induced by several different antigen preparations ranging from killed bacteria to endotoxin containing bacterial extracts.[71]

Although acute phase cytokines can cause shock and death if overproduced during the host response to infection,[72,73] they also have a protective effect which appears to be the case in *Legionella* infection. Initially it was shown that TNF mobilized in mice following *Legionella* infection activated polymorphonuclear leukocytes (PMNs) to restrict the growth of *Legionella* (Fig. 2)[74] and this activity was shown to also occur in cultures of human neutrophils.[75] Further studies showed that macrophage resistance to *Legionella* was linked to the production of TNF and IL-1 both in endotoxin activated mouse macrophages[76] and human monocytes cultured with recombinant TNF-α.[77] The latter study also showed that a portion of the anti-*Legionella* effect of IFN-γ in monocyte cultures was partly due to its ability to mobilize TNF in the cultures (Fig. 2). The mechanism of these anti-*Legionella* effects is not entirely clear at this time but may involve nitric oxide (Fig. 2). For example, studies in A/J mice[78] and rat lung alveolar macrophage cultures[79] suggested that nitric oxide enhanced production of TNF-α as well as the enhanced microbicidal activity of the phagocytes; in addition, the antimicrobial activity of IFN-γ was also linked to this system. Furthermore, it has been shown that nitric oxide induced by IFN-γ treatment and *Legionella* infection negatively regulates mouse macrophage production of IL-6 (Fig. 2), another of the acute phase cytokines.[80]

IL-1 is also induced following exposure to *Legionella* antigens, at least in mouse macrophages. This appears to be a generalized effect because macrophages of lung, spleen, and peritoneum produce large amounts of the cytokine[81] and IL-1 is mobilized along with IL-6 and TNF-α in mice infected with *Legionella*.[73] However, unlike TNF, IL-1 appears not to be directly involved in activating macrophages to kill *Legionella* in that GM-CSF-stimulated cells increase IL-1 production but are not resistant to *Legionella* infection[82] and IL-1 added to cultures of mouse peritoneal macrophages are not resistant.[83]

Cells other than phagocytes are involved in innate immunity to infection. One of these is the natural killer (NK) cell, which in addition to killing harmful target cells is now recognized as an important early source of cytokines. In this regard, it is of interest that the first report of cytokine induction by *Legionella* antigens in nonimmune cells described the production of IFN-γ by cultured splenocytes.[84] Initially, it was believed that T cells were the sole source of the IFN-γ however, it was shown later that NK cells also responded to *Legionella* antigen stimulation by not only producing IFN (Fig. 2) but also becoming activated to kill *Legionella* infected macrophage targets.[85,86] Other cytokines are induced during the early immune response to *Legionella* including IL-10,[87] IL-4 (Fig. 3), and IL-12 (Fig. 4). In addition,

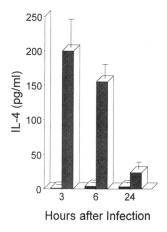

FIGURE 3. Production of IL-4 following *Legionella* infection. BALB/c mice were infected intravenously with 7 × 10⁶ *Legionella* and splenocytes collected at the times indicated. The splenocytes were cultured for 3 h and the supernatants tested for IL-4 by ELISA. ■ Noninfected mice. ▓ Infected mice.

cells such as γδ T (Fig. 2) cells may be involved in cytokine production along with NK cells and macrophages (unpublished observations). Clearly, cytokines of the innate as well as adaptive immune response are induced by *Legionella* antigens however, the role of these substances in host defense is still unclear.

Some of the antigens responsible for acute phase cytokine induction are known and include the LPS as cited previously as well as hsp60 and bacterial surface moieties. Treatment of cultured macrophages with cytochalasin D inhibits the uptake of added bacteria but not the binding to the cell surface.[88] Using cytochalasin D treated A/J macrophage cultures, it was shown that *Legionella*

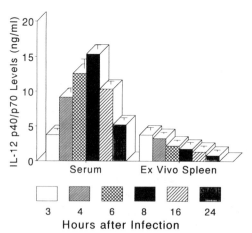

FIGURE 4. Production of IL-12 following *Legionella* infection. BALB/c mice were infected intravenously with 7 × 10⁶ *Legionella* and splenocytes and blood collected at the times indicated. The splenocytes were cultured and the supernatants along with blood serum samples tested for IL-12 p40/p70 proteins by ELISA.

organisms along with *Salmonella* and *Escherichia* induced IL-1α and -β, IL-6, TNF-α, and GM-CSF but did not induce IFN-β.[89] As a positive control, LPS induced all of the cytokines, whereas the negative control, bovine serum albumin-latex, had no effect. This suggested that surface antigens on microbes, including *Legionella*, interacted with the macrophage surface, inducing cytokine production. The surface antigens responsible for these effects included heat-labile antigens in addition to heat-stable endotoxin. In other studies, different types of macrophages responded differently to this type of stimulation and chemokines (Fig. 2) were shown to be induced along with TNF and IL-1.[90] Regarding the identity of the surface molecules, they appear to differ for the cytokine and chemokine responses. For example, the moiety involved in cytokine stimulation probably contains a mannose or other sugar residue because it is inhibited by α-methyl-d-mannoside; also, this moiety is linked to a different signaling protein kinase than the one involved in chemokine induction.[91] These studies suggest that acute phase cytokines and chemokines are induced by different *Legionella* surface antigens, but the chemical identity is unknown at this time.

The hsp60 of *Legionella* has also been shown to induce IL-1β similar to hsps from other bacteria.[92] The signaling mechanism involved in this response appears to involve protein kinase C (PKC) in that H7 pretreatment decreased the response and the PKC pseudosubstrate was phosphorylated following stimulation with the protein.[93] Whether hsp60 is one of the surface moieties discussed above is not known at this time; also, the identity of other active proteins awaits further study. All in all, it appears that *Legionella* organisms are powerful inducers of acute phase cytokines and that perhaps this response, along with developing T-cell immunity, is sufficient in some cases to attenuate the spread of infection and prevent pneumonia. The subsequent outcome would be either a subclinical infection, or, in the case of heavy exposure, a syndrome such as Pontiac fever.

4.2. Immune Cytokines

In addition to innate immune mechanisms involving acute phase cytokines, *Legionella* also stimulates cytokines of the adaptive immune response. As noted earlier, Horwitz was the first to report that cultured peripheral blood cells from Legionnaires' disease patients could be induced by *Legionella* organisms to produce soluble factors that activated monocyte cultures to restrict the intracellular growth of *Legionella*.[35] This study was followed by another showing that recombinant IFN-γ added to human monocyte cultures also restricted *Legionella* replication.[36] However, it was not until more recently that it was demonstrated that *Legionella* infection or exposure to *Legionella* antigens actually increases Th1 activity and the consequent production of IFN-γ (Fig. 2).[69,94] In these studies, mice infected 6 days previously with *Legionella* showed manifestations of Th1 activity and extensive splenocyte *ex vivo* production of IFN-γ.[69] The IFN-γ peak coincided with a mobilization of CD4⁺ cells in the mouse[95] and was only one of three peaks of IFN-γ activity observed following *Legionella* infection (Fig. 5). In addition to mouse, human CD4⁺ cells were shown to produce either IFN-γ or IL-4 depending on the type of antigen preparation used for stimulation,[94] a finding similar to that of Weeratna *et al.*,[24] who observed that in guinea pigs the OmpS protein appeared to be a more potent stimulator of CMI (Th1) whereas Hsp60 was more stimulatory for a humoral response (Th2).

5. CONCLUSION

Humans and animals are accidental hosts for *Legionella pneumophila*. In this situation, as is frequently the case, the microbial pathogen is an opportunist and causes disease by taking advantage of host weaknesses in immunity. The experimental evidence to date shows that humans and animals readily respond to *Legionella* antigens with vigorous humoral and cell-mediated immunity and that the latter leads to macrophage activation and elimination of the intracellular pathogen. It is also clear that exposure to *Legionella* induces the production of a variety of cytokines including IFN-γ, IL-1α, and -β, IL-4, IL-6, IL-12, IL-10, TNF-α, GM-CSF, and chemokines, and that NK cells, PMNs, and γδ T cells respond to these antigens in addition to T and B cells and macrophages. These cytokines serve to regulate both early (innate) and late (acquired) immunity and in the immunocompetent host this leads to resistance to infection and disease. However, many issues regarding the immune response to *Legionella* and other facultative intracellular pathogens need to be clarified. For example, the relative roles in immunity of the various cell populations stimulated by *Legionella* has yet to be fully defined. Are NK cells and γδ T cells important effector cells during the early stages of infection? In addition, the regulatory interaction between the acute

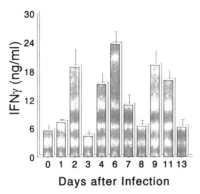

FIGURE 5. *Legionella* infection leads to three peaks of IFN-γ activity in spleen. BALB/c mice were injected with 7 × 10⁶ *Legionella* intravenously and the splenocytes collected at the times indicated. The splenocytes were cultured with anti-CD3 for 24 h and the level of IFN-γ measured by ELISA.

phase cytokines and the adaptive immune response needs further study and elucidation. Does the early production of IL-4 and IL-12 direct the production of TNF and IL-1 as well as direct the maturation of CD4$^+$ T cells? Finally, the immunomodulating potential of the various major antigens of *Legionella* requires continued definition and testing. Are some *Legionella* antigens Th1 dominant or Th2 dominant?

REFERENCES

1. Fraser, D. W., Tsai, T. R., Orenstein, W., Parkin, W. W., Beecham, H. J., Sharrar, R. G., Harris, J., Mallison, G. F., Martin, S. M., McDade, J. E., Shepard, C. C., Brachman, P. D., and Team, T. F. I., 1977, Legionnaires' disease: Description of an epidemic of pneumonia, *N. Engl. J. Med.* **297:**1189–1197.
2. McDade, J. E., Shepard, C. C., Fraser, D. W., Tsai, T. R., Redus, M. A., Dowdle, W. R., and Team, T. L. I., 1977, Legionnaires' disease: Isolation of a bacterium and demonstration of its role in othe respiratory disease, *N. Engl. J. Med.* **297:**1197–1203.
3. Kaufmann, A. F., McDade, J. E., Patton, C. M., Bennett, J. V., Skaliy, P., Feeley, J. C., Anderson, D. C., Potter, M. E., Newhouse, V. F., Gregg, M. B., and Brachman, P. S., 1981, Pontiac fever: Isolation of the etiologic agent *(Legionella pneumophila)* and demonstration of its mode of transmission, *Am. J. Epidemiol.* **114:**337–347.
4. Glick, T. H., Gregg, M. B., Berman, B., Mallison, G., Rhodes, W. W., and Kassanoff, I., 1978, Pontiac fever, an epidemic of unknown etiology in a health department. I. Clinical and epidemiologic aspects, *Am. J. Epidemiol.* **107:**149–160.
5. Adeleke, A., Pruckler, J., Benson, R., Rowbotham, T., Halablab, M., and Fields, B., 1996, Legionella-like amebal pathogens—phylogenetic status and possible role in respiratory disease, *Emerg. Infect. Dis.* **2:**225–230.
6. Jernigan, D. B., Hofmann, J., Cetron, M. S., Genese, C. A., Nuorti, J. P., Fields, B. S., Benson, R. F., Carter, R. J., Edelstein, P. H., Guerrero, I. C., Paul, S. M., Lipman, H. B., and Breiman, R. F., 1996, Outbreak of Legionnaires' disease among cruise ship passengers exposed to a contaminated whirlpool spa, *Lancet* **347:**494–499.
7. Thomas, D. L., Mundy, L. M., and Tucker, P. C., 1993, Hot tub legionnellosis: Legionnaires' disease and Pontiac fever after a point-source exposure to *Legionnella pneumophila*, *Arch. Intern. Med.* **153:**2597–2599.
8. Beaty, H. N., 1984, Clinical features of Legionellosis, in: *Legionella: Proceedings of the 2nd International Symposium* (C. Thornsberry, A. Balows, J. C. Feeley, and W. Jakubowski, eds.) American Society for Microbiology Press, Washington, D. C., pp. 6–10.
9. Finegold, S. M., 1988, Legionnaires' disease—still with us, *N. Engl. J. Med.* **318:**571–573.
10. Morley, J. N., Smith, L. C., Baltch, A. L., and Smith, R. P., 1994, recurrent infection due to *Legionella pneumophila* in a patient with AIDS, *Clin. Infect. Dis.* **19:**1130–1132.
11. Fields, B. S., Fields, S. R. U., Loy, J. N. C., White, E. H., Steffens, W. L., and Shotts, E. B., 1993, Attachment and entry of *Legionella pneumophila* in *Hartmannella vermiformis*, *J. Infect. Dis.* **167:**1146–1150.
12. Bozue, J. A., and Johnson, W., 1996, Interaction of *Legionella pneumophila* with *Acanthamoeba castellanii:* Uptake by coiling phagocytosis and inhibition of phagosome–lysosome fusion, *Infect. Immun.* **64:**668–673.
13. Nahapetian, K., Challemel, O., Beurtin, D., Dubrou, S., Gounon, P., and Squinazi, F., 1991, The intracellular multiplication of *Legionella pneumophila* in protozoa from hospital plumbing systems, *Institut. Pasteur.* **142:**677–685.

14. Winn, W. C., 1988, Legionnaires' disease: Historical perspective, *Clin. Microbiol. Rev.* **1:**60–81.
15. Edson, D. C., Stiefel, H. E., Wentworth, B. B., and Wilson, D. L., 1979, Prevalence of antibodies to Legionnaires' disease, *Ann. Intern. Med.* **90:**691–693.
16. Helms, C. M., Johson, W., Renner, E. D., Hierholzer, W. J., Wintermeyer, L. A., and Viner, J. P., 1980, Background prevalence of microagglutination antibodies to *Legionella pneumophila* serogroups 1, 2, 3, and 4, *Infect. Immun.* **30:**612–614.
17. McKinney, R. M., Wilkinson, H. W., Sommers, H. M., Fikes, B. J., Sasseville, K. R., Yungbluth, M. M., and Wolf, J. S. (1980), *Legionella pneumophila* serogroup six: Isolation from cases of legionellosis, identification by immunofluorescence staining, and immunological response to infection, *J. Clin. Microbiol.* **12:**395–401.
18. Wong, K. H., Schalla, W. O., Arko, R. J., Bullard, J. C., and Feeley, J. C., 1979, Immunochemical, serologic, and immunologic properties of major antigens isolated from the Legionnaires' disease bacterium, *Ann. Intern. Med.* **90:**634–638.
19. Sonesson, A., Jantzen, E., Bryn, K., Larsson, L., and Eng, J., 1989, Chemical composition of a lipopolysaccharide from *Legionella pneumophila, Arch. Microbiol.* **153:**72–78.
20. Wong, K. H., Moss, C. W., Hochstein, D. H., Arko, R. J., and Schalla, W. O., 1979, "Endotoxicity" of Legionnaires' disease bacterium, *Ann. Intern. Med.* **90:**624–627.
21. Johnson, W., Pesanti, E., and Elliott, J., 1979, Serospecificity and opsonic activity of antisera to *Legionella pneumophila, Infect. Immun.* **26:**698–704.
22. Elliott, J. A., Johnson, W., and Helms, C. M., 1981, Ultrastructural localization and protective activity of a high-molecular-weight antigen isolated from *Legionella pneumophila, Infect. Immun.* **31:**822–824.
23. Sampson, J. S., Plikaytis, B. B., and Wilkinson, H. W., 1986, Immunologic response of patients with legionellosis against major protein-containing antigens of *Legionella pneumophila* serogroup 1 as shown by immunoblot analysis, *J. Clin. Microbiol.* **23:**92–99.
24. Weeratna, R., Stamler, D. A., Edelstein, P. H., Ripley, M., Marrie, T., Hoskin, D., and Hoffman, P. S., 1994, Human and guinea pig immune responses to *Legionella pneumophila* protein antigens OmpS and Hsp60, *Infect. Immun.* **62:**3454–3462.
25. Keen, M. G., and Hoffman, P. S., 1989, Characterization of a *Legionella pneumophila* extracellular protease exhibiting hemolytic and cytotoxic activities, *Infect. Immun.* **57:**732–738.
26. Thomason, B. M., Chandler, F. W., and Hollis, D. G., 1979, Flagella on Legionnaires' disease bacteria: An interim report, *Ann. Intern. Med.* **91:**224–226.
27. Elliott, J. A., and Johnson, W., 1981, Immunological and biochemical relationships among flagella isolated from *Legionella pneumophila* serogroups 1, 2, and 3, *Infect. Immun.* **33:**602–610.
28. Horwitz, M. A., and Silverstein, S. C., 1981, Interaction of the Legionnaires' disease bacterium *(Legionella pneumophila)* with human phagocytes. Antibody promotes binding of *L. pneumophila* to monocytes but does not inhibit intracellular multiplication, *J. Exp. Med.* **153:**398–406.
29. Glavin, F. L., Winn, W. C., and Craighead, J. E., 1979, Ultrastructure of lung of Legionnaires' disease, *Ann. Intern. Med.* **90:**555–559.
30. Swanson, M. S., and Isberg, R. R., 1995, Association of *Legionella pneumophila* with the macrophage endoplasmic reticulum, *Infect. Immun.* **63:**3609–3620.
31. Horwitz, M. A., and Silverstein, S. C., 1980, Legionnaires' disease bacterium *(Legionella pneumophila)* multiplies intracellularly in human monocytes, *J. Clin. Invest.* **66:**441–450.
32. Horwitz, M. A., and Silverstein, S. C., 1981, Activated human monocytes inhibit the intracellular multiplication of Legionnaires' disease bacteria, *J. Exp. Med.* **154:**1618–1635.
33. Plouffe, J. F., and Baird, I. M., 1981, Lymphocyte transformation to *Legionella pneumophila, J. Clin. Lab. Immunol.* **5:**149–152.
34. Plouffe, J. F., and Baird, I. M., 1982, Lymphocyte blastogenic responses to *L. pneumophila* in acute legionellosis, *J. Clin. Lab. Immunol.* **7:**43–44.

35. Horwitz, M. A., 1983, Cell-mediated immunity in Legionnaires' disease, *J. Clin. Invest.* **71:**1686–1697.

36. Bhardwaj, N., Nash, T. W., and Horwitz, M. A., 1986, Interferon-γ-activated human monocytes inhibit the intracellular multiplication of *Legionella pneumophila*, *J. Immunol.* **137:**2662–2669.

37. Romagnani, S., 1997, The Th1/Th2 paradigm, *Immunol. Today* **18:**263–266.

38. Berendt, R. F., Young, H. W., Allen, R. G., and Knutsen, G. L., 1980, Dose–response of guinea pigs experimentally infected with aerosols of *Legionella pneumophila*, *J. Infect. Dis.* **141:**186–192.

39. Rolstad, B., and Berdal, B. P., 1981, Immune defenses against *Legionella pneumophila* in rats, *Infect. Immun.* **32:**805–812.

40. Baskerville, A., Fitzgeorge, R. B., Conlan, J. W., Ashworth, L. A. E., Gibson, D. H., and Morgan, C. P., 1983, Studies on protective immunity to aerosol challenge with *Legionella pneumophila*, *Zbl. Bakt. Hyg.* **255:**150–155.

41. Eisenstein, T. K., Tamada, R., Meissler, J., Flesher, A., and Oels, H. C., 1984, Vaccination against *Legionella pneumophila:* Serum antibody correlates with protection induced by heat-killed or acetone-killed cells against intraperitoneal but not aerosol infection in guinea pigs, *Infect. Immun.* **45:**685–691.

42. Friedman, H., Widen, R., Klein, T., Searls, L., and Cabrian, K., 1984, *Legionella pneumophila*-induced blastogenesis of murine lymphoid cells *in vitro*, *Infect. Immun.* **43:**314–319.

43. Friedman, H., Widen, R., Klein, T. W., and Johnson, W., 1984, Immunostimulation by *Legionella pneumophila* antigen preparations *in vivo* and *in vitro*, *Infect. Immun.* **43:**347–352.

44. Wong, K. H., McMaster, P. R. B., Feeley, J. C., Arko, R. J., Schalla, W. O., and Chandler, F. W., 1980, Detection of hypersensitivity to *Legionella pneumophila* in guinea pigs by skin test, *Curr. Microbiol.* **4:**105–110.

45. Friedman, H., Widen, R., Lee, I., and Klein, T., 1983, Cellular immunity to *Legionella pneumophila* in guinea pigs assessed by direct and indirect migration inhibition reactions *in vitro*, *Infect. Immun.* **41:**1132–1137.

46. Klein, T. W., Friedman, H., and Widen, R., 1984, Relative potency of virulent versus avirulent *Legionella pneumophila* for induction of cell-mediated immunity, *Infect. Immun.* **44:**753–755.

47. Breiman, R. F., and Horwitz, M. A., 1987, Guinea pigs sublethally infected with aerosolized *Legionella pneumophila* develop humoral and cell-mediated immune responses and are protected against lethal aerosol challenge, *J. Exp. Med.* **164:**799–811.

48. Blander, S. J., and Horwitz, M. A., 1991, Vaccination with the major secretory protein of *Legionella* induces humoral and cell-mediated immune responses and protective immunity across different serogroups of *Legionella pneumophila* and different species of *Legionella*, *J. Immunol.* **147:**285–291.

49. Blander, S. J., and Horwitz, M. A., 1993, Major cytoplasmic membrane protein of *Legionella pneumophila*, a genus common antigen and member of the hsp60 family of heat shock proteins, induces protective immunity in a guinea pig model of Legionnaires' disease, *J. Clin. Invest.* **91:**717–723.

50. Hoffman, P. S., Butler, C. A., and Quinn, F. D., 1989, Cloning and temperature-dependent expression in *Escherichia coli* of a *Legionella pneumophila* gene coding for a genus-common 60-kilodalton antigen, *Infect. Immun.* **57:**1731–1739.

51. Hoffman, P. S., Houston, L., and Butler, C. A., 1990, *Legionella pneumophila htpAB* heat shock operon: Nucleotide sequence and expression of the 60-kilodalton antigen in *L. pneumophila*-infected HeLa cells, *Infect. Immun.* **58:**3380–3387.

52. Hoffman, P. S., Seyer, J. H., and Butler, C. A., 1992, Molecular characterization of the 28- and 31-kilodalton subunits of the *Legionella penumophila* major outer membrane protein, *J. Bacteriol.* **174:**908–913.

53. Hoffman, P. S., Ripley, M., and Weeratna, R., 1992, Cloning and nucleotide sequencing of a

gene *(ompS)* encoding the major outer membrane protein of *Legionella pneumophila*, *J. Bacteriol.* **174:**914–920.

54. Constant, S. L., and Bottomly, K., 1997, Induction of TH1 and TH2 CD4⁺ T cell responses: The alternative approaches, *Annu. Rev. Immunol.* **15:**297–322.

55. Scott, D. E., Agranovich, I., Inman, J., Gober, M., and Golding, B., 1997, Inhibition of primary and recall allergen-specific T helper cell type 2-mediated responses by a T helper cell type 1 stimulus, *J. Immunol.* **159:**107–116.

56. Katz, S. M., and Poropatich, R., 1986, Susceptibility of LSH hamsters to intraperitoneal inoculation with *Legionella pneumophila*, *Ann. Clin. Lab. Sci.* **16:**62–66.

57. Skerrett, S. J., and Martin, T. R., 1991, Alveolar macrophage activation in experimental legionellosis, *J. Immunol.* **147:**337–345.

58. Yamamoto, Y., Klein, T. W., Newton, C. A., Widen, R., and Friedman, H., 1987, Differential growth of *Legionella pneumophila* in guinea pig versus mouse marcrophage cultures, *Infect. Immun.* **55:**1369–1374.

59. Yamamoto, Y., Klein, T. W., Newton, C. A., Widen, R., and Friedman, H., 1988, Growth of *Legionella pneumophila* in thioglycollate-elicited peritoneal macrophages from A/J mice, *Infect. Immun.* **56:**370–375.

60. Yamamoto, Y., Klein, T. W., Brown, K., and Friedman, H., 1992, Differential morphologic and metabolic alterations in permissive versus nonpermissive murine macrophages infected with *Legionella pneumophila*, *Infect. Immun.* **60:**3231–3237.

61. Yamamoto, Y., Klein, T. W., and Friedman, H., 1992, Genetic control of macrophage susceptibility to infection by *Legionella pneumophila*, *FEMS Microbiol. Immunol.* **89:**137–146.

62. Yoshida, S., Goto, Y., Mizuguchi, Y., Nomoto, K., Skamene, E., 1991, Genetic control of natural resistance in mouse macrophages regulating intracellular *Legionella pneumophila* multiplication *in vitro*, *Infect. Immun.* **59:**428–432.

63. Miyamoto, H., Maruta, K., Ogawa, M., Beckers, M., -C., Gros, P., and Yoshida, S., 1996, Spectrum of *Legionella* species whose intracellular multiplication in murine macrophages is genetically controlled by *Lgn1*, *Infect. Immun.* **64:**1842–1845.

64. Brieland, J., Freeman, P., Kunkel, R., Chrisp, C., Hurley, M., Fantone, J., and Engleberg, C., 1994, Replicative *Legionella pneumophila* lung infection in intratracheally inoculated A/J mice. A murine model of human Legionnaires' disease, *Am. J. Pathol.* **145:**1537–1546.

65. Brieland, J., McClain, M., Heath, L., Chrisp, C., Huffnagle, G., LeGendre, M., Hurley, M., Fantone, J., and Engleberg, C., 1996, Coinoculation with *Hartmannella vermiformis* enhances replicative *Legionella pneumophila* lung infection in a murine model of Legionnaires' disease, *Infect. Immun.* **64:**2449–2456.

66. Klein, T. W., Yamamoto, Y., Brown, H. K., and Friemand, H., 1991, Interferon-γ induced resistance to *Legionella pneumophila* in susceptible A/J mouse macrophages, *J. Leuk. Biol.* **49:**98–103.

67. Yamamoto, Y., Klein, T. W., Newton, C., and Friedman, H., 1992, Differing macrophage and lymphocyte roles in resistance to *Legionella pneumophila* infection, *J. Immunol.* **148:**584–589.

68. Fujio, H., Yoshida, S., Miyamoto, H., Mitsuyama, M., and Mizuguchi, Y., 1992, Investigation of the role of macrophages and endogenous interferon-γ in natural resistance of mice against *Legionella pneumophila* infection, *FEMS Microbiol. Immunol.* **89:**183–192.

69. Newton, C. A., Klein, T. W., and Friedman, H., 1994, Secondary immunity to *Legionella pneumophila* and Th1 activity are suppressed by delta-9-tetrahydrocannabinol injection, *Infect. Immun.* **62:**4015–4020.

70. Blanchard, D. K., Djeu, J. Y., Klein, T. W., Friedman, H., and Stewart, W. E., 1987, Induction of tumor necrosis factor by *Legionella pneumophila*, *Infect. Immun.* **55:**433–437.

71. Klein, T. W., Newton, C. A., Blanchard, D. K., Widen, R., and Friedman, H., 1987, Induction of interleukin 1 by *Legionella pneumophila* antigens in mouse macrophage and human mononuclear leukocyte cultures, *Zbl. Bakt. Hyg.* **A265:**462–471.

72. Heinrich, P. C., Castell, J. V., and Andus, T., 1990, Interleukin 6 and the acute phase response, *Biochem. J.* **265**:621–636.

73. Klein, T. W., Newton, C., Widen, R., and Friedman, H., 1993, Δ⁹-Tetrahydrocannabinol injection induces cytokine-mediated mortality in mice infected with *Legionella pneumophila*, *J. Pharmacol. Exp. Ther.* **267**:635–640.

74. Blanchard, D. K., Djeu, J. Y., Klein, T. W., Friedman, H., and Stewart, W. E., 1988, Protective effects of tumor necrosis factor in experimental *Legionella pneumophila* infection of mice via acativation of PMN function, *J. Leuk. Biol.* **43**:429–435.

75. Blanchard, D. K., Friedman, H., Klein, T. W., and Djeu, J. Y., 1989, Induction of interferon-gamma and tumor necrosis factor by *Legionella pneumophila:* Augmentation of human neutrophil bactericidal activity, *J. Leuk. Biol.* **45**:538–545.

76. Arata, S., Kasai, N., Klein, T. W., and Friedman, H., 1994, *Legionella pneumophila* growth restriction and cytokine production by murine macrophages activated by a novel *Pseudomonas* lipid A, *Infect. Immun.* **62**:729–732.

77. Matsiota-Bernard, P., Lefebre, C., Sedqui, M., Cornillet, P., and Guenoubou, M., 1993, Involvement of tumor necrosis factor alpha in intracellular multiplication of *Legionella pneumophila* in human monocytes, *Infect. Immun.* **61**:4980–4983.

78. Brieland, J. K., Remick, D. G., Freeman, P. T., Hurley, M. C., Fantone, J. C., and Engleberg, N. C., 1995, *In vivo* regulation of replicative *Legionella pneumophila* lung infection by endogenous tumor necrosis factor alpha and nitric oxide, *Infect. Immun.* **63**:3253–3258.

79. Skerett, S. J., and Martin, T. R., 1996, Roles for tumor necrosis factor alpha and nitric oxide in resistance of rat alveolar macrophages to *Legionella pneumophila*, *Infect. Immun.* **64**:3236–3242.

80. Yamamoto, Y., Klein, T. W., and Friedman, H., 1996, Immunoregulatory role of nitric oxide in *Legionella pneumophila*-infected macrophages, *Cell. Immunol.* **171**:231–239.

81. Widen, R. H., Newton, C. A., Klein, T. W., and Friedman, H., 1991, *Legionella pneumophila*-induced IL-1: Responses of murine peritoneal, splenic, and pulmonary macrophages, *Curr. Microbiol.* **22**:143–149.

82. Yamamoto, Y., Klein, T. W., Tomioka, M., and Friedman, H., 1997, Differential effects of granulocyte/macrophage colony-stimulating factor (GM-CSF) in enhancing macrophage resistance to *Legionella pneumophila* vs *Candida albicans*, *Cell. Immunol.* **176**:75–81.

83. McHugh, S. L., Newton, C. A., Yamamoto, Y., Widen, R., Friedman, H., and Klein, T. W., 1999, Tumor necrosis factor is a primary cytokine in controlling replication of *Legionella pneumophila* in A/J macrophage cultures, *Infect. Immun.* (submitted)

84. Blanchard, D. K., Klein, T. W., Friedman, H., and Stewart, W. E., 1985, Kinetics and characterization of interferon production by murine spleen cells stimulated with *Legionella pneumophila* antigens, *Infect. Immun.* **49**:719–723.

85. Blanchard, D. K., Stewart, W. E., Klein, T. W., Friedman, H., and Djeu, J. Y., 1987, Cytolytic activity of human peripheral blood leukocytes against *Legionella pneumophila*-infected monocytes: Characterization of the effector cell and augmentation by interleukin 2, *J. Immunol.* **139**:551–556.

86. Blanchard, D. K., Friedman, H., Stewart, W. E., Klein, T. W., and Djeu, J. Y., 1988, Role of gamma interferon in induction of natural killer activity by *Legionella pneumophila in vitro* and in an experimental murine infection model, *Infect. Immun.* **56**:1187–1193.

87. Park, D. R., and Skerrett, S. J., 1996, IL-10 enhances the growth of *Legionella pneumophila* in human mononuclear phagocytes and reverses the protective effect of IFN-γ, *J. Immunol.* **157**:2528–2538.

88. Elliott, J. A., and Winn, W. C., 1986, Treatment of alveolar macrophages with cytochalasin D inhibits uptake and subsequent growth of *Legionella pneumophila*, *Infect. Immun.* **51**:31–36.

89. Yamamoto, Y., Okubo, S., Klein, T. W., Onozaki, K., Saito, T., and Friedman, H., 1994, Binding of *Legionella pneumophila* to macrophages increases cellular cytokine mRNA, *Infect. Immun.* **62**:3947–3956.

90. Yamamoto, Y., Retzlaff, C., He, P., Klein, T. W., and Friedman, H., 1995, Quantitative reverse transcription-PCR analysis of *Legionella pneumophila*-induced cytokine mRNA in different macrophage populations by high-performance liquid chromatography, *Clin. Diagn. Lab. Immunol.* **2:**18–24.

91. Yamamoto, Y., Klein, T. W., and Friedman, H., 1996, Induction of cytokine granulocyte-macrophage colony-stimulating factor and chemokine macrophage inflammatory protein 2 mRNAs in macrophages by *Legionella pneumophila* or *Salmonella typhimurium* attachment requires different ligand–receptor systems, *Infect. Immun.* **64:**3062–3068.

92. Retzlaff, C., Yamamoto, Y., Hoffman, P. S., Friedman, H., and Klein, T. W., 1994, Bacterial heat shock proteins directly induce cytokine mRNA and interleukin-1 secretion in macrophage cultures, *Infect. Immun.* **62:**5689–5693.

93. Retzlaff, C., Yamamoto, Y., Okubo, S., Hoffman, P. S., Friedman, H., and Klein, T. W., 1996, *Legionella pneumophila* heat-shock protein-induced increase of interleukin-1B mRNA involves protein kinase C signalling in macrophages, *Immunol.* **89:**281–288.

94. Kitsukawa, K., Nakamoto, A., Koito, H., Matsuda, Y., Saito, A., and Yamamoto, H., 1995, Interferon-gamma (IFNγ) production by human T lymphocytes upon *Legionella pneumophila* stimulation *in vitro*, *Clin. Exp. Immunol.* **99:**76–81.

95. Newton, C. A., Widen, R., Friedman, H., and Klein, T. W., 1995, Lymphocyte subset changes following primary and secondary infection of mice with *Legionella pneumophila*, *Immunol. Infect. Dis.* **5:**18–26.

10

The Infectious/Pathogenic Processes Driven by *Listeria monocytogenes* in Laboratory Mice

G. MILON, M. LEBASTARD, and M.-B. HEVIN

1. INTRODUCTORY REMARKS

The term *infectious* or *parasitic* disease is used to define a local or systemic pathological state triggered by either viral, bacterial, fungal, or parasitic organisms in the hosts they have passively or actively invaded. Whereas parasites, viruses, and some bacteria, such as *Mycobacterium tuberculosis*, strictly depend on "their hosts" to achieve their so-called life cycle, other bacterial and fungal microorganisms are entirely independent of animal hosts for proliferation. For example, *Listeria monocytogenes* are Gram-positive bacteria commonly detected in the external environment, where they live as extracellular organisms.[1]

Thus, when *L. monocytogenes* are isolated from patients in whom local and/or systemic pathogenic processes do develop, they are recognized as "opportunistic bacteria."[1] Many different clinical syndromes are initiated by *L. monocytogenes* in humans who ingested heavily contaminated foods. Invasion by *L. monocytogenes* may take place at different sites along the digestive tract from its upper part to the intestines.[1] Once *Listeria* are released within the blood, the various tissues, namely the liver, the spleen, the brain, and the uteroplacental unit, can be invaded. In these sites the bacteria multiply rapidly. Steady-state conditions in the tissues

G. MILON, M. LEBASTARD, and M.-B. HEVIN • Unité d'Immunophysiologie Cellulaire, Institut Pasteur, 75724 Paris-Cedex 15, France.

Opportunistic Intracellular Bacteria and Immunity, edited by Lois J. Paradise *et al.* Plenum Press, New York, 1999.

are disturbed, leading to the development of short-term acute infectious/-inflammatory processes that first require urgent antibiotherapy and that would optimally require targeted antiinflammatory interventions. Human listeriosis remains a rare disease affecting mainly individuals with immune dysfunctions: systemic immune deficiency such as that triggered by leukemia, immunosuppressive interventions, or more local, naturally depressed immune functions such as those occurring within the uteroplacental unit in pregnant women.[1,2]

Laboratory mice are an invaluable resource for dissecting the different steps of *L. monocytogenes*–mammalian host interactions. Compared to domestic animals (such as cattle, and sheep, which develop listeriosis), laboratory mice are easy to handle in tightly controlled conditions at a relatively reasonable cost. In addition, many mouse genes have been assigned to specific chromosomal locations. Many of these genes are now known to operate at one or another step of (1) the development or (2) the expression of the constitutive and/or inducible functions of the immune system, that is, the multifocal systems that *L. monocytogenes* encounter when translocating from the digestive tract lumen to the extraintestinal tissues of their experimental hosts.[3]

The first cell populations that Mackaness used for studying the mechanisms of acquired resistance of mice to *L. monocytogenes* were"resident" and "activated" mouse macrophages. Nevertheless, considering the natural routes of entry and dissemination, many additional eucaryotic cells were expected to be and indeed are also host cells through which they translocate and/or wherein they multiply, including enterocytes and maybe the enterocyte-related M cells,[4] hepatocytes, endothelial cells, and later on during the infectious process, likely the epithelial cells of the choroid plexus within the central nervous system.[5]

2. PATHOGENIC PROCESSES DRIVEN BY INTRACELLULAR BACTERIA: GENERAL CONSIDERATIONS AND THE POSITION OF *L. MONOCYTOGENES*[6-11]

In the rapidly moving field of the analysis of bacterial pathogenesis, there is a need to consider both the infectious and pathogenic processes initiated by the bacteria under study, that is, (1) their local or systemic nature, (2) their duration, and (3) their connections with both the constitutive and inducible immune systems, as well as consequences of those on the fitness (persistence of the bacteria as live organisms). In addition, there is a need to distinguish the requirements for immunological resolution of the primary processes compared to the requirements for preventing a secondary infectious/pathogenic process from occurring or for rapidly stopping it, if the host is reexposed to the microorganisms under study. Within such a context, *L. monocytogenes* are "model" intracellular bacteria that remain relevant to study some of the processes they trigger within the host. Not only can they be used as models for studying early steps that are common to other intracellular bacteria able to exploit the machinery of resident mononuclear phagocytes for their growth/survival, but their use also offers new stimulating approaches for deciphering the biology of their host cells.[12] Nevertheless, there is a major restriction to the use of *L. monocytogenes* as model intracellular bacteria when addressing the different steps related to pathogenic processes driven by those intracellular bacteria that are—like parasites *stricto sensu*—tightly dependent on one host population for their persistence as live organisms, for example, *M. tuberculosis*. Indeed, for such strictly host-dependent bacteria, there is an urgent need to address properly the complex issues of pathogenesis in the control of host-to-host transmission.[11] Considering our present understanding of the life cycle of *L. monocytogenes* in nature, these bacteria will not allow us to properly address these critical questions related to host-to-host transmission.

3. CELL INVASION AND INTRACELLULAR LIFE STYLE OF *L. MONOCYTOGENES*

L. monocytogenes shares with *Shigella flexneri*, some *Rickettsia*, and *Trypanosoma cruzi* an unusual intracellular life style. These organisms are able to escape actively from the vacuolar compartments of the cells they invade and subsequently to multiply within the cytoplasm.[13] The *Listeria* genome has proved to be relatively easy to manipulate and, as a result, studies both *in vitro* and in mice have led to the identification of several candidate genes that operate during the very early steps of the infectious cycle and partly account for the resulting pathogenic processes. Using transposon mutagenesis, several *L. monocytogenes* genes involved in cell invasion, intracellular life cycle, cell-to-cell dissemination, and pathogenesis have been identified.[13]

3.1. *L. monocytogenes* and Host Molecules Used at the Step of Tissue/Cell Invasion

The surface proteins encoded by *inl* genes of *L. monocytogenes* confer tropism for different cell types such as enterocytes and heptatocytes (perhaps endothelial cells as well as some dendritic leukoctyes) the E-cadherin is at least one of the host molecules to which these bacterial internalins bind.[14] As far as tissue invasion is concerned, it is still not known whether *Listeria* use shuttle cells such as mucosa-associated dendritic leukocytes before being delivered to the blood.

The entry of *L. monocytogenes* within mononuclear phagocytes and likely within some dendritic leukocytes (those that do not express E-cadherin) depends upon other ligand–receptor pairs. The host molecules constitutively expressed by these leukocytes and exploited by *L. monocytogenes*, are, at least, either CR3[15] and/or scavenger receptors (SRs) (SR-AI/II as well as MARCO).[16-17] Although cell wall lipotechoic acid is the ligand that accounts for the binding of the bacteria to SR, the chemical nature of the molecules or motifs of *L. monoctyogenes* that confer binding properties to CR3 directly and/or through iC3b deserves further studies.[15]

3.2. The Intracellular Life Style and Cell-to-Cell Dissemination of *L. monocytogenes*

Once internalized, *L. monocytogenes* transiently resides within a vacuole, the characteristics of which have been clarified in only a limited number of cell types, namely mouse bone marrow derived macrophages[18] and J774-E.[19] This vacuole becomes acidified, allowing the bacteria to escape into the cytosol. This is achieved by the production of and activity of listeriolysin O (LLO) under the control of the *hly* gene.[13]

Within the cytosol, *L. monocytogenes* start to divide while moving at the tip of dynamic filamentous actin, the initial nucleation of which is under the control of the Acta protein that the *Listeria* export within the cytosol. This bacterial protein is able to direct the assembly of host cell actin and actin-binding proteins on the bacterial cell surface.[20] *Listeria* "riding on a comet" of actin filaments, form a projection when they reach the plasma membrane.[20] The neighboring cell can "phagocytose" these projections, thus becoming infected in the process. Secretion of lecithinase and phospholipase C by the bacteria results in lysis of the double membrane and release of bacteria into the cytosol.[13] Once in the cytosol, the process of intracytosolic replication and active movement begins again. All the *L. monocytogenes* genes mentioned earlier are optimally expressed at 37°C.[21]

4. THE IMMUNE SYSTEM: ITS CONSTITUTIVE AND INDUCIBLE ELEMENTS AND THE PROCESSES OF ITS REACTIVITY[22-24]

The immune system consists of resident and mobile cell populations whose functions are either constitutive (e.g., phagocytosis, recirculation) or more or less rapidly inducible (e.g., cytokine upregulation). The inducible functions could be triggered (1) very rapidly by any exogenous, signaling molecules acting on cells expressing constitutively the receptors that bind these signaling molecules (e.g., pattern recognition receptors that bind their ligands) or (2) more slowly because they result from a series of cell–cell interactions occurring in different locations from the lymphoid organs to the nonlymphoid compartments.

Thus, immune system reactivity is a dynamic process the basis and the regulation of which, under normal conditions, occur as a tightly controlled cascade of events involving (1) the constitutive renewal of mononuclear phagocytes known to reside in every tissue; (2) the constitutive renewal of neutrophils known to be transiently stored within the bone marrow exravascular compartment marginated along microvessels, or circulating within the blood vessels; (3) the still poorly understood production of natural killer (NK) and natural T (NT) cells;[22] (4) the constitutive sustained recirculation of both naive T and B lymphocytes between the blood and lymphoid organs using the still poorly defined lymphatic vasculature; and (5) the constitutive renewal of dendritic leukocytes that transiently operate as T-cell-stimulating leukocytes.[23][24] In considering T-cell expansion and differentiation, three issues have to be considered: (1) the generation of the ligands of their T cell receptor (TCR), (2) the conditions required for their activation by dendritic leukocytes, and (3) the pattern of cytokines they will be committed to produce once they will be reactivated. Indeed, it is now well documented that γδ T cells, CD4 and CD8 lymphocytes, can either be committed to secrete simultaneously many cytokines (type 0 pathway of differentiation), or committed to synthesize and to secrete type 1 [interleukin-2 (IL-2), interferon-γ (IFN-γ), tumor necrosis factor (TNF)] or type 2 (IL-4, IL-5, IL-10, IL-13) cytokines.[25,26]

Altogether these leukocytes and endothelial cells, their constitutive as well as inducible products (transmembrane or soluble cosignaling molecules such as cytokines and chemokines[27]) orchestrate the body's response to invading microorganisms through coordinated integrated mechanisms connecting constitutive and inducible elements of the immune system.[22]

5. THE KNOWN AND HYPOTHETICAL INFECTIOUS/PATHOGENIC PROCESSES DRIVEN BY *L. MONOCYTOGENES:* THEIR GENERAL AND UNIQUE CHARACTERISTICS

Within the field of bacterial pathogenesis, *L. monocytogenes* present a number of unique peculiarities. (1) As mentioned, they do not depend upon the hosts for persisting as living populations; (2) once ingested with contaminated food, they pass through the digestive tract lumen without triggering any inflammatory/pathogenic processes or immunological responses; and (3) their ability to initiate pathogenic processes, whether local (gastroenteritis) or systemic, is related to their ability to interact with the intestinal wall, to pass through the intestinal wall, and to reach the blood, a compartment from which they are first cleared by blood-filtering organs such as the liver, the spleen, and the bone marrow. The two last tissues are highly structured microenvironments in which the critical cell–cell interactions occur that lead to the production of immune effectors[22] and the renewal of blood cells, respectively.[28] If *L. monocytogenes* are not retained within the tissue of entry (digestive tract) and/or within the three tissues mentioned previously, a second wave of *L. monocytogenes* could be released into the blood. These bacteria are now able to invade tissues such as the brain and the uteroplacental unit, most likely as a consequence of the transient systemic release of cytokines known to act on endothelial cells of the microvasculature, including the blood–brain barrier.[5,29,30] While considering this later issue, again it is important to appreciate the needs for careful dissection of the sequence of events triggered either locally or systemically by the bacteria. These events are inducible synthesis of cytokines such as IL-12, TNF-α, IFN-α, -β, IL-6, IFN-γ, and chemokines, that together, within a complex network still to be clearly delineated, transiently change otherwise quiescent resident cells such as endothelial cells of macro- as well as microvessels, either locally or systemically. Thus, as intracellular bacteria, *L. monocytogenes* transiently exploit/subvert many host cells and molecules. The production of these host components is either constitutive, transiently inducible directly or indirectly by the live *Listeria* themselves, or through *Listeria*- derived products of their cell walls such as lipotechoic acid and peptidoglycan. Compared to other so-called facultative intracellular bacteria such as *Salmonella* spp., *L. monocytogenes* (once outside the digestive tract lumen, i.e., once released within the blood) trigger acute, short-term processes the resolution of which is achieved in 8 to 9 days in immunocompetent hosts,[3] pointing out the ability of the "hosts" to set up counterinflammatory processes rapidly. The molecular basis of these still deserves more studies. At present, at least IL-10 as well as "processed TGF-β1" will be the next cytokines for active study within such a context.[31]

6. THE INFECTIOUS/PATHOGENIC PROCESSES INITIATED BY THE INTRAVENOUS INOCULATION OF LETHAL OR SUBLETHAL DOSES OF *L. MONOCYTOGENES* TO LABORATORY MICE: METHODOLOGICAL ISSUES

6.1. The Laboratory Mice

Many inbred strains with known genetic features are available and allow precise genetic studies.[32] In addition, the ability to disrupt specific gene sequences by homologous recombination offers a powerful new tool to specify the role(s) of a given gene in infectious/pathogenic processes and related immune system reactivity, whether the latter reflects the functions of the innate or of the adaptive immune system. The availability and production of recombinant inbred strains and of recombinant congenic strains is also useful for mapping the gene(s) that could be participating in this bacteria–host interaction.

6.2. The Analysis of Virulence and Pathogenicity Processes in Experimental Systems: Readout Assays

Before proceeding, it is necessary to define the terms virulence and pathogenicity. Operationally, the *virulence* of microorganisms is quantified by the size of the dose required to infect (ID_{50}) or to kill (LD_{50}) 50% of the challenged laboratory mice. The terms virulence and pathogenicity are used interchangeably by many colleagues because while defining the molecular determinants of virulence, they include (1) the host and tissue specificity of the invading microorganisms (2) the nature of its "host dependence" (extracellular or intracellular life style) and (3) but still too rarely, the nature and extent of damage they directly or indirectly exert in the different host tissues they reach. Point (3) of the above definition actually refers to *pathogenicity*, that is, the ability of the microorganisms to disturb more or less severely the homeostasis of the tissues they reached, and where they create microenvironments in which they multiply, and/or from which they spread.

6.3. The Infectious Process: Operational Definition

The infectious process is monitored by estimating the load of live bacteria (colony-forming unit CFUs/tissue) recovered from tissues under study at different time points after inoculation of live *L. monocytogenes;* different doses of *L. monocytogenes* are given, lethal as well as sublethal ones. Another way to assess the infectious process is to determine the lethal dose in genetically different mice, an assessment generally translated by the LD_{50}, at a given period whatever the routes of inoculation, the most commonly used until recently being the intravenous route.

6.4. The Pathogenic Process: Operational Definition

The pathogenic process is less frequently addressed, except for signs such as aspect of the fur and decreased access to food and water no other clinical signs are systemically and carefully monitored. When the blood compartment is monitored, in addition to the transiently increased number of monocytes and the increased level of hepatic transaminases (a sign of hepatic damage), plasma and tissue bioactive or immunoreactive cytokines have been followed. IFN-α, -β, TNF-α, IL-6, IFN-γ, IL-10, and IL-12 have been the most regularly studied.[33,34]

It is important to note that the follow-up of cytokines has to be done very early after intravenous injection of *L. monocytogenes* (0 to 48 h). In addition, plasma level of these inflammatory cytokines strictly depends upon the initial size of the inoculum, the larger inoculum being the most effective one, and on the genetic background of the mice.[33]

6.5. New Tools and Reagents for Properly Addressing the Tissue-Dependent Pathogenic Processes Driven by *L. monocytogenes* in Mice

Although still too rare, data do document the existence of unique regulation of pathogen-driven processes depending on the steady-state properties of the tissue under study. Thus, there is an urgent need to properly address such issues by designing new readout assays such as *ex vivo* and *in situ* analysis, based on computerized imaging techniques.[35,36]

6.5.1. Manipulations of Laboratory Mice

6.5.1a. Nongenetic Manipulations. While Van Roijen *et al.* have carefully analyzed the optimal conditions for depleting resident mononuclear phagocytes of spleen and liver,[37] Rosen *et al.* have devised *in vitro* relevant adhesion assays for generating new monoclonal antibodies screened for inhibition of adhesive properties to substrata.[38] In brief, when given intravenously, multilamellar chlodronate liposomes are taken up by Küpffer cells and marginal zone macrophages of the spleen, allowing one to monitor the effect of depletion of these cell populations on the early fate of *L. monocytogenes*.[39] Once the rat monoclonal antibody 5C6 screened and raised by Rosen *et al.* was shown to immunoprecipitate mouse β2 integrin CR3, it was seen to be a powerful tool for preventing neutrophil and monocyte recruitment in many —although not all—inflammatory sites,[38] allowing studies to stress the role of neutrophils in the early containment of *L. monocytogenes* within the liver[34] for a review. It will be very important to properly screen other monoclonal antibodies using functional assays, for generating new tools. Inoculation of these reagents prior to or during the *L. monocytogenes* driven processes will be very helpful in delineating some of the events occurring within the unique architectural framework of the complex tissues invaded by this and other bacteria.

6.5.1b. Genetic Manipulations. As previously mentioned, with the development of gene cloning/sequencing and also of embryonic stem (ES) cell technology in the mouse, and with the advent of homologous recombination, it is now possible to inactivate, replace, or introduce subtle alterations to the endogenous genes of interest.[32] The resulting, mice which are homozygous for the genetic change, if still viable and maintained in specific pathogen-free conditions represent laboratory hosts for studying the host-gene-dependent processes driven by an exogenous live organisms such as *L. monocytogenes*. Of particular note is targeted transgenesis, as well as the more recently introduced conditional gene targeting, which also will be powerful additions to the currently available technology. *L. monocytogenes* are used as model bacteria to monitor the phenotypic characteristics of the absence of a given gene[40] or the presence of transgenes[41] as an example).

6.5.2. Quantitation of Transcripts of Cytokines, Chemokines, Adhesive/cosignaling Transmembrane Molecules. Immunocytochemistry and in Situ Hybridization on Tissue Sections

Progress in isolating genes and their products has also allowed production of numerous reagents such as oligonucleotide probes, primers, and monoclonal antibodies, rendering possible many *in vivo* and *ex vivo* studies. But curiously, very few studies so far are based on quantitative methods such as quantitative reverse-transcription polymerase chain reaction (RT-PCR)[42] to monitor cytokine and chemokine transcripts. Although microscopic computerized imaging of properly stained tissue sections is now available, its use for dissecting bacteria–host interactions is still too limited.[35,36]

6.5.3. Isolation of Extravascular Leukocytes from Nonlymphoid Tissues Such as the Liver

Characteristics of the processes driven by microorganisms are dependent on where they reside, reflecting the steady state and reactivity of the tissue they reach and where they establish the infectious/pathogenic processes. Within such a context, to have access to nonlymphoid tissues such as the liver[43] or the dermis[44] can be an interesting resource for getting qualitative as well as quantitative information on the dynamic nature of the processes driven by the microorganisms under study. Some methods are now available for addressing these issues. When they do not require any enzymatic digestion, they allow preparation of leukocytes in conditions suitable for direct phenotypic and *in vivo* as well as *in vitro* functional analyses, once the tissue has been properly perfused[43] or processed.[44]

7. THE PATHOGENESIS OF THE PROCESSES DRIVEN BY *L. MONOCYTOGENES* GIVEN INTRAVENOUSLY TO LABORATORY MICE

Vertebrates function through a complex of specialized interactive organs connected through *vascular beds* (blood as well as lymphatic vascular beds), which can act as routes for delivery of infectious/pathogenic organisms such as *L. monocytogenes*. Until now, the only one to which there is an easy access, at least in mice, remains the blood vascular bed.

7.1. The Blood-Filtering Tissues: Their Unique Features in Steady-State Conditions

7.1.1. The Liver and the Connected Lymphoid Tissues

The study of hepatogenesis during development as well as the study of hepatic regeneration allows us to understand the unique microarchitecture of the liver. In the hepatic lobule structured around fenestrated sinusoids (i.e., fenestrated endothelial cells without basement membrane) reside hepatocytes, the space of Disse being a loose extracellular matrix (ECM) where also reside or are slowly renewed Ito cells/NK cells and γδ T cells. Within sinusoids also reside Küpffer cells that represent the liver resident macrophages of the heterogenous mononuclear phagocyte system.

In addition, it recently became clear that dendritic leukocytes are also present within the liver.[45] Whether these leukocytes, once loaded with *L. monocytogenes*, will be mobilized in the draining celiac lymph nodes[46] and will be able to immunostimulate naive CD4 and CD8 T cells deserves studies, especially in the context of their ability to drive T cells along a type 1 differentiation pathway.

7.1.2. *The Spleen: A Complex Organ*[47]

The structure of the spleen varies between species. For example, ellipsoids otherwise known as the cord of Billroth are seen in the dog, cat, and chicken but not in rodents, which have marginal zones instead. The human spleen has both ellipsoids and marginal zones, the latter being located adjacent to periarterial lymphatic sheaths in continuation from terminals of central arteries. The pulp of the mouse spleen is divided into (1) white pulp consisting of lymphocytes (packed periarteriolar sheath, lymphoid follicle, and marginal zone) and (2) red pulp, which is composed of the splenic sinus and splenic cord and that surrounds the white pulp. The splenic sinus is not highly developed in the mouse spleen. In steady-state conditions, the relationship between the structure of the vascular bed and function remains one of the most debated problems, although the blood flow into the marginal zone and red pulp as well as its functional implications are critical points for consideration when studying the outcome of *L. monocytogenes* infection. Indeed, in steady-state conditions, the marginal zone is still regarded as an important passageway in which the disposal and/or distribution of exogenous substances or modified endogenous elements occur within the extravascular compartment. Thus, the spleen is recognized as an organ with both (1) a blood filtering/clearing function and (2) an immune function, two functions reflected in its complex vascular architecture. The blood either ends in sinuses of the marginal zone (MZ) where MOMA-2- and MARCO[17,47]-positive mononuclear phagocytes lie, or directly into the red pulp where sit F4/80-positive mononuclear phagocytes.[47] The lymphoid compartment, the white pulp, is the area where T and B lymphocytes constitutively recirculate/express their inducible program once they have left the blood at the level of the marginal zone.[47] Curiously, our present understanding of the entry of T and B cells within the white pulp extracellular matrix is still very poor. In other words, we do still ignore the number and nature of the ligand/counter ligands used by lymphocytes and cells of the marginal zone that allow T and B lymphocytes to exravasate from the blood and to migrate transiently within the T and B cell domains of the white pulp. In brief, the vascular addressin mucosaladdressin cell adhesive molecule-1 (MadCAM-1), a ligand used by T and B lymphocytes to recirculate within the mucosal immune system, is now known to be expressed on sinus endothelial lining cells in the marginal zone.[48] But it was recently shown that the absence of MadCAM-1 does not lead to recognizable alterations of the white pulp and the red pulp domains in steady-state conditions, thus it is necessary to search for other molecules present on resident cells within the marginal zone. Along that line, the MZ metallophil macrophages[47] that contact the white pulp side were, reasonably, considered as critical cells with which T and B lymphocytes can transiently interact before their further segregation toward T- and B-cell zones. This hypothesis was addressed following the elegant studies of Crocker et al.[49] documenting the presence of sialoadhesin on MOMA-1-positive metallophilic macrophages. This member of the immunoglobulin superfamily was first identified through functional criteria, namely the ability to bind sialic acid expressed by glycolipids of myeloid cells.[49] Later on, using the frozen mouse spleen section assay, T- and B-cell lines were shown to bind to these metallophilic macrophages through sialoadhesin, indicating that sialoadhesin could be one of the molecules involved in recirculation of T and B lymphocytes within the spleen.[50]

7.1.3. The Bone Marrow[51]

The hemopoietic cells (progenitors as well as differentiated cells) populate extravascular spaces between large venous sinusoids lying within a network of stromal cells and exracellular matrix components. Stromal cells include fibroblasts, endothelial cells, and macrophages. The stromal macrophages are uniformly distributed from the endosteum to the sinusoids and have elongated dendrites projecting within the sinusoid lumen, rendering it possible for their phagocytic functions to be expressed toward microorganisms present/released within the blood compartment. These stromal macrophages were the cells where the presence of sialoadhesin was first recognized,[49] allowing recognition that stromal macrophages residing within the bone marrow coexpress many different functions, such as phagocytosis as well as the ability to bind developing myeloid cells.

7.2. L. monocytogenes within Blood-Filtering Tissues: The Transient Pathogenic Processes Driven in the Spleen and Liver and their Connection with the Immune System Reactivity

7.2.1. Early Distribution of L. monocytogenes within the Liver, Spleen, and Bone Marrow

Following intravenous inoculation, L. monocytogenes are first found predominantly in those tissues containing large numbers of resident mononuclear phagocytes that are known to act as "filters of blood-borne pathogens," such as the liver, spleen, bone marrow, and, to a much lesser extent, the lungs. Within the liver, the very first cells to be invaded are the Küpffer cells, and about 80% of the overall bacterial load is found within these phagocytic cells within 30 min.

The other 20% are taken up mainly by the spleen and by the bone marrow if a large inoculum is injected. It is important to note that these populations of resident mononuclear phagocytes, especially those in the bone marrow, are much less susceptible to cytokine activation than the populations of young monocytes, which are more or less rapidly recruited in the *L. monocytogenes*-loaded microenvironments.

7.2.2. *The Complex Processes Driven in the Spleen*[52-54]

Within the spleen, bacteria are disseminated via the marginal sinus blood vessel and are rapidly taken up into marginal zone macrophages, that is, those macrophages contacting the red pulp domain.[47] The MOMA-1 positive/sialoadhesin-positive metallophilic macrophages, in contact with the external domain of the white pulp, do not appear to become infected following a sublethal inoculum, but further studies will be necessary concerning the distribution of the MARCO molecule (a member of the SR family) on some metallophilic macrophages.[17] That binding of *Listeria* to marginal zone macrophages is most probably mediated via scavenger receptors (SRA-I/II) on the cell surface has been indirectly documented recently using SRA-I/II KO mice.[55] It is interesting to note that we still do not know which cells within the white pulp of the *Listeria*-loaded spleen trigger/activate the *Listeria*-reactive CD8 and CD4 T lymphocytes. One reasonable candidate cell population is those immature dendritic leukocytes that sit transiently among the metallophilic macrophages and that are capable of phagocytosing *L. monocytogenes;* these cells can be mobilized within the T-cell-dependent area of the white pulp. It will be important to study carefully *in vivo* the outcome of viable *L. monocytogenes* within such dendritic leukocytes and to document the processes of listerial peptide loading of their major histocompatibility complex (MHC) class I and class II molecules and the further expression of these complexes at the membrane level. One consequence of this bacterial peptide processing within the white pulp of the spleen will be the activation, clonal expansion, and differentiation of *Listeria*-reactive CD8 and CD4 lymphocytes. Such activated T lymphocytes are expected to be released into the blood and to be recruited in the nonlymphoid tissues loaded with *L. monocytogenes*, such as the liver, if they have been committed to express adhesion molecules such as CD44, VLA-4, or the red pulp compartments of the spleen.

7.2.3. *The L. monocytogenes-Loaded Liver: A Nonlymphoid Tissue in which an Orchestrated Dynamic Recruitment of Different Leukocyte Subsets Occurs*

In the liver, the pattern of the infectious/pathogenic processes and the connected immune responses, reflecting the reactivity of both the innate and adaptive immune system, have been better characterized than in the spleen. In addition to Küpffer cells, neutrophils are also involved in the early killing of *L. monocytogenes*. Indeed, if prior to intravenous inoculation of *L. monocytogenes* mice are selectively depleted of Küpffer cells and neutrophils,[37-39] the bacterial load decrease observed in infected, nondepleted mice is difficult to detect and hepatocytes are very rapidly invaded, a process followed by their apoptotic death.[34] The other concomitant or slightly delayed stage is T-cell-independent generation of IFN-γ which probably involves mononuclear phagocytes and NK cells through a complex and still incompletely understood cytokine network.[39] One theoretical scenario is the following: macrophages by releasing TNF-α and IL-12 in the presence of a low level of IL-10 activate NK cells to produce IFN-γ.[39,58]

The significance of neutrophil recruitment in the early stage of the infectious process was first clearly demonstrated by the use of monoclonal antibodies to granulocytes,[34,38,56,57] it was also documented more recently through studies in mice whose granulocyte-colony-stimulating factor (G-CSF) or IL-6 or NF-IL-6 genes had been inactivated (see ref. 40 for a review). Until now the importance of NK cells has been demonstrated only by the use of too broadly reactive antibodies, namely anti-asialo GM1 ones. Another, and more sustained, wave also consists of CR3-positive monocytes, mainly young cells recruited from the blood, together with CD4, CD8, γδ T lymphocytes. The number of CD8 T cells is particularly high, with a high percentage of the cells being reactive to peptides processed from live *L. monocytogenes* at day 6 after inoculation (Goossens, P. L., Milon, G., unpublished data). It is likely that these cells recognize LLO and other listerial proteins, such as p60. The transient rise in the population of CD8 T cells is in contrast to the more sustained wave of CD4 T cells.[58] As yet, it remains to be established if all the recruited CD4 T lymphocytes show specific reactivity to *L. monocytogenes* and what role they have in resolution of primary infectious/-pathogenic processes. Certainly, they appear, along with CD8 T cells, to be important in the protective immune response triggered by a secondary infection. The presence within the liver extravascular compartment of primed CD8 and CD4 T cells reflects (1) the commitment to differentiation of their progenitors along the type 1 pathway within the lymphoid tissues (spleen and possibly the celiac lymph nodes), and (2) their delivery to the liver where they can express cytolytic functions or transiently release type 1 cytokines, namely IFN-γ, in the absence of type 2 cytokines (IL-4, IL-10, IL-13).[59,60] By acting in an inflammatory site where type 2 cytokines are absent, the type 1 cytokines efficiently deliver unique signals to the young CR3-positive mononuclear phagocytes that are recruited within the extravascular compartment. Curiously, it is not yet clear how IFN-γ, inhibits the intracellular life cycle of *L. monocytogenes* to kill them.[61]

Finally, the role of the γδ T cells (days 7 to 8) is also of interest. Although it is known that these cells play a part in the control of bacterial growth in the very early phase of infection, recent work suggests that γδ T cells may also be involved in the recovery process, which occurs 7 to 9 days after the *L. monocytogenes* inoculation. In the absence of γδ T cells, there is an extensive late recruitment of neutrophils to the liver. This second neutrophil wave is associated with hepatic tissue necrosis. Because some γδ T cells are known to recognize nonpeptidic bacterial cell-wall components, extensive destruction of *Listeria* on days 5 to 8 of the infectious process can lead to the release of large amounts of nonpeptidic cell wall components able to drive the recruitment and activation of γδ T cells into the extravascular space, and the subsequent secretion of counter-inflammatory cytokines such as IL-10, TGF-β allowing the rapid recovery to the initial steady-state conditions.[31,62]

7.3. *L. monocytogenes* within the Central Nervous System and the Uteroplacental Unit

7.3.1. L. monocytogenes within the Central Nervous System

As stated previously, it is not yet clear where *L. monocytogenes* enter the central nervous system (plexus choroid, blood–brain barrier?), but once within the brain parenchyma, an inflammatory reaction develops. This *L. monocytogenes*-driven inflammatory process, resulting in meningitis and encephalitis, is characterized by the presence of both cellular infiltrates and a cytokine network where TNF-α, INF-α, IL-6, IL-10, IFN-γ codominate first, the last cytokine likely reflecting the regulatory network counteracting inflammatory processes that would be detrimental to the neurons and glia.

7.3.2. L. monocytogenes within the Uteroplacental unit

During pregnancy, Th2-biased immune responses seem to predominate.[65] This shift in cytokine patterns provides one explanation for the increased susceptibility to a *L. monocytogenes* infectious / pathogenic-driven process developing within the uteroplacental unit. IL-10 and TGF-β may inhibit the production and action of macrophage-activating cytokines such as IFN-γ and TNF-α that otherwise shape the antibacterial properties of the *L. monocytogenes*-loaded tissues.

8. CONCLUDING REMARKS, PERSPECTIVES

Investigations of the experimental model of *L. monocytogenes*-driven immunological processes in laboratory mice have allowed elucidation of the roles of different leukocytes and cytokines in completely clearing these intracellular bacteria. From 1960 until 1990, mainly mononuclear phagocytes, NK, and T lymphocytes were studied, with TNF-α, IFN-γ, and CD8 T lymphocytes being recognized as the critical effectors for control and resolution of the primary bacterial load. More recently, action of neutrophils was also recognized as critical, especially within the liver. By inducing (1) apoptosis of the hepatocytes they invade and (2) the subsequent release of chemokines such as MIP-2α, *L. monocytogenes* initiate a response in which neutrophils act by eliminating the dead *L. monocytogenes*-loaded hepatocytes, killing the released bacteria. Later on, an antibacterial granuloma develops in which mononuclear phagocytes interact with *Listeria*-reactive αβ and γδ T lymphocytes, resulting in bacteria clearance and tissue homeostasis recovery.

Investigations on the pathogenic processes that develop within the spleen, brain, and uteroplacental unit are still very limited compared to those recently observed for the liver. To progress in this field, it is necessary to carefully follow the precise distribution and fate of *L. monocytogenes*, a step that could be achieved by the use of GFP-based fluorescent.[3] *L. monocytogenes* (wild-type as well as mutant *L. monocytogenes*), and imaging techniques applied to tissue sections.[35,36]

ACKNOWLEDGMENTS. In 1974, when G. M. joined the Unit of Cellular Immunophysiology, she was introduced to the field of *Listeria monocytogenes*/laboratory mouse interactions by Dr. Robert M. Fauve, to whom this review is dedicated. It is a pleasure to acknowledge Institut Pasteur, DGA (Contract no. 92/153), and the European Union (Grant TS3.CT.940319); their financial support is appreciated. Without M. Dehbi, who produced high-quality laboratory mice, the analyses performed in our Unit would have never been possible. Both M. Dehbi and Mrs. C. Brulé, who carefully edited this review, are deeply thanked.

REFERENCES

1. McLauchlin, J., 1997, The pathogenicity of *Listeria monocytogenes:* A public health perspective, *Rev. Med. Microbiol.* **8:**1–14.
2. Bortolussi, R., and Schlech, W. F., 1995, Listeriosis, in: *Infectious Diseases of the Foetus and the Newborn Infant*, 4th Ed. (J. S. Remington and J. O. Klein, eds.) W. B. Saunders, Philadelphia, pp. 1055–1073.
3. Goossens, P. L., Montixi, C., Saron, M. -F., Rodriguez, M., Zavala, F., and Milon, G., 1995, *Listeria monocytogenes:* A liver vector able to deliver heterologous protein within the cytosol and to drive a CD8 dependent T cell response, *Biologicals* **23:**135–143.
4. Savidge, T. C., 1996, The life and times of an intestinal M cell, *Trends Microbiol.* **4:**301–306.
5. Tuomanen, E., 1996, Entry of pathogens into the central nervous system, *FEMS Microbiol. Rev.* **18:**289–299.
6. Finlay, B. B., and Falkow, S., 1989, Common themes in microbial pathogenicity, *Microbiol. Rev.* **53:**210–230.
7. Salyers, A. A., and Whitt, D. D., 1994, *Bacterial Pathogenesis: A Molecular Approach*, 1st Ed., American Society for Microbiology Press, Washington, D. C.
8. Mims, C. A., Dimmock, N. J., Nash, A., and Stephen, J., eds., 1995, *Mims' Pathogenesis of Infectious Disease*, 4th Ed., Academic Press, New York.

9. Theriot, J. A., 1995, The cell biology of infection by intracellular bacterial pathogens, *Ann. Rev. Cell. Dev. Biol.* **11:**213–239.

10. Guiney, D. G., and Kagnoff, M. F., 1997, Host/pathogen interactions: Series introduction. *J. Clin. Invest.* **99:**155.

11. Lipsitch, M., and Moxon, E. R., 1997, Virulence and transmissibility of pathogens what is the relationship? *Trends Microbiol.* **5:**31–37.

12. Cossart, P., Boquet, P., Normark, S., and Rappuolli, R., 1996, Cellular microbiology emerging, *Science* **271:**325–326.

13. Sheehan, B., Kocks, C., Dramsi, S., Gouin, E., Klarsfeld, A. D., Mengaud, J., and Cossart, P., 1994, Molecuar and genetic determinants of the *Listeria monocytogenes* infectious process. *Curr. Top. Microbiol. Immunol.* **192:**187–216.

14. Mengaud, J., Ohayon, H., Gounon, P., Mege, R. M., and Cossart, P., 1996, E-cadherin is the receptor for internalin, a surface protein required for entry of *L. monocytogenes* into epithelial cells. *Cell* **84:**923–932.

15. Campbell, P. A., 1993, Macrophage-*Listeria* interactions, in: *Macrophage–Pathogen Interactions* (B. S. Zwilling and T. K. Eisenstein, eds.), Marcel Dekker, New York, pp. 313.

16. Pearson, A. M., 1996, Scavenger receptors in innate immunity, *Curr. Opin. Immunol.* **8:**20–28.

17. Elomaa, O., Kangas, M., Sahlberg, C., Tuukkanen, J., Sormunen, R., Liakka, A., Thesleff, I., Kraal, G., and Tryggvason, K., 1995, Cloning of a novel bacteria-binding receptor structurally related to scavenger receptors and expressed in a subset of macrophages, *Cell* **80:**603–609.

18. De Chastellier, C., and Berche, P., 1994, Fate of *Listeria monoctyogenes* in murine macrophages: Evidence for simultaneous killing and survival of intracellular bacteria, *Infect. Immun.* **62:**543–553.

19. Alvarez-Dominguez, C., Barbieri, A. M., Beron, W., Wandinger-Ness, A., and Stahl, P. D., 1996, Phagocytosed live *Listeria monocytogenes* influences Rab-5 regulated *in vitro* phagosome-endosome fusion, *J. Biol. Chem.* **271:**13834–13843.

20. Lasa, I., and Cossart, P., 1996, Actin-based bacterial motility: Towards a definition of the minimal requirements, *Trends Cell Biol.* **6:**109–114.

21. Kreft, J., Bohne, J., Gross, R., Kestler, H., Sokolovic, Z., and Goebel, W., 1995, Control of *Listeria monocytogenes* virulence by the transcriptional regulator PrfA, in: *Signal Transduction and Bacterial Virulence* (R. Rappuoli, V. Scarloto, and B. Arico, eds.), R. G. Landes, Springer-Verlag, Austin. pp. 129–142.

22. Fearon, D. T., and Locksley, R. M., 1996, The instructive role of innate immunity in the acquired immune response, *Science* **272:**50–54.

23. Cella, M., Sallusto, F., and Lanzavecchia, A., 1997, Origin, maturation and antigen presenting function of dendritic cells, *Curr. Opin. Immunol.* **9:**10–16.

24. Schuler, G., Thurner, B., and Romani, N., 1997, Dendritic cells: From ignored cells to major players in T cell-mediated immunity, *Int. Arch. Allergy Immunol.* **112:**317–322.

25. Arai, K., Lee, F., Miyajima, A., Miyatake, S., Arai, N., and Yokota, T., 1990, Cytokines: coordinators of immune and inflammatory responses, *Annu. Rev. Biochem.* **59:**783–836.

26. Cohen, M. C., and Cohen, S., 1996, Cytokine function, a study in biological diversity, *Am. J. Clin. Pathol.* **105:**589–598.

27. Premack, B. A., and Schall, T. J., 1996, Chemokine receptors: Gateways to inflamation and infection, *Nat. Med.* **2:**1174–1178.

28. Orkin, S. H., 1996, Development of the hematopoietic system, *Curr. Opin. Genet. Div.* **6:**597–602.

29. Cserr, H. F., and Knopf, P. M., 1992, Cervical lymphatics, the blood–brain barrier and the immunoreactivity of the brain: A new view, *Immunol. Today* **13:**507–512.

30. Merril, J. E., and Benveniste, E. N., 1996, Cytokines in inflammatory brain lesions: Helpful and harmful, *TINS* **19:**331–338.

31. Ferrick, D. A., Braun, R. K., Lepper, H. D., and Schrenzel, M. D., 1996, $\gamma\delta$ T cells in bacterial infections, *Res. Immunol.* **147:**532–541.

32. Wassarman, P. M., and de Pamphilis, M. L., 1993, Guide to techniques in mouse development, in *Methods in Enzymology*, Vol. 225, Academic Press, New York.
33. Mielke, M. E. A., Ehler, S., and Hahn, H., 1993, The role of cytokines in experimental listeriosis, *Immunobiology* **189**:285-315.
34. Unanue, E. R., 1996, Macrophages, NK cells and neutrophils in the cytokine loop of *Listeria* resistance, *Res. Immunol.* **147**:449-505.
35. Björk, L., Fehniger, T. E., Andersson, U., and Andersson, J., 1996, Computerized assessment of production of multiple human cytokines at the single cell level using image analysis, *J. Leuk. Biol.* **59**:287-295.
36. Savin, V. J., and Wiegmann, T. B., 1996, New *in vivo* and *in vitro* imaging techniques, *Int. Rev. Exp. Pathol.* **36**:1-220.
37. van Rooijen, N., 1996, Selective depletion of macrophages by liposome-encapsulated drugs, in: *Weir's Handbook of Experimental Immunology*, 5th Ed., Vol. IV: *The Integrated Immune System* (L. A. Herzenberg, L. A. Herzenberg, D. M. Weir, and C. Blackwell, eds.), Blackwell Science, Cambridge, England. pp. 165/1-165/5.
38. Rosen, H., and Hugues, D. A., 1996, Migration and adhesion *in vivo:* Myeloid cells, in: *Weir's Handbook of Experimental Immunology*, 5th Ed., Vol, IV: *The Integrated Immune System* (L. A. Herzenberg, L. A. Herzenberg, D. M. Weir, and C. Blackwell, eds.), Blackwell Science, Cambridge, England. pp. 161/1-161/10.
39. Pinto, A. J., Steward, D., van Rooijen, N., and Morahan, P. S., 1991, Selective depletion of liver and splenic macrophages using liposomes encapsulating the drug dichloromethylene diphosphonate: Effects on antimicrobial resistance, *J. Leuk. Biol.* **49**:579-586.
40. Brombacher, F. and Kopf, M., 1996, Innate versus acquired immunity in listeriosis, *Res. Immunol.* **147**:505-511.
41. Garcia, I., Miyazaki, Y., Araki, K., Araki, M., Lucas, R., Grau, G. E., Milon, G., Belkaid, Y., Montixi, C., Lesslauer, W., and Vassalli, P., 1995, Transgenic mice expressing high levels of soluble TNF-R1 fusion protein are protected from lethal septic shock and cerebral malaria, and are highly sensitive to *Listeria monocytogenes* and *Leishmania major* infections, *Eur. J. Immunol.* **25**:2401-2407.
42. Pannetier, C., Delassus, S., Darche, S., Saucier, C., and Kourilsky, P., 1993, Quantitative titration of nucleic acids by enzymatic amplification reactions run to saturation, *Nucleic Acids Res.* **21**:577-583.
43. Goossens, P., Jouin, H., Marchal, G., and Milon, G., 1990, Isolation and flow cytometric analysis of the free lymphomyeloid cells present in murine liver, *J. Immunol. Methods* **132**:137-144.
44. Belkaid, Y., Jouin, H., and Milon, G., 1996, A method to recover, enumerate and identify lymphomyeloid cells present in an inflammatory dermal site: A study in laboratory mice, *J. Immunol. Methods* **199**:5-25.
45. Wittmer-Pack, M. D., Crowley, M. T., Inaba, K., and Steinman, R. M., 1993, Macrophages but not dendritic cells accumulate colloidal carbon following administration in situ, *J. Cell Sci.* **105**:965-973.
46. Trutmann, M., and Sasse, D., 1994, The lymphatics of the liver—review article, *Anat. Embryol.* **190**:201-209.
47. Kraal, G., 1992, Cells in the marginal zone of the spleen, *Int. Rev. Cytol.* **132**:31-74.
48. Kraal, G., Schornagel, K., Streeter, P. R., Holzmann, and Butcher, E. C., 1995, Expression of the mucosal vascular addressin Mad CAM-1 on sinus lining cells in the spleen, *Am. J. Pathol.* **147**:763-771.
49. Crocker, P. R., Kelm, S., Hartnell, A., Freeman, S., Nath, D., Vinson, M., and Mucklow, S., 1996, Sialoadhesin and related cellular recognition molecules of the immunoglobulin superfamily, *Biochem. Soc. Trans.* **24**:150-156.
50. Van der Berg, T. K., Breve, J. J. P., Damoiseaux, J. G. M. C., Döpp, E. A., Kelm, S., Crocker,

P. R., Djikstra, C. D., and Kraal, G., 1992, Sialoadhesin on macrophages: Its identification as a lymphocyte adhesion molecule, *J. Exp. Med.* **176:**647–656.

51. Crocker, P. R., and Milon, G., 1992, Macrophages in control of haematopoiesis, in: *The Natural Immune System*, part II (C. Lewis, and J. O'D. McGee, eds.), Oxford Univerity Press, Oxford, pp. 115–156.

52. Amstrong, B. A., and Sword, C. P., 1966, Electron microscopy of *Listeria monocytogenes*-infected mouse spleen, *J. Bacteriol.* **91:**1346–1355.

53. Marco, A. J., Domingo, M., Prats, M., Briones, V., Pumarola, M., and Dominguez, L., 1991, Pathogenesis of lymphoid lesions in murine experimental listeriosis, *J. Comp. Pathol.* **105:**1–15.

54. Conlan, J. W., 1996, Early pathogenesis of *Listeria monocytogenes* infection with the mouse spleen, *J. Med. Microbiol.* **44:**295–302.

55. Susuki, H., Kurihara, Y., Takeya, M., Kamada, N., Kataoka, M., Jishage, K., Ueda, O., Sakagushi, H., Higashi, T., Suzuki, T., Takashima, T., Kawabe, Y., Cynshi, O., Wada, Y., Honda, M., Kurihara, H., Aburatani, H., Doi, T., Matsumoto, A., Azuma, S., Noda, T., Toyoda, Y., Itakura, H., Yazaki, Y., Horiuchi, S., Takahashi, K., Kruijt, J. K., Van Berkel, T. J. C., Steinbrecher, U. P., Ishibashi, S., Maeda, N., Gordon, S., and Kodoma, S., 1997, A role for macrophage scavenger receptors in atherosclerosis and susceptibility to infection, *Nature* **386:**292–296.

56. Gregory, S. H., Sagnimeni, A., and Wing, E. J., 1996, Bacteria in the bloodstream are trapped in the liver and killed by immigrating neutrophils, *J. Immunol.* **157:**2514–2520.

57. Unanue, E. R., 1997, Inter-relationship among macrophages, natural killer cells and neutrophils in early stages of *Listeria* resistance, *Curr. Opin. Immunol.* **9:**35–43.

58. Goossens, P., Marchal, G., and Milon, G., 1992, Transfer of both protection and delayed-type hypersensitivity against live *Listeria* is mediated by the CD8+ T cell subset: A study with *Listeria*-specific T lymphocytes recovered from murine infected liver, *Int. Immunol.* **4:**591–598.

59. Trinchieri, G., 1997, Cytokines acting on or secreted by macrophages during intracellular infection (IL10, IL12, IFNγ), *Curr. Opin. Immunol.* **9:**17–23.

60. Daugelat, S., and Kaufmann, S. H. E., 1996, Role of Th1 and Th2 cells in bacterial infections, in: *Chemical Immunology: Th1 and Th2 Cells in Health and Disease* Vol. 2 (S. Romagnani, ed.), Karger, Basel, pp. 66–97.

61. Fehr, T., Schvedon, G., Odermatt, B., Holtschke, T., Schneemann, M., Bachmann, M. F., Mak, T. W., Horak, I., and Zinkernagel, R. M., 1997, Crucial role of interferon consensus sequence binding protein, but neither of interferon regulatory factor 1 nor of nitric oxide synthesis for protection against murine listeriosis, *J. Exp. Med.* **185:**921–931.

62. Fu, Y. X., Roark, C. E., Kelly, K., Drevets, D., Campbell, P., O'Breen, R., and Born, W., 1994, Immune protection and control of inflammatory tissue necrosis by γδ T cells, *J. Immunol.* **153:**3101–3115.

63. Berche, P., 1995, Bacteremia is required for invasion of the murine central nervous system by *Listeria monocytogenes*, *Microbiol. Pathol.* **18:**323–336.

64. Fontana, A., Constam, D., Frei, K., Koedel, U., Pfister, W., and Weller, M., 1996, Cytokines and defense against CNS infection, in: *Cytokines and the CNS* (R. M. Ransohoff and E. N. Benveniste, eds.), CRC Press, Boca Raton, FL, pp. 187–219.

65. Weigmann, T. G., Hui, L., Guilbert, L., and Mossmann, T. R., 1993, Bidirectional cytokine interactions in the maternal-fetal relationship: Is successful pregnancy a Th2 phenomenon? *Immunol. Today* **14:**353–356.

66. Redline, R. W., and Lu, C. Y., 1987, Role of local immunosuppression in murine fetoplacental listeriosis, *J. Clin. Invest.* **79:**1234–1241.

67. Redline, R. W., and Lu, C. Y., 1988, Specific defects in the antilisterial immune response in discrete regions of the murine uterus and placenta account for susceptibility to infection, *J. Immunol.* **140:**3947–3955.

11

Rhodococcus equi: Pathogenesis and Replication in Macrophages

PATRICIA A. DARRAH, MARY K. HONDALUS, and
DAVID M. MOSSER

1. INTRODUCTION

Rhodococcus equi is a Gram-positive coccobacillus that is ubiquitous in nature. Infection with this bacterium can lead to the development of a pyogranulomatous pneumonia, primarily in immunocompromised hosts. Although first isolated nearly 75 years ago,[1] many aspects of *R. equi* infection, including bacterial pathogenesis and virulence and host immunity, are only recently being determined. *R. equi* is a well-recognized veterinary pathogen, and rhodococcal infection most commonly develops in newborn horses (foals) under the age of 3 months. In recent years, *R. equi* has emerged as an opportunistic pathogen of immunocompromised humans, such as persons with acquired immunodeficiency syndrome (AIDS) or those undergoing immunosuppressive drug therapy.[2] Upon inhalation, this facultative intracellular bacterium is phagocytized by host alveolar macrophages and resides and replicates in these cells. Inhibition of phagosome–lysosome fusion occurs following ingestion of *R. Equi* and is the mechanism proposed for survival of the organisms within macrophages.[3,4] It has been primarily through equine research and murine models of disease that we have

PATRICIA A. DARRAH and DAVID M. MOSSER • Department of Microbiology and Immunology, Temple University School of Medicine, Philadelphia, Pennsylvania 19140.   MARY K. HONDALUS • Howard Hughes Medical Research Institute, Albert Einstein College of Medicine, Bronx, New York 10461.

Opportunistic Intracellular Bacteria and Immunity, edited by Lois J. Paradise *et al.* Plenum Press, New York, 1999.

reached our present limited understanding of this organism. It is hoped that much of this information will be applicable to understanding human rhodococcal pneumonia, as this becomes a focus of further studies.

2. TAXONOMY, EPIDEMIOLOGY, AND INFECTION

Bacteria of the genus *Rhodococcus* ("red-pigmented coccus") are Gram-positive, aerobic, nonmotile, nonsporulating, catalase-positive, and partially acid fast. They belong to the phylogenic group known as nocardioform actinomycetes, which encompasses the genera *Caseobacter, Corynebacterium, Mycobacterium, Nocardia, Gordona,* and *Tsukmurella.*[5] As a group, the nocardioform actinomycetes synthesize peptidoglycan containing *meso*-diaminopimelic acid, utilize arabinose and galactose as their primary cell-wall sugars, and incorporate mycolic acids of varying lengths into their cell walls. In addition, the DNA of the actinomycetes is of high G + C content (>55 molar %).

R. equi emerged as a veterinary pathogen in 1923 when it was isolated from suppurative pulmonary lesions of an infected foal. It most likely became a pathogen of grazing animals because of its ubiquity in the environment. The growth requirements of this soil organism are fulfilled by the presence of herbivore manure, which provides the organic compounds on which this organism can thrive. Optimal soil pH (7.0 to 8.5) and temperate climates (optimally, 30°C) facilitate rhodococcal growth.[6] Thus, *R. equi* grows efficiently in manure-enriched soil. In addition, intraintestinal replication is possible and excretion of rhodococcus-contaminated feces is thought to promote the progressive increase of bacteria and infection on horse farms.[7] The prevalence of this bacterium has not been definitively determined, although it is endemic on some horse farms, sporadic on others, and unnoticed on most.[8] On endemic farms, most horses exhibit clinical symptomatology only during neonatal life. Adult horses are immune to the bacterium and only rarely experience clinically apparent infections.[9,10] Immunity to *R. equi* in adult horses may result from previous exposure to antigenically related bacteria, ingestion of bacteria,[11] or perhaps aerosol exposure to avirulent strains of rhodococcus itself.[12]

Initiation of infection in both animals and humans is thought to be due to acquisition of the bacterium via aerosol inoculation, commonly through inhalation of contaminated dust or soil.[13] Peak incidence of rhodococcal pneumonia in foals occurs within the second and third months of life, a window of time in which maternal antibody levels are declining yet the foal's own immune system is just beginning to develop. Human infections are primarily confined to those who are immunocompromised. The first documented case of human rhodococcal infection was in 1967 and involved a patient receiving corticosteriod therapy for chronic hepatitis.[14] A report in May 1995 cited 65 cases of rhodococcal infection in humans, 60 of which were immunosuppressed people with HIV infection, malignant neoplasms, or patients receiving immunosuppressive therapy.[2] Because *R. equi* is being isolated with increasing frequency from immunocompromised hosts, it is now considered to be an important opportunistic human pathogen.[15]

The most common clinical manifestation of *R. equi* infection is pneumonia. In both animals and humans the bacterium gains access to the lung, infects host alveolar macrophages, and replicates intracellularly.[16] The host immune response contributes to a granulomatous inflammation, which can lead to suppurative lung lesions and eventual tissue necrosis. In human and equine infections, the patient develops pulmonary abscesses with cavitation that can be observed by thoracic radiography. Many human rhodococcal infections go unreported, because *R. equi* cultured from sputum samples is often dismissed as a nonpathogenic diphtheroid contaminant.[15] In addition, misdiagnosis of rhodococcal infection for mycobacterial pneumonia can lead to incorrect drug treatment, thus prolonging clinical symptoms and increasing tissue damage.

3. BACTERIAL VIRULENCE DETERMINANTS

The ability of *R. equi* to cause disease depends not only on the immune status of the host (discussed below), but also on the pathogenic potential of the infecting organisms. A number of bacterial virulence factors have been proposed for *R. equi*. Naturally occurring and laboratory-derived strains, which lack the ability to cause infection in experimentally infected animals, have been exploited to study bacterial virulence factors. Unfortunately, many of the virulent culture-derived isolates of *R. equi* may lack several different virulence factors. A rational approach to the study of *R. equi* virulence awaits the development of molecular tools to permit the genetic manipulation of specific genes involved in the disease process.

Because *R. equi* is an encapsulated organism, the capsular polysaccharide has been considered a potential virulence determinant.[12] On other extracellular bacteria, the polysaccharide capsule often allows organisms to evade phagocytosis.[17] On *R. equi*, this capsule may contribute to resistance of bacteria to macrophage degradation. Serological examination has disclosed considerable variation among *R. equi* strains, and 27 capsular serotypes have been established.[18] Strains most often isolated from pulmonary lesions of diseased foals are primarily from two capsular serotypes. Although capsule-deficient organisms are avirulent, even in immunocompromised mice,[19] the necessity of capsular polysaccharide for *R. equi* virulence has not been definitively established.

The similarities in the clinical symptomatology between infections caused by *R. equi* and those caused by *Nocardia* spp. led researchers to investigate characteristics shared by those two bacteria as potential virulence factors. Incorporation of mycolic acid-containing glycolipid into the cell wall is one such characteristic.[20]

Upon extraction of the glycolipid, glucose monomycolate, from various *R. equi* strains, great heterogeneity was found in the lengths of the mycolic acid carbon chains. Using the mean lengths of these carbon chains, *R. equi* strains were segregated into three groups (types I, II, and III).[21] The correlation between mycolic acid carbon chain length and virulence was established, and rhodococcal strains having type III mycolic acids (C_{44} or C_{46}) were shown to be more virulent than those of type I (C_{32} or C_{34}) or type II (C_{34} or C_{36}) mycolic acids.[21] Longer length mycolic acids were associated with increased lethality and augmented granuloma formation in mice. These results were not attributable to bacterial strain differences, as injection of purified glycolipids of differing C-chain length yielded similar results.[21] Thus, the synthesis of long-chain mycolic acids by *R. equi* is one characteristic that may contribute to strain virulence. In addition, these molecules may also contribute to the host inflammatory response to *R. equi.*

The so-called "equi factors"[22] are another group of candidate *R. equi* virulence factors. These factors are membranolytic exoenzymes produced by the bacterium. Equi factors can act synergistically with sphingomyelinase C of *Staphylococcus aureus* (β toxin) or sphingomyelinase D of *Corynebacterium pseudotuberculosis* to induce hemolysis of sheep red blood cells (SRBCs). Cholesterol oxidase and a phospholipase C were determined to be the enzymatic components of equi factors.[23,24] Cholesterol oxidase killed a murine macrophage tumor cell line (RAW 264.7) in the absence of other enzymes such as phospholipases that are normally required to facilitate cholesterol oxidase binding to the membrane.[25] This direct lytic effect may be due to increased amounts of cholesterol in the membranes of RAW 264.7 cells as compared to native SRBCs. A choline phosphohydrolase isolated from *R. equi* supernatants was also found to exert a cytotoxic effect on macrophages.[25] Using a more sensitive assay for detection of hemolysis, two new enzymatic activities of *R. equi* have been reported to contribute to direct hemolysis of washed red blood cells.[26] A phosphatidylinositol-specific phospholipase C and a lecithinase exerted direct hemolytic activity that was independent of cholesterol oxidase. Thirteen of 14 rhodococcal strains examined possessed the ability to lyse RBCs. The one nonhemolytic strain studied exhibited lecithinase but not phosphatidylinositol-specific phospholipase C activity. It is tempting to speculate that the membranolytic capacity of these enzymes may confer some advantage to the bacterium. The lysis of primary phagosomes by *R. equi* has not been demonstrated, but the utilization of equi factors to lyse phagosome membranes would be a potential way for these organisms to access the macrophage cytoplasm. It should be noted that because equi factors are produced by both virulent and avirulent strains,[27] these factors may be necessary but not sufficient for bacterial virulence.

In 1987, an observation made by Chirino-Trejo and Prescott[28] changed the focus of rhodococcal virulence studies. Using sodium dodecyl sulfate-polyacrylamide gel electrophoresis (SDS-PAGE) in an effort to characterize bacterial proteins and their expression under differing culture conditions, they noticed the presence of a diffuse 15- to 17-kDa protein band from preparations of bacteria grown in nutritionally poor media. This band was lost upon repeated passage on blood agar at 42°C (50 and 100 passages) and was absent from a nonpathogenic strain preparation. Furthermore, this 15- to 17-kDa protein was expressed at 37°C but not at 30°C.[28] Using sera from naturally infected foals to immunoblot whole bacterial cell preparations, Takai and colleagues[29] identified rhodococcal protein antigens at molecular masses of 15- to 17-kDa, which were present in all clinical isolates tested.[29] A total of 102 environmental isolates were characterized with respect to expression of the 15- to 17-kDa antigens and, in each case, isolates expressing the antigens were virulent in mice, whereas those lacking the proteins were avirulent. This suggested that the presence of the 15- to 17-kDa bands could be used as a marker for virulence.[29] Because virulence determinants are often encoded by extrachromosomal DNA,[30] two groups independently examined virulent and avirulent strains of *R. equi* for possession of plasmid DNA and reported the isolation of plasmid from several rhodococcal isolates.[31,32] A plasmid of approximately 80 kb was associated with most equine clinical isolates and a 105-kb plasmid was described in some strains of porcine origin. Restriction enzyme analysis showed high similarity between these plasmids.[32] In addition, a correlation existed between plasmid possession, 15- to 17-kDa antigen expression, and virulence in both mice and horses. Plasmid-positive strains that were cured of the plasmid by repeated passage in culture at 38°C lost the 15- to 17-kDa protein and exhibited diminished virulence in mice.[31] These studies strongly suggested that the 15- to 17-kDa virulence-associated proteins were plasmid encoded.

Further characterization of the 15- to 17-kDa proteins using trypsin proteolysis and biotin–avidin western blotting revealed that they were localized to the cell surface.[33] Expression of the virulence-associated proteins was found to be temperature dependent. The antigens were expressed at higher temperatures (34 to 41°C), but not when bacteria were grown at temperatures between 25 and 32°C.[33] Optimal protein expression occurred at pH 6.5 and was absent at pH 8.9.[34] Using confocal immunofluorescence microscopy, we have shown that the virulence-associated antigen is expressed by bacteria within macrophages (Fig. 1). In 1995, the 15- to 17-kDa plasmid-encoded gene was cloned and termed *vapA* (virulence-associated protein A).[35,36] Variations in molecular weight of the protein encoded by *vapA* may be due to differential lipid modification of this single gene product or, alternatively, may be explained by differential peptide cleavage.[35,36] Gene sequencing data revealed a 570-bp gene encoding a protein of 189 amino acids with a predicted molecular weight of 16,245 Da (nonlipid modified).[35,36] The predicted VapA protein contains an alanine-rich signal sequence, which would allow the protein to be exported through the cell membrane.[36]

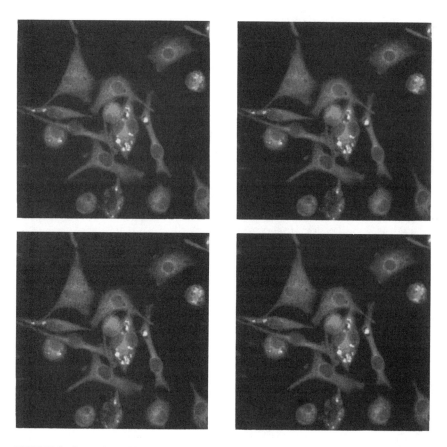

FIGURE 1. Expression of VapA by *R. equi* strain 103⁺ inside macrophages. A total of 7 × 10⁴ murine peritoneal macrophages were incubated for 30 min with the plasmid-positive *R. equi* strain 103⁺. After 24 h, macrophage monolayers were fixed with methanol and stained with a monoclonal antibody to VapA and a secondary FITC-conjugated antibody. Macrophages were counterstained with Evans blue. VapA-expressing bacteria were visualized via confocal microscopy. The absence of bacterial staining following paraformaldehyde fixation of parallel monolayers suggests that most, if not all, bacteria were intracellular.

Recent studies evaluated the role of virulence-associated plasmid in the pathogenesis of disease. Takai and colleagues[59] intravenously infected mice with isogenic strains of *R. equi*, presumably differing only with respect to plasmid possession. Injection of plasmid-positive *R. equi* resulted in bacterial replication, granuloma formation, and a specific antibody response. In contrast, plasmid-negative organisms were cleared quickly, with little evidence of granulomas or specific antibodies. Similarly, our laboratory studied the ability of three isogenic strain pairs, also differing only in terms of plasmid possession, to replicate following intravenous injection in mice. In agreement with Takai's work, we found that the plasmid-positive organisms grew efficiently in the livers and spleens of mice at 1, 3, 5, and 7 days following infection, during which time the plasmid-cured isogenic strains were cleared from mice (manuscript in preparation). In addition, intracellular replication of *R. equi* in macrophages was investigated. Plasmid-positive, VapA-positive bacteria exhibited a marked growth advantage over the plasmid-cured derivatives, which failed to replicate intracellularly. Thus, the possession of this large plasmid and synthesis of the VapA protein correlates with *R. equi* virulence and with intracellular replication in macrophages. Whether the *vapA* gene product is a true virulence determinant or simply a marker of virulence will require specific gene knockout and replacement experiments.

Although rhodococcal infection and the mechanisms of virulence in humans are less well studied, it would seem that the rules that govern rhodococcal virulence in mice and horses do not necessarily apply to human infection. Specifically, in contrast to equine infection, in which virtually all clinical isolates possess the virulence plasmid and express VapA, human clinical isolates have variable plasmid profiles.[37] Of 39 *R. equi* isolates from immunocompromised humans, only 8 contained an 85-kb virulence plasmid, expressed VapA, and were virulent in mice. None of the remaining isolates expressed the VapA antigens, although 19 contained plasmids of varying size and produced a plasmid-associated 20-kDa protein. Restriction endonuclease mapping and Southern blotting analysis showed that these plasmids were related to the original 85-kb virulence-associated plasmid. In addition, strains expressing the 20-kDa protein were determined to be of intermediate virulence in mice (10-fold higher LD_{50} than VapA-expressing strains). *R. equi* immune foal serum recognized both the novel 20-kDa and the original 15- to 17-kDa antigens.[37] These findings raise the possibility of shared virulence determinants among strains of *R. equi* isolated from foals and humans. However, some strains isolated from humans did not contain any plasmid, and thus it is possible that the severely immunocompromised status of HIV-infected individuals allows even relatively avirulent organisms to survive and cause disease.

Having shown that most human isolates of *R. equi* are resistant to β-lactam antibiotics, Nordmann and colleagues set out to analyze the mechanism of β-lactam resistance and its effect on virulence in a limited number of non-plasmid-containing human strains.[38] The resistant strains did not exhibit β-lactamase activity, nor were their penicillin-binding protein profiles different from those of β-lactam-susceptible strains. Phage-like particles (PLPs) were detected by electron microscopy in all strains exhibiting cell surface appendages. All β-lactam-resistant bacteria also displayed three additional protein bands via SDS-PAGE as compared to sensitive strains. PLP-positive isolates had lower LD_{50}s than did PLP-negative strains in euthymic and nude mice and, in culture,

PLP-positive strains grew much faster and showed higher bacterial numbers at the stationary phase. These experiments indicate a correlation between antibiotic resistance, phage-like particle production, and virulence of human *R. equi* isolates. Whether the PLPs actually confer β-lactam resistance is still questionable, as attempts to transfer resistance to susceptible strains via culture filtrates have been unsuccessful. Differences in cell-wall composition between resistance and susceptible strains may also contribute to some of the differences in their phenotype.

4. CELL BIOLOGY

In the infected host, *R. equi* reside primarily, if not exclusively, in tissue macrophages. A number of *in vitro* studies have demonstrated that the uptake of *R. equi* is restricted to professional phagocytic cells.[39] Optimal adherence of the bacteria to these cells generally requires opsonization with either antibody or complement. In the nonimmune host, complement appears to be the primary opsonin responsible for *R. equi* uptake by macrophages. *R. equi* fix complement by activating the alternative complement pathway,[39] a process that does not depend on antibody.[40] The binding of bacteria to macrophages in nonimmune serum is mediated primarily through ligation of the macrophage receptor MAC-1, also known as the complement receptor type 3.[39] *In vitro* the majority of bacterial binding to macrophages is blocked by monoclonal antibodies to MAC-1, provided that the assays are performed in serum that contains intact complement. In the immune host, antibody facilitates bacterial uptake, presumably via the macrophage Fc-γ receptors. In the absence of complement and antibody, bacterial adhesion to macrophages *in vitro* is much less efficient and occurs by as yet undetermined mechanisms. *In vitro*, opsonized *R. equi* also interacts with neutrophils,[41] cells that also express receptors for IgG and complement C3. However, bacterial survival and replication in neutrophils has never been demonstrated.

Several groups have shown that, following their adhesion to and phagocytosis by macrophages *in vitro*, *R. equi* can persist within the cells for extended periods. Electron microscopic ultrastructural studies[15,17] demonstrated that the bacteria are located within membrane-enclosed vacuoles. Many of the vacuoles containing intact *R. equi* have the appearance of primary phagosomes to which cellular lysosomes have not yet fused.[3,4] This finding is reminiscent of studies involving other intracellular bacteria that reside in macrophages, including *Mycobacteria* spp., *Nocardia asteroides*, and *Legionella pneumophila*. In all of these organisms there is evidence for a lack of normal phagolysosomal fusion following macrophage infection.[42–45] Interestingly, the opsonization of *R. equi* with antibody prior to their addition to equine alveolar macrophages results in increased phagolysosomal fusion[4] and enhanced intracellular killing. This work suggests that the mechanism of bacterial entry into macrophages can influence both the intracellular location of the bacteria and their intracellular survival within macrophages.

Within resident nonactivated macrophages, *R. equi* not only persist, they also replicate. Recent *in vitro* studies measured the replication of virulent *R. equi* in resident macrophages taken from several different species and from different anatomical locations.[46] *R. equi* grew intracellularly in large clusters within macrophages, and the organisms appeared to be confined to membranous organelles. The number of morphologically intact bacteria within macrophages increased over time, and those organisms incorporated progressively more tritiated uracil, indicating that they were viable and metabolically active. Following an initial lag phase of several hours, the intracellular doubling time of *R. equi* in macrophages was found to be approximately 6 to 8 h.[46]

Several isolates of *R. equi,* obtained following repeated passage in culture, are avirulent in experimental animals. In contrast to clinically derived virulent strains of *R. equi,* which multiply intracellularly in macrophages *in vitro,* avirulent strains fail to replicate efficiently in macrophages.[46] The most widely distributed avirulent type strain is ATCC 6939.[47] This organism is able to persist within macrophages *in vitro,* but it does not give rise to the large clusters of replicating bacteria. Within macrophages, bacterial numbers reman relatively constant over the first several days in culture and then gradually decrease. Thus, although avirulent isolates of *R. equi* are not able to grow in macrophages, these organisms retain the ability to resist the rapid and efficient killing that typically occurs when macrophages encounter avirulent extracellular bacteria. It is not clear whether the low levels of bacterial persistence in these cells represent a balance between killing and intracellular replication, or whether the avirulent bacteria are truly resistant to macrophage-mediated killing. Importantly, the cellular site of these avirulent organisms within macrophages has not yet been determined. The efficiency with which avirulent organisms are able to prevent phagolysosomal fusion merits further study. The lack of intramacrophage growth by these avirulent strains has been taken to explain their failure to cause infections in experimental animals.

Treatment of macrophages *in vitro* with (IFN-γ) and low levels of lipopolysaccharide converts them into activated macrophages. These cells inhibit intracellular bacterial growth, even when infected by virulent clinical isolates of *R. equi* (Darrah *et al,* submitted). These studies suggest that the activated macrophage is a primary effector cell in rhodococcal infections. We have begun to examine the mechanism of bacterial killing by activated murine macrophages, and have implicated macrophage-derived reactive nitrogen and oxygen species in bacterial killing. When exposed to *R. equi,* activated murine macrophages produce both nitric oxide and superoxide (O_2^-) (Fig. 2). These two molecules can combine to form the potent bactericidal compound, peroxynitrite.[49] Exposure of virulent strains of rhodococcus to peroxynitrite in a cell-free system efficiently

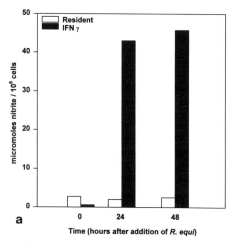

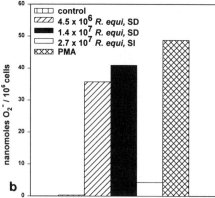

FIGURE 2. The production of nitric oxide and superoxide by activated macrophages. (a) 1 × 10⁵ untreated or IFN-γ-primed murine macrophages were infected with 2 × 10⁶ *R. equi* for 30 min. Total nitrite content in cell supernatants was determined at 0, 24, and 48 h postinfection using the Griess reaction.[60] (b) *R. equi* or phorbol myristate acetate (PMA, 0.5 μg/ml) was added to 1 × 10⁵ activated murine bone marrow derived macrophages in the presence (SD) or absence (SI) of 5% fresh normal mouse serum. Control monolayers received neither *R. equi* nor PMA. The reduction of cytochrome *c* following a 30 min incubation was determined by the increase in absorbance at 550 nm, which then was converted to nanomoles of superoxide per 10⁶ macrophages as described.[48]

kills the bacteria (Fig. 3). Thus, the failure of resident murine macrophages to produce nitric oxide may account for their susceptibility to *R. equi* infection.

5. IMMUNITY

The mechanism of immunity to *R. equi* has not yet been fully resolved. In humans and mice, cell-mediated immunity appears to be the primary mechanism for clearing infection with rhodococcus. Studies in immunodeficient mice demonstrated that an intact cellular immune system is necessary for disease resolution.[19] Severe combined immunodeficient (SCID) mice and T-cell-deficient *nu/nu* (nude) mice are more susceptible to infection by *R. equi* than are normal, immunocompetent mice.[19] The administration of immunosuppressive agents such as steroids or

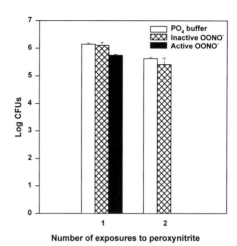

FIGURE 3. Killing of *R. equi* by peroxynitrite. 10^6 *R. equi* were exposed to 1 mM peroxynitrite (OONO) in potassium phosphate buffer (pH 7.4) at 37°C for 3 min as described.[50] Bacteria were then centrifuged, resuspended, and exposed a second time. Control cells were either untreated (PO_4 buffer) or treated with decomposed peroxynitrite (Inactive OONO). Cell viability was determined by a colony-forming unit assay.

cyclophosphamide also results in exacerbated disease.[51] Nordmann and colleagues[52] demonstrated that adoptive transfer of immune splenocytes protected mice from subsequent challenge with *R. equi*. Several groups have performed *in vitro* depletion experiments to identify the lymphocyte subsets responsible for protection. A clear consensus has not yet emerged from these studies, but the indications are that both CD4+ and CD8+ T cells contribute to *R. equi* immunity. Some studies suggest that the CD4+ subset may play a more important role than the CD8+ subset. Kanaly and coworkers[53] examined pulmonary clearance of *R. equi* in mice lacking either functional CD8+ or CD4+ T cells. They observed a significant degree of clearance in both groups of mice, relative to control SCID mice. However, CD8-deficient mice exhibited complete pulmonary clearance of *R. equi* at a time when the CD4-deficient mice had low but detectable levels of *R. equi*. Ross and colleagues[54] transferred immune CD8+ or CD4+ T cells into naive SCID mice and examined bacterial clearance following infection. Adoptively transferred mice, receiving either CD8+ or CD4+ T cells, had reduced bacterial burdens relative to those of normal nontransferred mice, 2 weeks after infection. Mice receiving CD4+ T cells had slightly lower bacterial burdens than did mice receiving CD8+ T cells. Nordmann and colleagues performed T-cell depletion studies and demonstrated that both CD4+ and CD8+ T cells are required for optimal clearance of *R. equi*, with the CD8+ subset playing a significant role.[52] Recent studies have demonstrated that efficient resolution of experimental *R. equi* disease in mice correlated with the development of a Th1-type immune response.[55] Treatment of mice with anti-IFN-γ exacerbated disease, whereas treatment with anti-IL-4 resulted in accelerated bacterial clearance. Furthermore, adoptive transfer of a CD4+ Th1 T cell line into nude mice conferred resistance to infection.[56] Taken together, all of these studies demonstrate the importance of the CD4+ T-cell subset in immunity to *R. equi*. However, they also indicate an important role for CD8+ T cells, which may relate to the ability of these cells to produce IFNγ. Therefore, although *R. equi* pneumonia in AIDS patients is rarely seen before the CD4+ lymphocyte count declines below 200,[57] a role for CD8+ lymphocytes in host defense to *R. equi* cannot be dismissed. The involvement of the CD4+ subset of T cells in immunity to *R. equi* is predictable, given the intracellular location of *R. equi* in macrophages and the importance of CD4+ T cells in producing macrophage-activating cytokines. A direct role of CD8+ T cells in this disease is intuitively less obvious, given the *in vitro* studies that indicate that *R. equi* reside enclosed within macrophage membranous vacuoles and not free in the cytoplasm. The importance of cytotoxic T-cells lines and/or clones to host defense against *R. equi* has not been systematically examined, and the nature of the peptide(s) presented to major histocompatibility complex class I-specific CD8+ T cells is not known.

In contrast to the experimental studies in the murine model, there are several lines of evidence that point to a significant role for antibody in the protection of horses against the development of *R. equi* pneumonia. First, the age at onset of disease in foals temporally coincides with the decline of cololstrum-derived maternal antibody. Second, adult horses are resistant to infection by *R. equi* and most have measurable titers of antibody to the bacterium.[9] Finally, passive administration of *R. equi*-immune sera to foals protects them, against experimental aerosol administration of *R. equi*,[58] and is currently being used prophylactically on some horse farms in which *R. equi* is endemic.

In conclusion, there is compelling experimental and clinical evidence that an intact cell-mediated immune response is important for host defense to *R. equi*. In horses, the passive immunization with plasma-containing antibodies to *R. equi* may supplant this requirement and confer a measure of protection that is adequate until natural immunity is initiated. Studies on the nature of the immune response to *R. equi* are important for development of specific vaccines.

6. FUTURE STUDIES

The difficulty with describing future studies to be pursued on this relatively understudied organism is that so much work remains to be done. Studies to define more closely the epidemiology of *R. equi* infection are needed. Despite increased awareness by physicians of the pathogenic potential of *R. equi* in the immunocompromised, there are little hard data on the prevalence of this organism in this population. Both retrospective and prospective studies to determine the prevalence of disease are needed. In addition, the risk factors for exposure to this bacterium should be determined.

There is a clear need for a vaccine to this organism, especially in the equine population. However, the development of an effective vaccine depends on determination of the nature of the immune response that is responsible for clearing *R. equi*. Attention is necessary to elucidate the role of CD8$^+$ cells in bacterial clearance, the epitopes recognized by cytotoxic T cells, and the mechanism whereby this organism gains access to the major histocompatibility complex class I pathway. With respect to the bacterium, virulence factors that permit their intracellular growth in macrophages must continue to be analyzed, in particular by development of molecular reagents that are functional in *R. equi*. The time and cost of developing these tools are investments that must be made before the mysteries of this organism will reveal themselves. Because *R. equi* utilize strategies to escape macrophage killing that may be common to other bacteria, such as *Mycobacterium* spp., answers developed in this model may apply to other bacterial pathogens. Thus, genetic analysis of *R. equi* pathogenesis is merited not only for itself but also because it may reveal general lessons about bacterial virulence and intracellular survival within macrophages.

ACKNOWLEDGMENT. This work was supported in part by the Grayson-Jockey Club Research Foundation.

REFERENCES

1. Magnusson, H., 1923, Spezifische infedktiose pneumonie beim fohlem. Ein neuer eitererreger beim pferde, *Arch. Wiss Praktise Tierheilkd.* **506:**22–38.
2. Scott, M. A., Graham, B. S., Verrall, R., Dixon, R., Schaffner, W., and Tham, K. T., 1995, *Rhodococcus equi* – an increasingly recognized opportunistic pathogen, *Clin. Microbiol. Infect. Dis.* **103:**649–655.
3. Zink, M. C., Yager, J. A., Prescott, J. F., and Fernando, M. A., 1987, Electron microscopic investigation of intracellular events after ingestion of *Rhodococcus equi* by foal alveolar macrophages, *Vet. Microbiol.* **14:**295–305.
4. Hietala, S. K., and Ardans, A. A., 1987, Interaction of *Rhodococcus equi* with phagocytic cells from *R. equi* exposed and non-exposed foals, *Vet. Microbiol.* **14:**307–320.
5. Goodfellow, M., 1987, Taxonomic status of *Rhodococcus equi, Vet. Microbiol.* **14:**205–209.
6. Hughes, K. L., and Sulaiman, I., 1987, the ecology of *Rhodococcus equi* and physiochemical influences on growth, *Vet. Microbiol.* **14:**241–250.
7. Prescott, J. F., Travers, M., and Yager-Johnson, J. A., 1984, Epidemiological survey of *Corynebacterium equi* infections on five Ontario horse farms, *Can. J. Com. Med.* **48:**10–13.
8. Rooney, R. J., 1966, Corynebacterial infections in foals, *Mod. Vet. Pract.* **47:**43–45.
9. Hietala, S. K., Ardans, A. A., and Sansome, A., 1985, Detection of *Corynebacterium equi*-specific antibody in horses by enzyme-linked immunosorbent assay, *Am. J. Vet. Res.* **46:**13–15.
10. Prescott, J. F., Ogilvie, T. H., and Markham, R. J. F., 1980, Lymphocyte immunostimulation in the diagnosis of *Corynebacterium equi* pneumonia of foals, *Am. J. Vet. Res.* **41:**2073–2075.
11. Chirino-Trejo, J. M., Prescott, J. F., and Yager, J. A., 1987, Protection of foals against experimental *Rhodococcus equi* pneumonia by oral immunization, *Can. J. Vet. Res.* **51:**444–447.
12. Prescott, J. F., 1991, *Rhodococcus equi:* An animal and human pathogen, *Clin. Microbiol. Rev.* **4:**20–34.

13. Martens, R. J., Fiske, R. A., and Renshaw, H. W., 1982, Experimental subacute foal pneumonia induced by aerosol administration of *Corynebacterium equim Equine Vet. J.* **14:**111–116.

14. Golub, B., Falk, G., and Spink, W. W., 1967, Lung abscess due to *Corynebacterium equi.* Report of first human infection, *Ann. Intern. Med.* **66:**1174–1177.

15. Mosser, D. M., and Hondalus, M. K., 1996, *Rhodococcus equi:* An emerging opportunistic pathogen, *Trends Microbiol.* **4:**29–33.

16. McNeil, M., and Brown, J., 1994, The medically important aerobic actinomycetes: Epidemiology and microbiology, *Clin. Microbiol. Rev.* **7:**357–417.

17. Densen, P., and Mandell, G. L., 1980, Effects of capsule on phagocytosis, *Rev. Infect. Dis.* **2:**817–838.

18. Nakazawa, M., Kubo, M., Sugimoto, C., and Isayama, Y., 1983, Serogrouping of *Rhodococcus equi, Microbiol. Immunol.* **27:**837–846.

19. Yager, J. A., Prescott, C. A., Kramer, D. P., Hannah, H., Balson, G. A., and Croy, B. A., 1991, The effect of experimental infection with *Rhodococcus equi* on immunodeficient mice, *Vet. Microbiol.* **28:**363–376.

20. Kaneda, K., Sumi, Y., Kurano, F., Kato, Y., and Yano, I., 1996, Granuloma formation and hematopoiesis induced by C^{36-48} mycolic acid-containing glycolipids from *Nocardia ruba, Infect. Immun.* **54;**869–875.

21. Gotoh, K., Mitsuyama, M., Imaizumi, S., Kawamura, I., and Yano, I., 1991, Mycolic acid-containing glycolipid as a possible virulence factor of *Rhodococcus equi* for mice, *Microbiol. Immunol.* **35:**175–185.

22. Fraser, G., 1964, The effect on animal erythrocytes of combinations of different diffusible substances produced by bacteria, *J. Pathol. Bacteriol.* **88:**49–53.

23. Linder, R., and Bernheimer, A. W., 1982, Enzymatic oxidation of membrane cholesterol oxidase in relation to lysis of sheep erythrocytes by corynebacterial enzymes, *Arch. Biochem. Biophys,* **213:**395–404.

24. Bernheimer, A. W., Linder, R., and Aviged, L., 1980, Stepwise degradation of membrane sphigomyelin by corynebacterial phospholipases, *Infect. Immun.* **29;**123–131.

25. Machang'u, R. S., and Prescott, J. F., 1991, Purification and properties of cholesterol oxidase and choline phosphohydrolase from *Rhodococcus equi, Can. J. Vet. Res.* **55:**332–340.

26. Katerov, V., and Schalen, C., 1994, Haemolytic and phosholipase C (PLC) activities of *Rhodococcus equi, J. App. Bacteriol.* **77:**325–333.

27. Prescott, J. F., Lastra, M., and Barksdale, L., 1982, Equi factors in the identification of *Corynebacterium equi, J.Clin. Microbiol.* **16:**988–990.

28. Chirino-Trejo, J. M., and Prescott, J. F., 1987, Polyacrylamide gel electrophoresis of whole-cell preparations of *Rhodococcus equi, Can. J. Vet. Res.* **51:**297–300.

29. Takai, S., Koike, K., Ohbushi, S., Izumi, C., and Tsubaki, S. 1991, Identification of 15- to 17-kilodalton antigens associated with virulent *Rhodococcus equi, J. Clin. Microbiol.* **29:**439–443.

30. Smith, H., 1989, The mounting interest in bacterial pathogenicity, *Annu. Rev. Microbiol.* **43:**1–22.

31. Takai, S., Sekizaki, T., Ozawa, T., Sugawara, T., Watanabe, Y., and Tsubaki, S., Sekizaki, T., Ozawa, T., Sugawara, T., Watanabe, Y., and Tsubaki, S., 1991, Association between a large plasmid and 15- to 17-kilodalton antigens in virulent *Rhodococcus equi, Infect. Immun.* **59:**4056–4060.

32. Tkachuk-Saad, I., and Prescott, J., 1991, *Rhodococcus equi* plasmids: Isolation and partial characterization, *J. Clin. Microbiol.* **29:**2696–2700.

33. Takai, S., Iie, M., Watanabe, Y., Tsubaki, S., and Sekizaki, T., 1992, Virulence-associated 15- to 17-kilodalton antigens in *Rhodococcus equi:* Temperature-dependent expression and location of the antigens, *Infect. Immun.* **60:**2995–2997.

34. Takai, S., Fukunaga, N., Kamisawa, K., Imai, Y., Sasaki, Y., and Tsubaki, S., 1996, Expression of virulence-associated antigens of *Rhodococcus equi* is regulated by temperature and pH, *Microbiol. Immunol.* **40:**591–594.

35. Tan, C., Prescott, J. R., Patterson, M. C., and Nicholson, V. M., 1995, Molecular characterization of a lipid-modified virulence-associated protein of *Rhodococcus equi* and its potential in protective immunity, *Can. J. Vet. Res.* **55:**51–59.

36. Sekizaki, T., Takai, S., Egawa, Y., Ikedo, T., Ito, H., and Tsubaki, S., 1995, Sequence of the *Rhodococcus equi* gene encoding the virulence-associated 15-17 kDa antigens, *Gene* **115:**135–136.

37. Takai, S., Sasaki, Y., Ikeda, T., Uchida, Y., Tsubaki, S., and Sekizaki, T., 1994, Virulence of *Rhodococcus equi* isolates from patients with and without AIDS, *J. Clin. Microbiol.* **32:**457–460.

38. Nordmann, P., Keller, M., Espinasse, F., and Ronco, E., 1994, Correlation between antibiotic resistance, phage-like particle presence, and virulence in *Rhodococcus equi* human isolates, *J. Clin. Microbiol.* **32;**377–383.

39. Hondalus, M. K., Diamond, M. S., Rosenthal, L. A., Springer, T. A., and Mosser, D. M., 1993, The intracellular bacterium *Rhodococcus equi* requires MAC-1 to bind to mammalian cells, *Infect. Immun.* **61:**2919–2929.

40. Fearon, D. T., 1978, Regulation by membrane sialic acid of β1H-dependent decay-dissolution of amplification C3 convertase of the alternative complement pathway, *Proc. Natl. Acad. Sci. USA* **75:**1971–1975.

41. Yager, J. A., Duder, C. K., Prescott, J. F., and Zink, M. C., 1987, The interaction of *Rhodococcus equi* and foal neutrophils *in vitro*, *Vet. Microbiol.* **14:**287–294.

42. Armstrong, J. A., and D'Arcy Hart, P., 1971, Response of cultured macrophages to *Mycobacterium tuberculosis*, with observations of fusion of lysosomes with phagosomes, *J. Exp. Med.* **143:**713–740.

43. Horowitz, M. A., 1983, The Legionnaires' disease bacterium (*Legionella Pneumophila*) inhibits phagosome-lysosome fusion in human monocytes, *J. Exp. Med* **158:**2108–2126.

44. Davis-Scibienski, C., and Bearman, B. L., 1980, Interaction of *Nocardia asteroides* with rabbit alveolar macrophages: Effect of growth phase and viability on phagosome–lysosome fusion, *Infect. Immun.* **29:**24–29.

45. Frehel, C., de Chastellier, C., Lang, T., and Rastogi, N., 1986, Evidence for inhibition of fusion of lysosomal and prelysosomal compartments with phagosomes in macrophages infected with pathogenic *Mycobacterium avium*, *Infect. Immun.* **52:**242–262.

46. Hondalus, M. K., and Mosser, D. M., 1994, Survival and replication of *Rhodococcus equi* in macrophages, *Infect. Immun.* **62:**4167–4175.

47. Hondalus, M. K., Sweeney, C. R., and Mosser, D. M., 1992, An assay to quantitate the binding of *Rhodococcus equi* to macrophages, *Vet. Immunol. Immunopathol.* **32:**339–350.

48. Mosser, D. M., and Edelson, P. J., 1987, The third component of complement (C3) is responsible for the intracellular survival of *Leishmania major*, *Nature* **327:**329–331.

49. Ischiropoulous, H., Zhu, L., and Beckman, J. S., 1992, Peroxynitrite formation from macrophage-derived nitric oxide, *Arch. Biochem. Biophys.* **298:**446–451.

50. Zhu, L., Gunn, C., and Beckman, J. S., 1992, Bactericidal activity of peroxynitrite, *Arch. Biochem. Biophys.* **298:**452–457.

51. Bowles, P. M., Woolcock, J. B., and Mutimer, M. D., 1989, The effect of immunosuppression on resistance to *Rhodococcus equi* in mice, *Vet. Immunol. Immunopathol.* **22:**369–378.

52. Nordmann, P., Ronco, E., and Nauciel, C., 1992, Role of T-lymphocyte subsets in *R. equi* infection, *Infect. Immun.* **60:**2748–2752.

53. Kanaly, S. T., Hines, S. A., and Palmer, G. H., 1993, Failure of pulmonary clearance of *Rhodococcus equi* infection in CD4+ T-lymphocyte-deficient transgenic mice, *Infect. Immun.* **61:**4929–4932.

54. Ross, T. L., Balson, G. A., Miners, J. S., Smith, G. D., Shewen, P. E., Prescott, J. F., and Yager, J. A., 1996, Role of CD4+, CD8+ and double negative T-cells in the protection of SCID/beige mice against respiratory challenge with *Rhodococcus equi*, *Can. J. Vet. Res.* **60:**186–192.

55. Kanaly, S. T., Hines, S. A., and Palmer, G. H., 1995, Cytokine modulation alters pulmonary

clearance of *Rhodococcus equi* and development of granulomatous pneumonia, *Infect. Immun.* **63:**3037–3041.

56. Kanaly, S. T., Hines, S. A., and Palmer, G. H., 1996, Transfer of CD4⁺ Th1 cell line to nude mice effects clearance of *Rhodococcus equi* from the lung, *Infect. Immun.* **64:**1126–1132.

57. Sane, D. C., and Durrack, D. T., 1986, Infection with *Rhodococcus equi* in AIDS, *N. Engl. J. Med.* **314:**56–57.

58. Martens, R. J., Martens, J. G., Fiske, R. A., and Hietala, S. K., 1989, *Rhodococcus equi* foal pneumonia. Protective effects of immune plasma in experimentally infected foals. *Equi Vet. J.* **21:**249–255.

59 Takai, S., Madarame, H., Matsumoto, C., Inoue, M., Sasaki, Y., Hasegawa, Y., Tsubaki, S., and Nakane, A., 1995, Pathogenesis of *Rhodococcus equi* infection in mice: roles of virulence plasmids and granulomagenic activity of bacteria, *FEMS Immunol. Med. Microbiol.* **11:**181–190.

60. Ding, A. H., Nathan, C. F., and Stuehr, D. J., 1988, Release of reactive nitrogen intermediates and reactive oxygen intermediates from mouse peritoneal macrophages, *J. Immunol.* **141:**2407–2412.

12

Bartonella Infections in the Immunocompromised Host

ANDREW W. O. BURGESS, DAVID JOHNSON,
and BURT E. ANDERSON

1. INTRODUCTION

The spectrum of diseases associated with *Bartonella* infections in patients who are immunocompromised by acquired immunodeficiency syndrome (AIDS), chronic alcoholism, or immunosuppressive therapy is broader than in immunocompetent individuals. Reports of *Bartonella* infections in adult AIDS patients have increased. The roles of *Bartonella* species as modern day pathogens were first recognized in immunocompromised patients with bacillary angiomatosis (BA). Since the initial association of *Bartonella* species with BA, this genus has been implicated in a diverse array of clinical manifestations. Clinical syndromes associated with infection of immunocompromised patients include cutaneous BA, bacillary peliosis of the liver (bacillary peliosis hepatis) and spleen, fever with bacteremia, endocarditis, and intracerebral bacillary angiomatosis.

ANDREW W. O. BURGESS and BURT E. ANDERSON • Department of Medical Microbiology and Immunology, University of South Florida, College of Medicine, Tampa, Florida 33612. DAVID JOHNSON • Infectious Diseases Section, Department of Veterinary Affairs Medical Center, Bay Pines, Florida 33744.

Opportunistic Intracellular Bacteria and Immunity, edited by Lois J. Paradise *et al.* Plenum Press, New York, 1999.

2. INTRACELLULAR LOCATION OF *BARTONELLA*

The genus *Bartonella* was created by merging the genus *Rochalimaea* with the genus *Bartonella*, which had only one existing member, *B. bacilliformis*. The genus *Bartonella* belongs to the α-2 subgroup of the class Proteobacteria.[1] Recent data support the ability of *Bartonella* to survive and replicate intracellularly in several cell types.[2-4] By electron microscopy, erythrocytes obtained from two cats with *B. henselae* bacteremia showed organisms within erythrocytes in 2.9% of red blood cells in one cat and in 6.2% in the second cat.[4] *B henselae* cocultivated with Vero cells were seen intracellularly as shown by fluorescent microscopy and confirmed by electron microscopy.[2] In this study, organisms were observed in the cytoplasm mainly around the nuclei. *B. henselae* and *B. quintana* adhere to and invade human epithelial cells (Hep-2) *in vitro*.[3] *B. henselae*, however, is able to invade Hep-2 cells several hundred to several thousand times more efficiently than *B. quintana*. Furthermore, piliated *B. henselae* strains enter Hep-2 cells to a much greater extent than nonpiliated strains, suggesting that specific attachment is a prerequisite for subsequent entry. Large clumps of *B. henselae* present in vacuoles as well as occasional single intracellular bacteria were observed.

Although *in vitro* studies demonstrate enhancement of phagocytosis and subsequent production of oxygen radicals in the presence of *B. henselae* previously opsonized with immune sera, persistent bacteremia has been described.[5] This suggests that a *B. henselae* reservoir persists intracellularly.[6] The observation that AIDS patients have defective phagocytosis and oxidative burst by polymorphonuclear leukocytes may explain the higher susceptibility of these patients to disseminated and persistent *Bartonella* infections.[6]

3. THE GENUS *BARTONELLA* AND DISEASE

Human pathogens in the genus *Bartonella* include *B.henselae, B. bacilliformis, B. quintana, and B. elizabethae*. The genus also contains several members that have not yet been associated with human disease.

Both *B. henselae* and *B. quintana* have been implicated as causative agents in many of the disease syndromes associated with immunocompromised individuals. Both species are associated with bacillary angiomatosis[7] and bacteremia.[5] To date, *B. henselae* is the only confirmed agent of bacillary peliosis hepatis.[8,9] Although *B. henselae*[10] and *B. elizabethae*[11] have been isolated form immunocompetent patients with endocarditis, *B. quintana* is the only *Bartonella* species reported to be associated with endocarditis in immunocompromised patients.[12,13] In the 1990s, *B. quintana* infections have emerged among the homeless population.[14] It is likely that host factors such as altered immunity due to alcoholism or other existing health problems are important risk factors for the development of clinical infections following exposure of the homeless to *B. quintana*.[14] Identity of the bacilli causing intracerebral bacillary angiomatosis has not been established. *B. henselae* also has been associated with dementia in human immunodeficiency virus (HIV)-infected individuals.[15]

4. CLINICAL PRESENTATIONS IN THE IMMUNOCOMPROMISED PATIENT

4.1. Bacillary Angiomatosis

Bacillary angiomatosis, also referred to as epithelioid angiomatosis or bacillary epithelioid angiomatosis, associated with *B. henselae* or *B. quintana* infections is characterized by vascular lesions. BA usually occurs in immunocompromised patients, most commonly those infected with HIV, as well as transplant patients receiving immunosuppressive therapy. BA was first described by Stoler *et al.* in 1983 in a patient with AIDS and involved the skin and regional lymph nodes.[16] Since then BA has been observed in many internal organs including the liver, spleen, bone, brain, larynx, lung, tongue, intestine, and subcutaneous fat.[17]

There have been reports of BA both in healthy individuals without HIV infection[18,19] and in HIV-infected patients with disseminated *Bartonella* infections without evidence of BA.[20] It is not known whether the latter are due to strain variation within *Bartonella* species, to host differences, or to stage differences of *Bartonella* infection associated with AIDS.[17] It is also not known why BA occurs primarily in patients with compromised cell-mediated immunity.

4.1.1. Clinical Manifestations

BA usually involves the skin, although other organ systems may be involved. Cutaneous lesions are either solitary or multiple and may be superficial, dermal, or subcutaneous.[1,21] BA primary lesions are papules that gradually increase in size to form nodules.[22] Superficial lesions may be red, purple, or skin colored. Figure 1 illustrates the clinical appearance of an AIDS patient with BA.[23] A widespread distribution of reddish purple, vascular papules and nodules over the face can be seen. Figure 2 illustrates the clinical appearance of cutaneous BA lesions.[24] Deeper lesions are usually skin colored and may be mobile or fixed to underlying structures. When first recognized, lesions are usually peasized. When multiple lesions are present, distribution may be widespread and there may be several hundred to thousands of pinpoint papules on the skin. Individual lesions may be ulcerated with crusting or they may have a smooth surface. The consistency of lesions is usually rubbery to firm. When BA lesions are punctured, they tend to bleed profusely. Resolved lesions are usually slightly hyperpigmented and slightly indurated.

In a recent systematic study of the clinical features of 42 HIV-1 patients with histologically confirmed BA and/or bacillary parenchymal peliosis (discussed

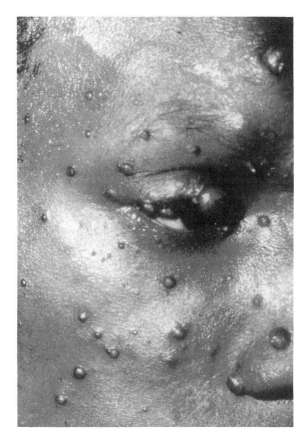

FIGURE 1. Clinical appearance of a patient with cutaneous bacillary angiomatosis. (From Cockerell, C. J., *et al.*, 1991, *J. Invest. Dermatol.* **97**:812–817, with permission.)

later), 55% presented with cutaneous or subcutaneous lesions, 21% had lymph-adenopathy alone, and 24 presented with fever and abdominal symptoms.[25] These patients were compared to 84 HIV-1-infected patients without BA. BA patients were more severely immunocompromised with a median CD4 lymphocyte count of 21/mm³ (range of 1 to 228/mm³) when compared to controls (median of 186/mm³ and a range of 0 to 910/mm³). Only 6% of BA patients had CD4 lymphocyte counts of ≥200/mm³. These data suggest that BA and/or bacillary parenchymal peliosis occur late in the course of HIV infection, when there is severe immunosuppression, and should be considered an AIDS-defining opportunistic infection.[25]

BA resembles other vascular processes such as pyogenic granuloma, Kaposi's sarcoma, epithelioid hemangioma, and angiosarcoma.[22] Clinically, it may

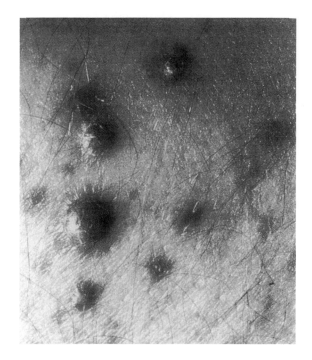

FIGURE 2. Clinical appearance of lesions of cutaneous bacillary angiomatosis. (From Adal, K. A., *et al.*, 1994, *N. Engl. J. Med.* **330:**1509–1515, with permission.)

be impossible to distinguish the solitary form of BA from pyogenic granuloma. The absence of macules, patches, and plagues in BA aids in its differentiation from Kaposi's sarcoma. When multiple lesions are present, BA usually can be easily differentiated from these other disease processes. However, diagnosis of BA can be made definitively on the basis of histological features.[26] Therefore, a skin biopsy is an important part of the diagnostic evaluation.

4.1.2. Histological Features

The most prominent feature of a cutaneous BA lesion is vascular proliferation composed of plump endothelial cells.[24,27] Both superficial and deeper lesions are lobular capillary proliferations.[22] The lobules are aggregates of capillaries, usually with more mature capillaries toward the center and less mature vessels around the periphery. The stroma around early lesions is edematous and fibrotic around late ones. There may be only a slight protrusion of the endothelial cells into the vascular lumina, or there may be dramatic endothelial cell swelling leading to complete blockage of the blood vessels. Lesions also consist of a mixed inflammatory cell infiltrate consisting predominantly of neutrophils and leukocytes with fragmented nuclei. The neutrophils are scattered throughout the lesions and are frequently clustered around aggregates of bacteria, except when there is an extremely high bacterial load.

Endothelial cell necrosis also may be present.[22] The necrotic foci are often small and contain neutrophils and sometimes macrophages. Large necrotic areas are sometimes observed in the centers of vascular lobules.

4.1.3. Bacteria

Bacteria in BA lesions can be seen by Warthin–Starry staining or by electron microscopy. The organisms appear as dark aggregates in the interstitia within the lesions.[23] Isolation of *Bartonella* typically requires incubation for 2 to 6 weeks or longer for primary isolation. The isolate must then be identified by genetic or biochemical methods. Isolation of *B. henselae* and *B. quintana* from the blood of immunocompromised patients, chronic alcoholics, or patients with systemic disease is usually possible. This method of isolation is not difficult and does not require special media or equipment not usually found in a clinical laboratory. Alternatively, the polymerase chain reaction (PCR) can be used to detect *Bartonella* DNA extracted from skin lesions. This method is more rapid and allows the specific detection of the organism directly from the clinical sample. PCR, however, requires special equipment and is technically more difficult than isolation.

4.1.4. Treatment

The length of treatment for cutaneous bacillary angiomatosis varies according to the immune status of the patient.[24] In immunocompetent patients, treatment for 2 to 4 weeks is usually sufficient, depending on the clinical response. In HIV-positive patients, treatment may be needed for weeks to months or longer, if relapses occur. In immunosuppressed, HIV-negative patients, treatment for 4 weeks is usually sufficient. The optimal lengths of time of treatment in patients with BA in conjunction with bacillary peliosis hepatis, fever, and bacteremia, or extracutaneous manifestations are not yet well defined. As a general rule, duration of therapy should be extended. Erythromycin appears to be the antibiotic of choice for treatment of BA. For patients who are not able to tolerate erythromycin, doxycycline may be an alternative.

4.2. Bacillary Peliosis

Peliosis is a rare pathological condition appearing as multiple, blood-filled spaces in parenchyma that are randomly distributed and variable in size.[28] *B. henselae* is the etiological agent of parenchymal bacillary peliosis hepatis (BPH), so termed because it was first observed in the liver. Because bacilli also can be found in the spleen[8,29] and in the interstitium of abdominal lymph nodes of AIDS patients with bacillary peliosis, the term "parenchymal bacillary peliosis" has been adopted for the general condition.[8]

BPH is being recognized more frequently in immunocompromised individuals, especially HIV-positive patients. Perkocha *et al.* in 1990, first reported an association between BPH and HIV infection.[29] In that report, bacteria were found within lesional tissue of all eight HIV-infected patients with peliosis hepatis. Histological features present in patients with BPH, but not in patients with non HIV-associated peliosis hepatis, include peliotic spaces separated from surrounding liver cells by fibromyxoid stroma containing a mixture of inflammatory cells, dilated capillaries, and clumps of granular material. Warthin–Starry staining and electron microscopy showed that the clumps were clusters of bacteria. Leong *et al.* observed that the bacilli may be present extracellularly as well as intracellularly in the cytoplasm of hepatic sinusoidal endothelial cells.[21] As is the case with BA, BPH lesions are lined by stimulated vascular endothelium.[29]

Symptoms of BPH include fever, nausea, vomiting, diarrhea, and abdominal distension. Upon physical examination, hepatosplenomegaly is usually present. Laboratory findings typically demonstrate a mild-to-moderate elevation of serum aminotransferase level and a moderate-to-severe elevation of alkaline phosphatase levels.[29] Bilirubin levels may be normal or only slightly elevated.

BPH may also affect a patient's hematological status.[28] BPH was reported to have caused an anemia not responsive to blood transfusions in an HIV-infected patient.[28] This anemia was due to the sequestration of blood in the liver. Although BPH can occur as an isolated condition, it also may coexist with BA.[8,29]

In BPH, it also appears that *B. henselae* can induce several different pathological responses depending on the immunocompromised status of the patient.[8] In patients in whom the cell-mediated immune response is incompletely abrogated, as in the case of transplant patients receiving immunosuppressive therapy, a pyogranulamatous response can occur. This response appears to be associated with morphological disruption of *B. henselae* present in the pyogranulomatous lesions as organisms showed varying stages of disintegration.[8] However, in the case of HIV-infected patients with BA and/or BPH, the more profound suppression of cell-mediated immunity may limit or prevent granuloma formation.[8]

BPH resolves after treatment with antibiotics, especially erythromycin.[29] Inadequate treatment of HIV-associated BPH can be progressive and may be fatal.

4.3. Bacteremia

B. henselae and *B. quintana* cause bacteremia in immunocompromised patients, as well as in immunocompetent patients. In 1990, Slater *et al.*, first reported *Bartonella*-associated bacteremia.[5] They isolated the previously unrecognized species *B. henselae* after extended incubation of blood cultures from three immunocompromised patients and two immunocompetent patients. Two of the immunocompromised patients were HIV-infected and the other was a bone marrow transplant recipient. There was no evident portal of infection. There appear to be two distinct clinical syndromes associated with bacteremia due to infection with *B. henselae*.[5,30] Patients infected with HIV have a developing syndrome of generalized fatigue, malaise, weight loss, and increasing temperatures.These symptoms last for weeks to months before being diagnosed.

To eradicate the fever and prevent relapses, patients must be treated for 1 month or more. Because organisms may no longer be cultured after the beginning of antimicrobial therapy, when this syndrome is suspected it is important to emphasize that cultures be obtained before the start of antimicrobial therapy, On the other hand, immunocompromised patients not infected with HIV, as well as immunocompetent patients, tend to have a sudden onset of febrile illness that lasts only several days. With short courses of antimicrobial treatment (no longer than 10 days), there is rapid resolution of the bacteremia and no subsequent clinical recurrences.[9]

The most complete study of bacteremia caused by *B. quintana* was reported by Spach *et al.* who followed ten patients at a single hospital in Seattle, WA. within a 6-month period.[31] All ten patients were chronic alcoholics, eight were homeless, and the six who were tested for HIV infection were HIV-negative.[31] Although the authors did not state the immune status of the patients, it has been reported that chronic alcoholism is a factor contributing to an immunocompromised state.[32] In these patients, physical examination did not reveal any consistent symptoms other than fever and weight loss. In three patients for whom follow-up data were available, antimicrobial treatment for at least 3 weeks resulted in negative blood cultures. One patient who did not comply with antimicrobial therapy had persistent (relapsing) bacteremia for 8 weeks until he finally completed treatment. Bacteremia due to *B. quintana* has also been reported in HIV-infected individuals with BA[33] and endocarditis.[13]

4.4. Endocarditis

Spach *et al.* were the first to report *Bartonella* as a cause of endocarditis.[13] The patient was a 50-year-old HIV-positive homosexual man who presented with a swollen, erythematous left palm. The patient complained of fatigue, weight loss, and night sweats. Physical examination revealed a holosystolic heart murmur, a palpable spleen, and left palmar erythema and swelling. An echocardiogram revealed a small echogenic mass on the aortic valve and another on the mitral valve. *B. quintana* was isolated from blood cultures after 28 to 42 days of incubation and was identified by DNA relatedness studies. Further supporting *B. quintana* as the cause for this patient's endocarditis was the negative serology tests for

Coxiella burnetii, Brucella sp., and *Francisella tularensis* and failure to isolate an organism other than *B. quintana* from blood cultures. *B. quintana* endocarditis was also reported in three homeless men.[12] All three were not infected with HIV, but had histories of chronic alcoholism.

To date, there have been 33 reported cases of *Bartonella* endocarditis, with the most comprehensive study being a report of 22 cases by Raoult *et al.*[34] Because *Bartonella* spp. are fastidious organisms and cannot be isolated from blood by routine methods, they may cause "culture-negative" infections. It has been estimated that *Bartonella* species causes 3% of all cases of endocarditis and that many of the previously reported cases of blood culture-negative endocarditis may be due to *Bartonella* species.[34] Blood culture-negative endocarditis accounts for 5% to 30% of cases of endocarditis, and remains a diagnostic and therapeutic problem.[34]

Serological cross-reactivity between *B. quintana* and *Chlamyida* species has been observed.[12] Because both *Bartonella* and *Chlamydia* species are implicated in infectious endocarditis, this may confuse the diagnosis. Presumptive diagnosis of endocarditis caused by *Bartonella* or *Chlamydia* species may be supported by serological studies, but definitive diagnosis requires demonstration of the organism in blood or a cardiac valve. Although *B. henselae, B. elizabethae,* and *B. quintana,* are etiologic agents of endocarditis, only *B. quintana,* thus far, has been associated with an immunocompromised state. *B. henselae* is associated with exposure to cats and *B. quintana* with homelessness, alcoholism, and poor hygiene.[35]

4.5. Central Nervous System Involvement

In 1992, the first case of intracranial bacillary angiomatosis was described by Spach *et al.*[26] A 49-year-old HIV-positive man presented with a lesion (1.5 cm) in the left temporal lobe with no evidence of vascular proliferation or malignancy. Clinical signs 4 months later included headaches, blindness in his right visual field, and difficulty speaking. At this time there was an increase in the size of the lesion to 2 cm, with lymphocytic infiltration, prominent microvasculature with plump endothelial cells, and an overgrowth of astrocytes. No evidence of malignancy was present. Four months later, a new 2.2 cm temporal mass surrounded by edema presented in the right antecubital fossa. The lesion showed signs of vascular proliferation, pleomorphic bacilli by Warthin–Starry staining, and trilaminar cell-walled organisms by electron microscopy. Warthin–Starry staining of the second brain biopsy specimen also showed pleomorphic bacilli. Additional evidence that the intracranial lesion was due to the BA bacilli was the resolution of the skin lesions and the nearly complete resolution of the brain lesions in response to erythromycin treatment. Extensive histological and microbiological examination of the brain tissue did not reveal an alternative cause. The specific *Bartonella* species responsible for the intracerebral bacillary angiomatosis was not identified.

An association between onset of neuropsychological decline or dementia in HIV-infected individuals and serum IgM antibodies to *B. henselae* was reported.[15] In this study, the dementia or neuropsychological decline observed in 4% of HIV-seropositive patients was attributed to *B. henselae* infection. It was reported that the evidence suggested that these patients responded to antimicrobial treatment. This is of clinical importance, as *B. henselae* is one of the few treatable causes of dementia.

4.6. Other Clinical Manifestations

Other clinical manifestations due to *Bartonella* in immunocompromised individuals include *B. henselae*-associated aseptic meningitis, regional lymphadenitis, and neuroretinitis in HIV-infected patients.[36] In the case of aseptic meningitis, prolonged bacteremia was also observed. For patients with neuroretinitis, especially if a stellate lesion is present, *B. henselae* infection should be considered in the differential diagnosis because it is a treatable cause of this disease.

5. CONCLUSIONS

Bartonella spp. have been recently identified as emerging infectious agents. A variety of clinical manifestations have been associated with *B. henselae* and *B. quintana*, with the spectrum of illnesses still expanding. In light of this, especially in the immunocompromised host, it is possible that *Bartonella* spp. thought to be nonpathogenic for humans will be shown to cause human disease and that new species within the genus *Bartonella* will be identified. In general, patients who are immunocompromised by having AIDS, chronic alcoholism, immunosuppression, or other compromising health problems tend to have systemic disease. As our knowledge of *Bartonella* as infectious agents in immunocompromised, as well as immunocompetent, individuals increases, better diagnosis treatment, and prevention of diseases caused by these organisms will be developed.

REFERENCES

1. Brenner, D. J., O'Connor, S. P., Winkler, H. H., and Steigerwalt, A. G., 1993, Proposals to unify the genera *Bartonella* and *Rochalimaea*, with descriptions of *Bartonella quintana* comb. nov., *Bartonella vinsonii* comb. nov., Bartonella henselae comb. nov., and *Bartonella elizabethae* comb. nov., and to remove the family *Bartonellaceae* from the order *Rickettsiales*, *Int. J. Syst. Bact.* **43:**777–786.
2. Zbinden, R., Hochli, M., and Nadal, D., 1995, Intracellular location of *Bartonella henselae* cocultivated with Vero cells and used for an indirect fluorescent-antibody test, *Clin. Diagn. Lab. Immunol.* **2:**693–695.
3. Batterman, H. J., Peek, J. A., Loutit, J. S., Falkow, S., and Tompkins, L. S., 1995, *Bartonella henselae* and *Bartonella quintana* adherence to and entry into cultured human epithelial cells, *Infect. Immun.* **63:**4553–4556.

4. Kordick, D. L., and Breitschwerdt, E. B., 1995, Intraerythrocytic presence of *Bartonella henselae, J. Clin. Microbiol.* **33:**1655–1656.
5. Slater, L. N., Welch, D. F.,Hensel, D., and Coody, D. W., 1990, A newly recognized fastidious gram-negative pathogen as a cause of fever and bacteremia. *N. Engl. J. Med.* **23:**1587–1593.
6. Rodriguez-Barradas, M. C., Bandres, J.U., Hamill, R. J., Trial, J., Clarridge, J. E., III, Baughn, R. E., and Rossen, R. D., 1995, *In vitro* evaluation of the role of humoral immunity against *Bartonella henselae, Infect. Immun.* **63:**2367–2370.
7. Koehler, J. E., Quinn, F. D., Berger, T. G., LeBoit, P. E., and Tappero, J. W., 1992, Isolation of *Rochalimaea* species from cutaneous and osseous lesions of bacillary angiomatosis, *N. Engl. J. Med.* **327:**1625–1631.
8. Slater, L. N., Welch, D. F., and Min, K. W., 1992, *Rochalimaea henselae* causes bacillary angiomatosis and peliosis hepatis, *Arch. Intern. Med.* **152:**602–606.
9. Welch, D. F., Pickett, D. A., Slater, L. N., Steigerwalt, A. G., and Brenner, D. J., 1992, *Rochalimaea henselae* sp. nov., a cause of septicemia, bacillary angiomatosis, and parenchymal bacillary peliosis, *J. Clin. Microbiol.* **30:**275–280.
10. Hadfield, T. L., Warren, R., Kass, M., Brun, E., and Levy, C., 1993, Endocarditis caused by *Rochalimaea henselae, Hum. Pathol.* **24:**1140–1141.
11. Daly, J. S., Worthington, M. G., Brenner, D. J., Moss, C. W., Hollis, D. G., Weyant, R. S., Steigerwalt, A. G., Weaver, R. E., Daneshvar, M. I., and O'Connor, S. P., 1993, *Rochalimaea elizabethae* sp. nov. isolated from a patient with endocarditis, *J. Clin. Microbiol.* **31:**872–881.
12. Drancourt, M., Mainardi, J. L., Brouqui, P., Vandenesch, F., Carta, A., Lehnert, F., Etienne, J., Goldstein, F., Acar, J., and Raoult, D., 1995, *Bartonella (Rochalimaea) quintana* endocarditis in three homeless men, *N. Engl. J. Med.* **332:**419–423.
13. Spach, D. J., Callis, K. P., Paauw, D. S., Houze, Y. B., Schoenknecht, F. D., Welch, D. F., Rosen, H., and Brenner, D. J., 1993, Endocarditis caused by *Rochalimaea quintana* in a patient infected with human immunodeficiency virus, *J. Clin. Microbiol.* **31:**692–694.
14. Jackson, L. A., and Spach, D. H., 1996, Emergence of *Bartonella quintana* infection among homeless persons, *Emerg. Infect. Dis.* **2:**141–143.
15. Schwartzman, W. A., Patnaik, M., Angulo, F. J., Visscher, B. R., Miller, E. N., and Peter, J. B., 1995, *Bartonella (Rochalimaea)* antibodies, dementia, and cat ownership among men infected with human immunodeficiency virus, *Clin. Infect. Dis.* **21:**954–959.
16. Stoler, M. H., Bonfiglio, T. A., Steigbigel, R. T., and Pereira, M., 1983, An atypical subcutaneous infection associated with acquired immune deficiency syndrome, *Am. J. Clin. Pathol.* **80:**714–718.
17. Schwartzman, W. A., 1996, (Editorial) Bacillary angiomatosis and parenchymal peliosis: Frequent absence of mucocutaneous lesions, *Clin. Infect. Dis.* **22:**801–802.
18. Tappero, J. W., Koehler, J. E., Berger, T. G., Cockerell, C. J., Lee, T. H., Busch, M. P., Stites, D. P., Mohle-Boetani, J., Reingold, A. L., and LeBoit, P. E., 1993, Bacillary angiomatosis and bacillary splenitis in immunocompetent adults, *Ann. Intern. Med.* **118:**363–365.
19. Smith, K. J., Skelton, H. G., Tuur, S., Larson, P. L., and Angritt, P., 1996, Bacillary angiomatosis in an immunocompetent child, *Am. J. Dermatopathol.* **18:**597–600.
20. Slater, L. N., Pitha, J. V., Herrera, L., Hughson, M. D., Min, K. W., and Reed, J. A., 1994, *Rochalimaea henselae* infection in acquired immunodeficiency syndrome causing inflammatory disease without angiomatosis or peliosis: Demonstration by immunocytochemistry and corroboration by DNA amplification, *Arch. Pathol. Lab. Med.* **118:**33–38.
21. Leong, S. S., Cazen, R. A., Yu, G. S. M., LeFevre, L., and Carson, J. W., 1992, Abdominal visceral peliosis associated with bacillary angiomatosis, *Arch. Pathol. Lab. Med.* **116:**866–871.
22. Cockerell, C. J., and LeBoit, P. E., 1990, Bacillary angiomatosis: A newly characterized, pseudo-neoplastic infectious, cutaneous vascular disorder, *J. Am. Acad. Dermatol.* **22:**501–512.
23. Cockerell, C. J., Tierno, P. M., Friedman-Kien, A. E., and Kim, K. S., 1991, Clinical, histologic,

microbiologic, and biochemical characterization of the causative agent of bacillary (epitheliod) angiomatosis: A rickettsial illness with features of bartonellosis, *J. Invest. Dermatol.* **97:**812–817.

24. Adal, K. A., Cockerell, C. J., and Petri, W. A., 1994, Cat scratch disease, bacillary angiomatosis, and other infections due to *Rochalimaea*, *N. Engl. J. Med.* **330:**1509–1515.

25. Mohle-Boetani, J. C., Koehler, J. E., Berger, T. G., LeBoit, P. E., Plikaytis, B. D., Wenger, J. D., and Tappero, J. W., 1996, Bacillary angiomatosis and bacillary peliosis in patients infected with human immunodeficiency virus: Clinical characteristics in a vase-control study, *Clin. Infect. Dis.* **22:**794–800.

26. Spach, D. H., Panther, L. A., Thorning, D. R., Dunn, J. E., Plorde, J. J., and Miller, R. A., 1992, Intracerebral bacillary angiomatosis in a patient infected with human immunodeficiency virus, *Ann. Intern. Med.* **116:**740–742.

27. Anderson, B. E., and Neuman, M. A., 1997, *Bartonella* spp. as emerging human pathogens, *Clin. Microbiol. Rev.* **10:**203–219.

28. Garcia-Tsao, G., Panzini, L., Yoselevitz, M., and West, A. B., 1992, Bacillary peliosis hepatis as a cause of acute anemia in a patient with the acquired immunododeficiency syndrome, *Gastroenterology* **102:**1065–1070.

29. Perkocha, L. A., Geaghan, S. M., Benedict Yen, T. S., Nishimura, S. L., Chan, S. P., Garcia-Kennedy, G., Honda, A. C., Stoloff, H. Z., Klein, R. L., Goldman, S., Van Meter, L. D., Ferrell, R., LeBoit, P. E., 1990, Clinical and pathological features of bacillary peliosis hepatis in association with human immunodeficiency virus infection, *N. Engl. J. Med.* **323:**1581–1586.

30. Schwartzman, W. A., 1992, Infections due to *Rochalimaea:* The expanding clinical spectrum, *Clin. Infect. Dis.* **15:**893–902.

31. Spach, D. H., Kanter, A. S., Dougherty, M. J., Larson, A. M., Coyle, M. B., Brenner, D. J., Swaminathan, B., Matar, G. M., Welch, D. F., Root, R. K., and Stamm, W. E., 1995, *Bartonella (Rochalimaea) quintana* bacteremia in inner-city patients with chronic alcoholism, *N. Engl. J. Med.* **332:**424–428.

32. Roschmann, R. A., and Bell, C. L., 1987, Septic bursitis in immunocompromised patients, *Am. J. Med.* **83:**661–665.

33. Maurin, M., Roux, V., Stein, S., Ferrier, F., Viraben, R., and Raoult, D., 1994, Isolation and characterization by immunofluorescence, sodium dodecyl sulfate-polyacrylamide gel electrophoresis, Western blot, restriction fragment length polymorphism PCR, 16S rRNA gene sequencing, and pulsed field gel electrophoresis of *Rochalimaea quintana* from a patient with bacillary angiomatosis, *J. Clin. Microbiol.* **32:**1166–1171.

34. Raoult, D., Fournier, P. E., Drancourt, M., Marrie, T. J., Etienne, J., Cosserat, J., Cacob, P., Poinsignon, Y., Leclercq, P., and Sefton, M., 1996, Diagnosis of 22 new cases of *Bartonella* endocarditis, *Ann. Intern. Med.* **125:**646–652.

35. Breathnach, A. S., Hoare, J. M., and Eykyn, S. J., 1997, Culture-negative endocarditis: Contribution of *Bartonella* infections, *Hearst* **77:**474–476

36. Wong, M. T., Dolan, M. J., Lattuada, C. P., Jr., Regnery, R. L., Garcia, M. L., Mokulis, E. C., LaBarre, R. C., Ascher, D. P., Delmar, J. A., Kelly, J. W., Leigh, D. R., McRae, A. C., Reed, J. B., Smith, R. E., and Melcher, G. P., 1995, Neuroretinitis, aseptic meningitis, and lymphadenitis associated with *Bartonella (Rochalimaea) henselae* infection in immunocompetent patients and patients infected with human immunodeficiency virus type I, *Clin. Infect. Dis.* **21:**352–360.

13

Chlamydia trachomatis Infections

JULIUS SCHACHTER

1. THE ORGANISM

Chlamydiae are unusual in that they are obligate intracellular parasites (characteristic of viruses), but they have other characteristics of bacteria. In fact, for many years they were thought to be viruses. However, it became clear that they had a complex cell wall (somewhat similar to that of Gram-negative bacteria in composition), both DNA and RNA, prokaryotic ribosomes, and metabolic enzymes that would permit independent existence, except that they lack energy-production mechanisms. Moulder thus termed the chlamydiae "energy parasites" and credited their obligate intracellular parasitism to this trait.[1]

Chlamydiae are presently placed in their own order, the *Chlamydiales*, family *Chlaydiaceae*, with one genus, *Chlamydia*.[2] There are four species—*C. trachomatis, C. psittaci, C. pecorum,* and *C. pneumoniae*. All are important pathogens of humans or animals. *C. trachomatis*, the subject of this chapter, includes the organisms causing trachoma, inclusion conjunctivitis, lymphogranulam venereum (LGV) and the other sexually transmitted chlamydial infections, and some rodent pneumonia strains. *C. trachomatis* strains are sensitive to the action of sulfonamides and produce a glycogen-like material within an inclusion vacuole, which stains with iodine. The mouse pneumonitis, LGV, and the trachoma strains are representative of the three biovars in this species.

The LGV and trachoma biovars are exclusively human pathogens. Both can be sexually transmitted, with the LGV biovar causing oculogenital infections.

JULIUS SCHACHTER • Department of Laboratory Medicine, University of California, San Francisco, San Francisco, California 94110.

Opportunistic Intracellular Bacteria and Immunity, edited by Lois J. Paradise *et al.* Plenum Press, New York, 1999.

They differ significantly in their biological activity. LGV strains (three serovars) are more invasive and can invade many tissues in addition to epithelial cells (e.g., lymph-node invasion, forming the characteristic bubo). The oculogenital strains, comprising the trachoma biovar, consist of 12 serovars. They are not highly invasive in cell culture (they require mechanical assistance for infection whereas the LGV biovar does not). *In vivo*, the trachoma biovar grows only in columnar and squamocolumnar epithelial cells (conjunctivae, respiratory tract, urethra, cervix, gastrointestinal tract, and rectal mucosa). Within *C. trachomatis* the chlamydiae are usually referred to by serovar or biovar.

The organism is about 40% to 50% lipid, 35% protein, and there are small amounts (1% to 2%) of carbohydrate. Chlamydiae have a cell wall structure that is in some ways similar to that of Gram-negative bacteria, although the peptidoglycan layer appears to be lacking. The major outer membrane protein (MOMP or omp1) is generally in the molecular weight range of 39,000 to 45,000 daltons and comprises approximately 60% of the weight of the outer membrane.[3] Chlamydiae also contain a rough lipopolysaccharide (LPS).[4]

2. REPLICATION

The unique characteristic of the chlamydiae is their reproductive cycle. The extracellular form of the organism is the elementary body (EB), and it alone is infectious. Following attachment, the EB enters the host cell, apparently by a receptor-mediated endocytosis process.[5] If the particles are live, or do not have antibody attached, they prevent phagolysosomal fusion and undergo replication in the phagosome. The phagocytic process is directly influenced by the chlamydiae as ingestion of organisms is specifically enhanced.[6] Uptake of many organisms has been shown to be associated with tyrosine phosphorylation of host cell and outer membrane proteins and evidence has been presented to suggests that the same is true for chlamydiae.[7] It is obvious that the EB would be vulnerable to the action of neutralizing or bactericidal antibody action prior to entering a susceptible host cell. Chlamydiae also have specific sites involved in attachment to the susceptible host cell and conceivably antibody could prevent infectivity by blocking the attachment sites, or perhaps even steric hindrance by attached antibody might be an effective way of preventing infection. It appears that heparan-like compounds are involved in attachment of *C. trachomatis* to susceptible host cells.[8] These highly charged sulfated polysaccharides appear to attach both the chlamydiae and to a cell site involved in triggering endocytosis on the part of the mammalian cell. Thus, the heparan-like compounds act as a bridge between the EB and the cell.

Following attachment, the EB enters the cell in an endosome where the entire growth cycle is completed. Once the EB (diameter 0.25 to 0.35 μm) has entered the cell, it reorganizes into a reticulate body (RB or initial body) that is larger (0.51 to 1 μm) and richer in RNA. There does appear to be trafficking between the Golgi apparatus and the chlamydial inclusion as lipids are transferred to the inclusion from the cell.[9] After about 8 h, the RB begins dividing by binary fission. Approximately 18 to 24 h after infection, these RBs start to become EBs by a poorly understood reorganization or condensation process. These intracytoplasmic collections of elementary bodies constitute the inclusions that may be seen in cytological smears stained by Giemsa or immunofluorescence methods.

Typically the host cell is lysed at the end of the cycle, but occasionally the inclusion is extruded and the host cell survives. The full cycle takes about 40 h for the LGV biovar, and 72 to 96 h for the trachoma biovar.

The EBs released may then initiate another cycle of infection. The EBs are specifically adapted for extracellular survival and are the infectious form, whereas the intracellular metabolically active and replicating form, the RB, does not survive well outside the host cell and is adapted for an intracellular milieu.

3. ANTIGENIC COMPOSITION

All chlamydiae share a common complement-fixing antigen. This antigen is the LPS. It is soluble in either, stable to boiling and sensitive to periodate. It is antigenically similar to the LPS of *Acinetobacter calcoaceticus* and Re mutants of *Salmonella*.[4] There are also protein antigens of genus, species, and subspecies specificity.[3,10]

C. trachomatis may be divided by the microimmunofluorescence (micro-IF) technique into 15 serovars.[11] These serovars fall into two major complexes (the B and C complexes). The endemic trachoma strains are in the A, B, Ba, and C serovars, whereas the D through K serovars are typically sexually transmitted. The LGV biovar forms another group of three serovars–L1, L2, and L3—that fall within the B complex and are broadly cross reactive.

The best studied chlamydial surface and structural protein is the major outer membrane protein. Much of the serovar reactivity (as well as the species-specific reactions) is due to epitopes on MOMP.[10] MOMP is a highly crosslinked cysteine-rich protein that appears to contribute to the structural rigidity of the organism through disulfide bonds with other MOMP molecules as well as two other proteins (Omp2 and Omp3) of approximately 60 kDa and 13 kDa. Animals immunized with purified elementary bodies of *C. trachomatis* respond by making large quantities of antibodies to MOMP. The nucleotide sequences of the MOMP genes of different serovars of *C. trachomatis* have been elucidated. There are five conserved regions bounding four variable regions. The four variable regions are encoded for peptides of serovar, serogroup, and species-specific antigens.[12] Amino acid changes in two of these regions appear responsible for serovar specificity. Serovar-specific and neutralizing responses have been shown to usually reside in variable regions 1 and 2 in peptide fragments as small as six to ten amino acids.[13] The species-specific reactivity is in variable region 4.

It is assumed that this protein has a multiple looped structure with three of the variable domains appearing at the surface of the organism as protruding loops. That there is considerable variation within these domains suggests that they may have undergone a selection process by neutralizing antibody. This has added to the speculation that this protein is a good candidate antigen for a vaccine and that neutralizing antibody may be important in immunity to chlamydial infection. It must be stressed that although it is fairly easy to demonstrate neutralization *in vitro*, the actual mechanism of immunity to chlamydial infection is not clear. Still, MOMP has been considered the likely candidate for a chlamydial vaccine.

The observation that many MOMP variants are found in a single sexually transmitted disease (STD) high-risk core group suggests that there is active antigenic selection in a highly exposed, that is, assumed to be highly immune, population.[14] This suggests that a MOMP vaccine may be of questionable value. In fact, the presence of serum neutralizing antibody has been found not to correlate with resistance to reinfection with that same serovar.[15] It is possible that the serovars could be very closely related because escape variants that appear to be very similar to the original serovars have been shown to escape neutralization by polyclonal human sera.[16] However, in endemic trachoma in The Gambia there was relatively little evidence of antigenic drift or genovar variation over an approximate 2-year period. MOMP variation was quite limited.[17]

Chlamydiae have a number of other antigenic properties that may be assayed. These include a hemagglutinin for murine and certain fowl erythrocytes, and mouse toxicity (intravenous inoculation of large quantities of viable chlamydia results in rapid death in mice and this can be neutralized by specific antisera).

4. CLINICAL ASPECTS AND EPIDEMIOLOGY

4.1. Genital Tract Infections

C. trachomatis is currently considered to be the most common sexually transmitted bacterial pathogen.[18] In men, it is a major cause of nongonococcal and postgonococcal urethritis and epididymitis. In women, the organism may cause mucopurulent endocervicitis, urethritis, and endometritis. Chlamydiae have been shown to be important causes of acute salpingitis and are responsible for many of the complications associated with this condition. Thus, the organism is now known to be an important cause of Fitz–Hugh–Curtis syndrome (perihepatitis), tubal factor infertility, and ectopic pregnancy. Rectal infections and proctitis can occur in either sex. Mild and subclinical infections with these organisms are common. The organism may persist in the genital tract for years in the absence of anti-microbial therapy. Treatment is usually with doxycycline (100 mg b.i.d. × 7 d), or azithromycin as single-dose (1 g) therapy.

4.2. Trachoma

Trachoma is a chronic keratoconjunctivitis caused by *C. trachomatis*. It may begin as mucopurulent conjunctivitis and is often complicated by secondary bacterial infection. Marked follicular reaction and papillary hypertrophy develop. In hyperendemic areas most active disease is seen in young children. As the follicular reaction resolves, some focal necrosis may occur and scarring of the upper conjunctivae can develop. Over time, these scars contract and cause in-turning of the upper eyelids, so that the eyelashes abrade the cornea. These lesions (trichiasis and entropion) represent the blinding lesions of trachoma. It takes many years for sufficient contraction of scars to occur to cause lid distortion and this blindness is generally seen more that 25 to 30 years after the peak of active inflammatory processes. Mild cases of trachoma rarely lead to visual loss.

The main reservoir for infection is young children with severe inflammatory disease. Trachoma is a family disease and is spread from child to child by direct personal contact. Flies can act as mechanical vectors, as they feed on ocular discharges. Occasionally adults may have active disease or be inapparent shed-ders and a source of infection for children in the household.

Trachoma may be effectively treated with systemic antibiotics. Tetracycline is the drug of choice, although contraindicated for those less than 8 years old. Thus, sulfonamides and erythromycin have been used. In the endemic area, however, systemic therapy is difficult to manage and most trachoma control programs are based on mass treatment with topical tetracycline.

It should be noted that although trachoma occurs in parts of Asia and Africa where acquired immunodeficiency syndrome (AIDS) is a problem, there is no evidence that the course of trachoma is affected by the immunocompromised status of those with human immunodeficiency virus (HIV) infection. Similarly, there is no evidence that sexually transmitted chlamydial infections have a differ-ent course of infection in AIDS as compared to that found in individuals with intact immune systems. There is no evidence for a broader spectrum of disease attributed to *C. trachomatis* in the presence of HIV. Efforts to identify *C. trachomatis* as a possible pathogen in respiratory tracts of those with AIDS have found very low rates of infection in lung biopsies or bronchoalveolar lavages.[19]

5. PATHOGENESIS

There is little information on the molecular basis of chlamydial virulence. Studies in cell cultures have identified a number of virulence factors that appear to be important in establishing infection. These include the ability to recognize specific attachment sites, the ability to induce phagocytosis, and the ability to avoid phagolysosomal fusion.

In the early stages trachoma is a follicular conjunctivitis with hyperemia, edema, and distortion of the vascular pattern of the conjunctiva. This is accompanied by papillary hypertrophy of the conjunctiva. The follicles are, in fact, lymphoid germinal centers. Such conjunctival follicles can develop as a response to a number of stimuli, both infectious and toxic. The infant conjunctiva cannot so respond for a number of weeks, and thus chlamydial ocular infection of the newborn (inclusion conjunctivitis) is not follicular, even though the organisms are biologically indistinguishable from those causing trachoma. The chronic follicular conjunctivitis of trachoma heals by scarring.

These signs of trachoma have all been duplicated in subhuman primates infected with isolated *C. trachomatis*. However, the initial infection in subhuman primates is typically a self-limited follicular conjunctivitis. The long-term sequelae as signs of a chronic disease found in humans are seen only in the experimental disease after repeated infection. Pannus (corneal neovascularization) is only a result of reinfection (exogenous reinfection or endogenous relapse).[20] Whether this is true for human disease has never been substantiated. If it is, then the disease that is characterized as trachoma (with pannus) is never a primary infection. It definitely is clear in human disease that the serious sequelae leading to blindness occur only as a result of many reinfections, made worse by the many other causes of corneal diseases in hyperendemic trachomatous populations including bacterial infections and various environmental factors such as dust and sunlight.

Members of the trachoma biovar of *C. trachomatis* are essentially parasites of columnar epithelial cells and appear to cause disease in most anatomical sites where these cells are found. These organisms are primarily pathogens of the conjunctivae and genital tract, where these cells predominate. They can also cause disease in the gastrointestinal and respiratory tracts. The LGV biovar has a broader cell range, involving lymphoid and endothelial cells. It is more invasive and apparently can cause more tissue destruction as a result of the infectious process.

Because the trachoma biovar does not appear to be capable of infecting enough cells to cause the tissue damage that appears in some of the diseases, immunological mechanisms for pathogenesis have been postulated. More severe disease is often seen in secondary infection and in reinfection with heterolgous biovars. It has been shown that a triton extract of chlamydial particles can induce conjunctival inflammation in guinea pigs sensitized by a prior chlamydial infection.[21] An active component within the triton extracts has been identified as the chlamydial homolog of the GroEL heat-shock protein (hsp).[22] This 57-kDa (usually called hsp 60) antigen shares epitopes with *Escherichia coli* and *Mycobacterium tuberculosis*.[23]

It has been postulated that hypersensitivity reaction to specific chlamydia heat-shock proteins may be responsible for the inflammation seen on reinfection. The same extract (hsp 60) shown to induce inflammation when dropped onto the eyes of guinea pigs previously infected with guinea pig inclusion conjunctivitis will cause inflammation in the eyes of monkeys that have been previously infected by *C. trachomatis.*[24]

High titers of antibody to the heat-shock protein have also been detected in women suffering the consequences of pelvic inflammatory disease (ectopic pregnancy and tubal factor infertility),[23,25] and in scarring trachoma. It has long been known that women with repeated episodes of PID are more likely to suffer these kinds of consequences of PID. More recent studies have documented that young women who have repeated episodes of chlamydial infection of the cervix are also more likely to suffer these consequences. Presumably, many of these are due to subclinical PID. Epidemiological studies performed in the state of Wisconsin found that women with three diagnosed chlamydial infections between the years 1985 and 1992 had a relative risk of 5 for ectopic pregnancy as compared to women with a single infection. The crude rates for those are 250 ectopic pregnancies per 100,000 for those with one infection; 446 per 100,000 for two infections, and 939 per 100,000 for three or more infections.[26]

It has been suggested, although not yet proven, that local hyperreactivity to this antigen may be responsible for some of the severe inflammation, scarring, and ultimate consequences of disease due to *C. trachomatis.* However, individuals from a trachoma endemic area who had severe conjunctival scarring were actually found to have lower cell-mediated immune responses to chlamydial elementary bodies, MOMP, or hsp 60 than were matched controls who were free of scarring. The individuals with scarring had higher antibody levels. This of course is inconsistent with the theory that scarring results from enhanced cell-mediated immunity (CMI) to hsp 60.[27]

Scarring is a common endpoint in the pathological sequence of these infections for it is that which ultimately leads to blindness in trachoma and to infertility or ectopic pregnancy in salpingitis. LGV also has scarring as a prominent consequence. The currently prevailing theory is that the severe disease outcome, which is typified at the end-stage level by scarring of target sites [conjunctiva in the case of trachoma, fallopian tubes in the case of salpingitis, rectal mucosa in the case of LGV (although this mechanism may be different)] is due to enhanced cell-mediated immune responses to heat-shock proteins, largely hsp 60.

6. IMMUNITY

If reinfection is a necessary factor for severe trachoma, what is the role of immunity? In the experimental animal, after infections for a short period there is immunity to reinfection with homologous strains (but no immunity to heterologous rechallenge). In studies that were made with what are now recognized as relatively crude and antigenically weak vaccines, there was transient immunity to rechallenge. When this immunity waned, not only were experimental animals susceptible to reinfection, but also the severity of disease produced by such rechallenge was enhanced (a phenomenon similar to that seen in other early and crude experimental vaccines, such as those for *Mycoplasma pneumoniae* and respiratory syncytial virus). Whether such a period of hyperreactivity exists in natural human infection has not been determined, but immunity in nature is fleeting. Infection in humans and in experimental animals produces both local and circulatory immune responses, but these antibodies do not appear to be protective. One epidemiological fact continues to kindle interest in the prospect of producing an effective vaccine for trachoma—the observation that in all endemic situations studied, active trachoma decreases with age. Although the age at which this occurs will vary with the intensity of disease in the population, ultimately the older segment of the population no longer has active disease, suggesting that immunity eventually prevails. It is the aim of proponents of vaccine development to create a vaccine that would mimic the natural occurrence.

The assumption that protective immunity to *C. trachomatis* infection develops after naturally occurring infection is supported by other epidemiological studies of chlamydial disease. It has long been known that age-specific prevalence of infections drops quickly after the peak age of prevalence. This occurs regardless of mode of transmission. For example, in trachoma hyperendemic areas, virtually all individuals in the endemic area are infected before they reach age 2. Age-specific prevalence peaks somewhere between 2 and 5 years and then falls fairly dramatically until age 10. Infection rates in adults are seldom higher than 5% to 10%, whereas infection in preschool children is often 50% to 60% or higher. In sexually transmitted chlamydial infections, it has long been recognized that the highest prevalence occurs in sexually active adolescents and that rates drop to much lower levels between the ages of 20 and 30 years. Although some of the observations could be explained on behavioral grounds, it is far likelier that an immunological component is dominant.

Because trachoma is the leading preventable cause of blindness, with hundreds of millions of people living in trachoma endemic areas and millions blinded as a result of disease, it became highly attractive to develop a vaccine for prevention of blinding trachoma or blindness due to trachoma. Shortly after the organism was first isolated in the late 1950s, a number of research teams attempted to develop vaccines. These were relatively crude preparations of partially purified elementary bodies grown in yolk sac (tissue culture was not successfully used at that time.) In addition, these experimental vaccines could protect subhuman primates from infection or disease after challenge. The studies were extended into human field trials and they showed that a short-lived protective effect could be demonstrated.

Unfortunately, those early vaccine trials were compromised by also providing evidence of worse clinical outcome for some of those who developed infection after natural exposure. These observations—the short-lived protective effect and presumed sensitization for worse outcome—led to the abandonment of vaccine studies until more recent times when recombinant technology and research allowed researchers to attempt separation of protective and sensitizing antigens in experimental vaccines.

In part, much of the evidence for immunity in chlamydial infection reflects biases of researchers and prophecies. It must be stated that the actual mechanism of protection or clearance is not known with certainty nor are the protective antigens. However, there is considerable evidence for both protective antibody responses and cell-mediated immune responses for clearance of established infection. Both responses appear to be aimed at reactive sites on chlamydial MOMP. Here too, a body of evidence suggests but does not prove that this is the protective antigen. Clearly the demonstration of considerable serovar specificity and antigenic variation in variable regions of the MOMP supports the concept of immune selection and pressure and, by inference, the importance of these responses in protection.

Other lines of evidence suggest that when high levels of antibody are present, either in ocular or cervical secretions (particularly secretory IgA antibody) there is an inverse correlation between level of antibody and shedding of chlamydiae.[28] In the laboratory it appears fairly easy to demonstrate neutralizing antibody directed against surface exposed antigenic sites in the variable regions of the MOMP. However, it also appears fairly simple to demonstrate neutralizing antibody to a variety of other proteins, including heat-shock proteins, and it is difficult to accept that all of this neutralization seen in laboratory systems is biologically relevant in terms of protection.

7. MEASURING IMMUNE RESPONSES TO *CHLAMYDIA*

As with other microorganisms, the immune responses to chlamydiae often differ according to whether they result from infections induced by natural routes, whether in nature or in the laboratory, or from inoculations of whole organisms or purified antigens. Here, we consider primarily responses to natural infection. Because of wide variations in methods, types of chlamydiae, and study populations reported by various workers, this short account is necessarily generalized.

7.1. Antibody Responses

Chlamydia-specific antibodies of the IgM, IgG, and IgA classes appear both in serum and in local secretions, including tear fluid in the case of eye infections;

the nature and magnitude of the responses vary with the type and duration of infection.

7.2. Antibody Classes

Specific IgA is more constantly demonstrable in secretions from infected mucous membranes than in serum, whereas the reverse is true of IgM antibody. Some or all of the IgG antibody detectable in secretions may be derived by transudation from the blood. IgM and IgG serum antibody titers are liable to be higher in generalized diseases such (as LGV) than in localized infections (such as trachoma). IgM antibody appears early in the serum, but may persist alongside IgG for relatively long periods, especially if reinfections occur. Individuals with complicated infections tend to have higher levels of antibody (that may persist for years) than do individuals with uncomplicated localized infections. For example, women with salpingitis have higher levels of antibody than women with cervical infection; and men with epididymitis have higher levels of antibody than men with uncomplicated urethritis.

It is much easier to measure chlamydia-specific antibodies than to define their role in protection and recovery from infection. In the sera of patients with proven chlamydial infections of the genital tract, IgG, IgM, and IgA antibodies are directed against the MOMP and various other polypeptides of elementary and reticulate bodies.[29] Serotype-specific epitopes on some of these polypeptides elicit neutralizing antibodies, that if produced at mucous surfaces, may play some part in protecting against reinfection, at least in the short term. Antibodies against a variety of specific chlamydial proteins are capable of neutralizing infectivity in cell culture systems, but it has not been possible to relate them to protection against infections *in vivo*. The presence of antichlamydial IgG antibody in tears of individuals living in trachoma endemic areas was not protective—and actually appears to be predictive of an onset of trachoma.[30] There is an inverse correlation between the presence of specific secretory IgA (sIgA) in cervical secretion and the amount of chlamydiae shed.

8. CELL-MEDIATED IMMUNE RESPONSES

C. trachomatis binds to and causes polyclonal stimulation of murine B lymphocytes *in vitro*. The effector molecule does not appear to be the LPS; but rather, it may be the MOMP. By contrast with B lymphocytes, T cells showed specific clonal stimulation by *C. trachomatis* (serotype L2) with class II HLA restriction[31]; in these experiments primed blood monocytes served as antigen presenting cells. The role of T-cell-mediated cytoxicity in chlamydial infection may depend upon the species.

An effective cell-mediated immune response appears, in animal models, to be critical in resolution of chlamydial infection. In owl monkeys, resolution of ocular infection appears to coincide with development of CMI while in chronic mouse pneumonitis infection in nude mice, treatment with antigen-specific T cells was shown to enhance resolution.[32] Attempts to determine whether the same is true in humans with resolved ocular chlamydial infection in trachoma endemic areas showed that the individuals who cleared the chlamydial infection had greater lymphoproliferative response to EB suspensions, a MOMP preparation, or hsp 60.[33]

It has become obvious in a number of experimental systems that resistance to reinfection and the ability to clear primary infection is, in large part, dependent on T-cell functions. Both CD4 and CD8 cells have been shown to have a protective role. Cytotoxic T cells (CTLs) could be important in immunity to chlamydial infection. Nonspecific lysis of infected cells by natural killer (NK) cells has been a fairly common observation. It has been shown that earlier reports indicating that there was no cytotoxic action against infected target cells were flawed on technical grounds and specific lysis of chlamydia-infected cells has now been demonstrated.[34,35] NK cell activity may also play a role.

CD4 and CD8 cells both appear to play important roles in either protection or clearance of chlamydial infection. In animal experiments using the mouse pneumonitis model, depletion of CD4 cells leads to a dramatic decrease in chlamydia-specific antibody levels and interferon-γ (INF-γ). These changes were accompanied by a significant increase in mortality. CD8 cells, in some systems, appear to be important as well. In some strains of mice, both CD4 and CD8 cells produce INF-γ. Higher infectious leads were found with depletion of either CD4 or CD8 cells.[36]

The induction of cytokines by infection may play an important role in determining the outcome of chlamydial infection, and may be important not only in defensive and protective responses but also in pathogenesis. Interferons are active against chlamydiae and the most important one appears to be INF-γ. Chlamydial infections induce the production of INF-γ and the organisms are sensitive to its action. In the presence of INF-γ chlamydial replication is inhibited at the RB stage. INF-γ inhibits chlamydial growth by inducing indolemine dioxygenase (IDO), which degrades tryptophan.[37] This may functionally result in dramatic reduction in chlamydial infection and as some infected cells may be sloughed, the infection may be abrogated. However, the infected cells may also be excreting chlamydial antigen that can induce further sensitization and contribute to pathogenic mechanisms. It is likely then, that delayed-type hypersensitivity reactions to chlamydia represent a double-edged sword with both protective and immunopathological implications. Tumor necrosis factor may also play a role, either independently or by enhancing INF-γ.

The role that cytokines play here is even more speculative. A case can be made for INF-γ to be an important cytokine, both in the context of downregulating chlamydial infection, that is, a protective response, or one that may have immunopathological consequences because of the potential for perhaps leading to low-level persistence which may be correlated with hypersensitivity reactions. Thus, cytokines can play an inflammatory role or a protective role.

Little is known about the respective roles of helper T and suppressor T cells in chlamydial infections. Lymphocytes from monkeys repeatedly reinfected with trachoma proliferated weakly *in vitro* when exposed to *C. trachomatis* antigen.[38] Depletion of suppressor T cells significantly increased proliferation, from which it was inferred that such cells might impair the cell-mediated immune response to infection, but later experiments did not support this supposition. Both helper T and suppressor/cytotoxic T cells, the latter predominating, appeared in large numbers in the conjunctival follicles of monkeys inoculated with *C. trachomatis*.[39] It is clear that the roles of the various T-cell subsets also need further exploration.

In animal studies, both humoral and cell-mediated immune responses have been shown to play some role in either resistance to reinfection or clearance of infection. Athymic mice will not readily clear chlamydial genital tract infection, but rather develop a chronic infection, whereas competent mice clear the infection in less than 3 weeks. B-cell-deficient mice are capable of resolving genital infection. Immunization is capable of protecting against genital challenge and there is evidence suggesting the a sIgA antibody response may have some protective effect.

9. ARTIFICIAL IMMUNIZATION

The wide prevalence of trachoma, its major role as a cause of visual disability, and the difficulties of mass treatment led to several attempts to produce an effective vaccine. The results of experiments in animals gave encouraging results, but those of field trials were disappointing.[40] Different vaccines either conferred short-term protection, had no discernible effect, or were actually deleterious. Some appeared to enhance the severity of trachoma in those who subsequently acquired the infection, whereas others increased (rather than diminished) the attack rate. There seems little doubt that some of these vaccines induced hypersensitivity rather than protection and field trials have been abandoned pending the development of safer antigens for use in humans. Using genetic engineering, it has been possible to insert chlamydial genes into a poliovirus vaccine.[41] The virus had surface exposure of serovar-specific portions of the chlamydial MOMP and it has been possible to induce neutralizing antibodies in mice and subhuman primates.

Antibodies directed against different variable segments have been shown to be responsible for neutralization in different serovars. The neutralizing antibodies have been found in variable segment (VS) 2 as well as variable segments 1 and 4. Chimeric synthetic peptides that basically included the VS1 and VS4 of serovars B and E, respectively, are capable of eliciting serovar-specific antibodies to both serovars.

Thus, models have been created that allow for development of vaccines that present potentially protective chlamydial antigens while deleting the sensitizing antigens that may contribute to disease. Such vaccines have been targeted for prevention of PID as well as trachoma. None have been evaluated in humans, but these vaccines have not produced the degree of protection against chlamydiae that was seen with cruder vaccines in the monkey studies for trachoma vaccine.

10. SEROLOGICAL DIAGNOSIS

Although many different serological tests are available, only the following two are widely used in diagnosis.

The most widely used serological test for diagnosing chlamydial infections is the complement-fixation (CF) test. This is useful in diagnosing psittacosis, in which paired sera often show fourfold or greater increases in titer. It may also be useful in diagnosing LGV, in which single-point titers of >1:64 are highly supportive of this clinical diagnosis. With LGV it is difficult to demonstrate rising titers, as the nature of the disease results in the patient being seen by the physician after the acute stage. Any titer above 1:16 is considered significant evidence of exposure to chlamydiae. The CF test is not particularly useful in diagnosing trachoma-inclusion conjunctivitis or the related genital tract infections, and it plays no role in diagnosing neonatal chlamydial infections.

The microimmunofluorescence (MIF) method is a much more sensitive procedure for measuring antichlamydial antibodies.[42] Trachoma, inclusion conjunctivitis, and the genital tract infections may be diagnosed by the MIF technique if appropriately timed, paired, acute, and convalescent sera can be obtained. However, it is difficult to demonstrate rising antibody titers, particularly in sexually active populations. Many of these individuals will be seen for chronic or repeat infections. The background rate of seroreactors in venereal disease clinics may be >60%, making it particularly difficult to demonstrate seroconversion. Individuals with systemic infection (epididymitis, salpingitis) usually have much higher antibody levels than those with superficial infections, and women tend to have higher antibody levels than men.

Serology is particularly useful in diagnosing chlamydial pneumonia in neonates. High levels of IgM antibody are regularly found in association with disease.[43] IgG antibodies are not useful because the infants are being seen when they have high levels of circulating maternal IgG (these infections are acquired from the infected mother, who is almost always seropositive). It takes from 6 to 12 months for maternal antichlamydial antibodies to disappear. Infants with inclusion conjunctivitis or respiratory tract carriage of chlamydia without pneumonia usually have low levels of IgM antibodies. Thus, a single IgM titer of >1:32 may support the diagnosis of chlamydial pneumonia.

The MIF technique uses many serotypes of chlamydiae and the procedure, as simplified by Wang *et al.*, is recommended.[44] Because the IgM antibody responses can be markedly specific, the use of single, broadly reacting antigens will miss at least 15% to 25% of the results that would be positive by a multiple-antigen MIF. Inclusion fluorescence assays will also measure genus-specific reactions because of the LPS in the inclusion.

Enzyme immunoassay (EIA) techniques have been described that measure antichlamydial antibodies. Most of these procedures have been successful in measuring IgG antibody, but are often less sensitive than the MIF technique. They have been less successful in measuring IgM antibody. Some tests are commercially available, yet there is inadequate published experience with those tests to recommend them.

There are also commercially available preparations that measure antibody reactivity to chlamydial inclusions in cell culture. Some have attempted to use reactivity with these antigens as diagnostic of chlamydial infection based on single-point antibody determination. For the most part, these efforts are ill conceived. Antibody reactions are also purported to be species-specific for the species used to prepare the antigen (usually *C. trachomatis*). Unfortunately, inclusions contain considerable amounts of LPS and thus staining activity will include genus-specific antibodies. Thus, there is a constant problem of confounding due to high levels of background antibody to *C. pneumoniae*.

Some manufacturers claim detection of IgA antibody is diagnostic of current infection. It is not. IgG antibodies also will persist for long periods of time and it is a disservice to patients to treat on the basis of antibody levels with the intention of continuing treatment until antibodies disappear.

11. COMMENTARY

Many of the studies of either immunopathology or protection have used proxies for what the researchers assumed was the actual effect or mechanism. For example, antibodies to heat-shock proteins are often measured because it is technically easier and researchers assume that high levels of antibody are predictive of high levels of CMI and thus the conclusions are reached that there are greater cell-mediated immune responses to hsp 60 associated with disease. Consequently, a number of theories have evolved; some may actually turn out ultimately to be true. Some of the theories are so well accepted today that they have virtually become dogma in the field, but they are not yet proven. The simplest explanations are that:

1. Clearance of chlamydial infection is dependent on cell-mediated immune responses and that both CD4 and CD8 cells can participate but it is likelier that the CD4 cell's role is dominant.
2. Protection against reinfection is likely to be due to sIgA neutralizing antibody directed against sites on the MOMP.

Because all initial interactions here occur at mucosal surfaces, and there are some data to support this, it is possible that sIgA antibodies are dominant in this role, but it is also possible that IgG antibodies are more important.

Diseases caused by chlamydiae tend to run chronic and relapsing courses. If untreated, the same serovar of *C. trachomatis* can be found in the eye or genital tract of an individual for 2 to 5 years or longer, suggesting continued infection rather than reinfection. Clinically inapparent infections occur in virtually all chlamydial diseases. Healthy carriers can be important in the spread of infection. This chronicity in turn implies that chlamydiae do not usually evoke a thoroughly effective immune response. Nevertheless, the natural history of chlamydial diseases, as well as some early trachoma vaccine trials, indicate that short-lived protective effects can be induced.

Chlamydial infection or immunization results in abundant humoral, secretory, and cell-mediated immune responses, but their role in resistance to infection is not clear. In primates, eye infection with *C. trachomatis* can induce solid immunity of a few months' duration.

There are several useful unifying principles in regard to the oculogenital infections caused by *C. trachomatis:*

1. The organism infects superficial columnar epithelial cells in various sites (endocervix, urethra, epididymis, endometrium, salpinx, conjunctiva, nasopharynx, lower respiratory tract) and appears to have little propensity for invasion or destruction of deeper tissue.
2. The clinical features of chlamydial infection seem to be produced by the host inflammatory response, rather than by the inherent destructiveness of the organism.
3. *C. trachomatis* infections may be present and asymptomatic (latent or "silent" infection) for prolonged periods of time. For example, infants have been documented to shed organisms from conjunctivae for up to 2 years postdelivery. Similarly, women with cervical infection have been culture positive for at least 18 months.
4. The stimuli that convert latent infection to chronic disease, or that determine symptomatic vs. asymptomatic primary infection, are unknown.
5. Infection can occur, recur, and persist even in the presence of serum

antibody. Cell-mediated immune responses (as measured by lymphocyte blastogenic response) appear to be associated with clearing infection, although the evidence is far from clear.

One important concept related to naturally occurring chlamydial infection is that of latency. It is very clear that chlamydial infections in their natural hosts do not induce severe disease. This probably reflects a long-term adaptation in evolutionary terms, as the intracellular life cycles and mode of replication of these organisms would suggest. Some of the assumptions of latency have reflected an inability to recover organisms in individuals who are infected. This inability may be due in part to the poor sensitivity of many diagnostic tests and inadequate sampling of appropriate infected cell sites. In other instances, it is possible that there is a low-level, chronic infection that involves replication of the organism that is controlled, but not cleared, by the host's defense mechanisms. There are several proposed models for latency. Most are based on an effective metabolic retardation of chlamydial metabolism or maturation within the inclusions. On microscopy each of these inclusions show an abnormal form of the organism within the inclusion that may go on to develop normally once the suppression is removed. This can happen in the presence of interferon, penicillins, and amino acid deprivation. The sensitivity of the organism to INF-γ has been widely touted as the most likely immune suppressive function that is capable of causing a latent infection. The biological relevance of this hypothesis is still uncertain.

REFERENCES

1. Moulder, J. W., 1996, The relation of the psittacosis group (Chlamydiae) to bacteria and viruses, *Annu. Rev. Microbiol.* **20:**107–130.
2. Moulder, J. W., 1984, Order Chlamydiales and family Chlamydiaceae, in: *Bergey's Manual of Systematic Bacteriology*, Vol. 1 (N. R. Krieg, ed.), Williams Wilkins, Baltimore, pp. 729–739.
3. Caldwell, H. D., Kromhout, J., and Schachter, J., 1981, Purification and partial characterization of the major outer membrane protein of *Chlamydia trachomatis*, *Infect. Immun.* **33:**1161–1176.
4. Nurminen, M., Leinonen, M., Saikku, P., and Makela, P. H., 1983, The genus-specific antigen of Chlamydia: Resemblance to the lipopolysaccharide of enteric bacteria, *Science* **220:**1279–1281.
5. Hodinka, R. L., and Wyrick, P. B., 1986, Ultrastructural study of mode of entry of *Chlamydia pssittaci* into L-929, *Infect. Immun.* **54:**855–863.
6. Byrne, G. I., and Moulder, J. W., 1978, Parasite-specific phagocytosis of *Chlamydia psittaci* and *Chlamydia trachomatis* by L and HeLa cells, *Infect. Immun.* **19:**598–606.
7. Birkelund, S., Johnsen, H., and Christiansen, G., 1994, Entry of *Chlamydia trachomatis* L2 into HeLa cell induces tyrosine phosphorylation of HeLa cell proteins [Abstract], in: *Chlamydial Infections: Proceedings of the Eighth International Symposium on Human Chlamydial Infections* (Orfila, J., Byrne, G. I., Chernesky, M. A., Grayston, J. T., Jones, R. B., Ridgway, G. L., Saikku, P., Schachter, J., Stamm, W., and Stephens, R. S., eds.), Societa Editrice Esculapio, Bologne, pp. 395–398,
8. Stephens, R. S., 1994, Molecular mimicry and *Chlamydia trachomatis* infection of eukaryotic cells, *Trends Microbiol.* **2:**99–101.

9. Hackstadt, T., Scidmore, M., and Rockey, D. D., 1994, A fluorescent sphingolipid analog is transported from the Golgi apparatus and incorporated into the chlamydial cell wall [Abstract], in: *Chlamydial Infections* (Orfila, J., Byrne, G. I., Chernesky, M. A., Grayston, J. T., Jones, R. B., Ridgway, G. L., Saikku, P., Schachter, J., Stamm, W., and Stephens, R. S., eds.), Societa Editrice Esculapio, Bologne, pp. 407–410.

10. Caldwell, H. D., and Schachter, J., 1982, Antigenic analysis of the major outer membrane protein of Chlamydia spp. *Infect. Immun.* **35:**1024–1031.

11. Wang, S. P., and Grayston, J. T., 1970, Immunologic relationship between genital TRIC, LGV, and related organisms in a new microtiter indirect immunofluorescence test, *Am. J. Ophthalmol.* **70:**367–374.

12. Stephens, R. S., Mullenback, G., Sanchez-Pescador, R., and Agabian, N., 1986, Sequence analysis of the major outer membrane protein gene from *Chlamydia trachomatis* serovar L2, *J. Bacteriol.* **168:**1277–1282.

13. Villeneuva, A., Brossay, L., Paradis, G., and Herbert, J., 1994, Characterization of neutralizing epitopes in variable domain 1 of B and C complex serovars of *Chlamydia trachomatis* [Abstract], in: *Chlamydial Infections: Proceedings of the Eighth International Symposium on Human Chlamydial Infections* (Orfila, J., Byrne, G. I., Chernesky, M. A., Grayston, J. T., Jones, R. B., Ridgway, G. L., Saikku, P., Schachter, J., Stamm, W., and Stephens, R. S., eds.), Societa Editrice Esculapio, Bologne, pp. 122–125.

14. Yang, C. L., Maclean, I., and Brunham, R. C., 1993, DNA sequence polymorphism of the *Chlamydia trachomatis* Omp1 gene, *J. Infect. Dis.* **168:**1225–1230.

15. Jones, R. B., and Van der Pol, B., 1994, Lack of correlation between acquisition of infection and ability of serum to neutralize chlamydial infectivity *in vitro* [Abstract], in: *Chlamydial Infections: Proceedings of the Eighth International Symposium on Human Chlamydial Infections* (Orfila, J., Byrne, G. I., Chernesky, M. A., Grayston, J. T., Jones, R. B., Ridgway, G. L., Saikku, P., Schachter, J., Stamm, W., and Stephens, R. S., eds.), Societa Editrice Esculapio, Bologna, pp. 95–98.

16. Lampe, M. F., Kuehl, L. M., Wong, K. G., and Stamm, W. E., 1994, *Chlamydia trachomatis* major outer membrane protein variants escape nutralization by polyclonal human immune sera [Abstract], *Chlamydial Infections: Proceedings of the Eighth International Symposium on Human Chlamydial Infections* (Orfila, J., Byrne, G. I., Chernesky, M. A., Grayston, J. R., Jones, R. B., Ridgway, G. L., Saikku, P., Schachter, J., Stamm, W., and Stephens, R. S., eds.), Societa Editrice Esculapio, Bologne, pp. 91–94.

17. Hayes, L. J., Pecharatana, S., Bailey, R. L., Hampton, T. J., Pickett, M. A., Mabey, D. C., Watt, P. J., and Ward, M. E., 1995, Extent and kinetics of genetic change in the omp1 gene of *Chlamydia trachomatis* in two villages with endemic trachoma, *J. Infect. Dis.* **172:**268–272.

18. Centers for Disease Control, 1993, Recommendations for the prevention and management of *Chlamydia trachomatis* infections, 1993, *MMWR Morb. Mortal. Wk. Rep.* **42:**1–39.

19. Moncada, J. V., Schachter, J., and Wofsy, C., 1986, Prevalence of *Chlamydia trachomatis* lung infection in patients with acquired immune deficiency syndrome, *J. Clin. Microbiol.* **25:**986.

20. Grayston, J. T., Wang, S. P., Yeh, L. J., Kuo, C. C., 1985, Importance of reinfection in the pathogenesis of trachoma, *Rev. Infect. Dis.* **7:**717–725.

21. Watkins, N. G., Hadlow, W. J., Moos, A. B., and Caldwell, H. D., 1986, Ocular delayed hypersensitivity: A pathogenetic mechanism of chlamydial-conjunctivitis in guinea pigs, *Proc. Natl. Acad. Sci. USA* **83:**7480–7484.

22. Morrison, R. P., Belland, R. J., Lyng, K., and Caldwell, H. D., 1989, Chlamydial disease pathogenesis. The 57-kD chlamydial hypersensitivity antigen is a stress responses protein, *J. Exp. Med.* **170**1271–1283.

23. Wagar, E. A., Schachter, J., Bavoil, P., and Stephens, R. S., Differential human serologic response to two 60,000 molecular weight *Chlamydia trachomatis* antigens, *J. Infect. Dis.* **162:**922–927.

24. Taylor, H. R., Johnson, S. L., Schachter, J., Caldwell, H. D., and Prendergast, R. A., 1987, Pathogenesis of trachoma: The stimulus for inflammation, *J. Immunol.* **138:**3023 3027.

25. Toye, B., Laferriere, C., Claman, P., Jessamine, P., and Peeling, R., 1993, Association between antibody to the chlamydial heat-shock protein and tubal infertility, *J. Infect. Dis.* **168:**1236 1240.

26. Hillis, S. D., Owens, L. M., Marchbanks, P. A., Amsterdam, L. F., and MacKenzie, W. R., 1997, Recurrent chlamydial infections increase the risks of hospitalization for ectopic pregnancy and pelvic inflammatory disease, *Am. J. Obstet. Gynecol.* **176(Pt 1):** 103 107.

27. Holland, M. J., Bailey, R. L., Hayes, L. T., Whittle, H. C., and Mabey, D. C., 1993, Conjunctival scarring in trachoma is associated with depressed cell-mediated immune responses to chlamydial antigens, *J. Infect. Dis.* **168:**1528 1531.

28. Brunham, R. D., Kuo, C.-C., Cles, L., and Holmes, K. K., 1983, Correlation of host immune response with quantitative recovery of *Chlamydia trachomatis* from the human endocervix, *Infect. Immun.* **39:**1491 1494.

29. Cevenini, R., Sarov, I., Rumpianesi, F., Donati, M., Melega, C., Varotti, C., and Laplaca, M., 1984, Serum specific IgA antibody to *Chlamydia trachomatis* in patients with chlamydial infections detected by ELISA and an immunofluorescence test, *J. Clin. Pathol.* **37:**686 691.

30. Bailey, R. L., Kajbaf, M., Whittle, H. C., Ward, M. E., and Mabey, D. C., 1993, The influence of local antichlamydial antibody on the acquisition and persistence of human ocular chlamydial infection: IgG antibodies are not protective, *Epidemiol. Infect.* **111:**315 324.

31. Qvigstad, E., and Hirschberg, H., 1984, Lack of cell-mediated cytotoxicity towards *Chlamydia trachomatis* infected target cells in humans, *Acta. Pathol. Micorbiol. Immunol. Scand. [C]* **92:**153 159.

32. Ramsey, K. H., and Rank, R. G., 1991, Resolution of chlamydial genital infection with antigen-specific T-lymphocyte lines, *Infect. Immun.* **59:**925 931.

33. Bailey, R. L., Holland, M. J., Whittle, H. C., and Mabey D. C., 1995, Subjects recovering from human ocular chlamydial infection have enhanced lymphoproliferative responses to chlamydial antigens compared with those of persistently diseased controls, *Infect. Immun.* **63:**389 392.

34. Pavia, C. S., and Schachter, J., 1983, Failure to detect cell-mediated cytotoxicity against *Chlamydia trachomatis*-infected cells, *Infect. Immun.* **39:**1271 1274.

35. Beatty, P. R., and Stephens, R. S., 1994, CD8+ T lymphocyte-mediated lysis of Chlamydia-infected L cells using an endogenous antigen pathway, *J. Immunol.* **153:**4588 4595.

36. Magee, D. M., Williams, D. M., Smith, J. G., Bleicker, C. A., Grubbs, R. G., Schachter, J., and Ranka, R. G., 1995, Role of CD8 T cells in primary Chlamydia infection, *Infect. Immun.* **63:**516 521.

37. Byrne, G. I., Lehmann, L. K., Landry, G. J., 1986, Introduction of tryptophan catabolism is the mechanism for gamma-interferon-mediated inhibition of intracellular *Chlamydia psittaci* replication, *Infect. Immun.* **53:**347 351.

38. Young, E., and Taylor, H. R., 1984, Immune mechanisms in chlamydial eye infection: Cellular immune responses in chronic and acute disease, *J. Infect. Dis.* **150:**745 751.

39. Whittum-Hudson, J. A., Taylor, H. R., Farazdaghi, M., and Prendergast, R. A., 1986, Immunohistochemical study of the local inflammatory response to chlamydial ocular infection, *Invest. Ophthalmol. Vis. Sci.* **27:**64 69.

40. Schachter, J., and Dawson, C. R., 1978, *Human Chlamydial Infections*, PSG, Littleton, MA.

41. Murdin, A. D., Su, H., Manning, D. S., Klein, M. H., Parnell, M. J., and Caldwell, H. D., 1993, A poliovirus hybrid expressing a neutralization epitope from the major outer membrane protein of *Chlamydia trachomatis* is highly immunogenic, *Infect. Immun.* **61:**4406 4414.

42. Wang, S. P., and Grayston, J. R., 1974, Human serology in *Chlamydia trachomatis* infection with microimmunofluorescence, *J. Infect. Dis.* **130:**388 397.

43. Schachter, J., Grossman, M., and Azimi, P. H., 1982, Serology of *Chlamydia trachomatis* in infants, *J. Infect. Dis.* **146:**530–535.
44. Wang, S. P., Grayston, J. T., Alexander, E. R., and Holmes, K. K., 1975, Simplified microimmunofluorescence test with trachoma-LGV (*Chlamydia trachomatis*) antigens for use as a screening test for antibody., *J. Clin. Microbiol.* **1:**250–255.

14

Chlamydia Infection and Pneumonia

MURAT V. KALAYOGLU, DAVID L. HAHN,
and GERALD I. BYRNE

1. INTRODUCTION

A wide spectrum of human diseases can result from chlamydial infections. Psittacosis is an infectious disease of avians caused by *Chlamydia psittaci* that can manifest in severe systemic disease in humans.[1] *Chlamydia trachomatis* infections are the leading cause of sexually transmitted genital tract disease, the only cause of classic trachoma, and also result in perinatal infant pneumonia and conjunctivitis acquired from the infected mother during childbirth.[2] *Chlamydia pneumoniae* causes a variety of acute respiratory illnesses, including pharyngitis, sinusitis, bronchitis, and pneumonia, and has been associated with chronic cardiopulmonary diseases including adult-onset asthma[3] and atherosclerosis.[4] Although *C. psittaci*, *C. trachomatis*, and *C. pneumoniae* each have been associated with a distinct array of human diseases, pneumonia is common to all three. Pneumonias caused by each species have both unique and shared features and consideration of these differences and similarities may provide insight into mechanisms of these chlamydial diseases. For this reason, the current chapter examines the epidemiology, pathogenesis, clinical symptoms, and immune response to chlamydial pneumonias.

MURAT V. KALAYOGLU and GERALD I. BYRNE • Department of Medical Micriobiology and Immunology, University of Wisconsin Medical School, Madison, Wisconsin 53706. DAVID L. HAHN • Arcand Park Clinic, Dean Medical Center, Madison, Wisconsin 53705.

Opportunistic Intracellular Bacteria and Immunity, edited by Lois J. Paradise *et al.* Plenum Press, New York, 1999.

2. CHLAMYDIAL BIOLOGY

Chlamydiae are intracellular bacteria with unique morphology and a biphasic life cycle.[5] Two functionally and morphologically distinct forms can be identified during the growth cycle: the infectious elementary body (EB) and the replicative reticulate body (RB). The EB is a small (0.1 to 0.2 μm), metabolically inert form that can survive extracellularly, contains no peptidoglycan, and instead may maintain structural integrity via a network of disulfide crosslinkages involving two cysteine-rich proteins and/or the major outer membrane protein (MOMP). In contrast, the RB is larger (0.8 to 1 μm) and noninfectious, but synthesizes DNA, RNA, and proteins to divide by binary fission. As chlamydiae cannot synthesize adenosine triphosphate (ATP) or nucleotides de novo, RBs must acquire host cell energy and nutrients to replicate and the bacterium must parasitize a eukaryotic host cell to survive and multiply.

The life cycle begins when the EB binds a host membrane receptor and becomes endocytosed by unknown mechanisms. Once internalized, the organisms are detectable in membrane-bound phagosomes and incorporate host-cell sphingolipids into the inclusion membrane[6][8] without interfering with Golgi-mediated exocytosis of glycoproteins.[9] Chlamydiae block phagolysosomal fusion and begin to reorganize EBs into RBs. RBs multiply by binary fission within phagosomes and revert back to EBs before the EB-filled phagosome ruptures. Chlamydial EBs then exit the cell to begin another round of replication. In vitro incubation and replication periods vary with different chlamydial species, serovars, and host cell types.

All chlamydiae can infect and multiply within epithelial cells, and Chlamydia–epithelial cell interactions have been extensively characterized.[10] Other cell types are less permissive to growth of most chlamydial species. Polymorphonuclear leukocytes (PMNs) ingest and destroy most C. psittaci and C. trachomatis EBs,[10] and growth within mononuclear phagocytes (Mφs) is restricted for C. trachomatis.[11] C. pneumoniae and some strains of C. psittaci can replicate within Mφs, and C. pneumoniae is unique in that it also can replicate in endothelial cells and smooth muscle cells.[12,13] This broad tropism may contribute to the diversity of diseases associated with C. pneumoniae. Importantly, the Mφ has been proposed to mediate persistence and spread of chlamydiae in vivo,[14] and the alveolar macrophage may be a primary target cell in chlamydial pneumonias caused by all three species. The alveolar macrophage also may act as a vehicle to transport the organism to extrapulmonary sites, such as the liver for C. psittaci[15] and coronary arteries for C. pneumoniae.[16]

3. PSITTACOSIS

Psittacosis is a systemic zoonosis that can cause an atypical pneumonia in humans.[1] Disease severity and duration are variable, but mortality may be as high as 30% in untreated cases.

3.1. Epidemiology

C. psittaci normally infects birds and some domestic animals but can be transmitted to humans by aerosol droplets. Approximately 5% to 8% of birds are carriers for *C. psittaci* but 100% of birds may be infected in overcrowded or other stress-inducing environments.[1,17] Any bird is a potential hazard, as over 130 bird species have been shown to carry *C. psittaci;* infections acquired from turkeys or parrots are particularly virulent to humans. Severe illness is thought to result rarely from human-to-human transmission. The infection is most common in young and middle-aged adults, and most epidemiological studies do not find prevalence differences between genders. Although fewer than 200 cases of psittacosis are reported to the Centers for Disease Control each year, the severity of disease makes psittacosis a significant concern to poultry farmers, abattoir workers, and veterinarians.[1,17]

3.2. Pathogenesis and Symptoms

The onset of symptoms follows a 1- to 3-week incubation period. The organism initially establishes infection in the lung as most patients present with an atypical pneumonia characterized by fever, cough, and severe headache, and less frequently with sore throat and chest soreness.[1,18,19] Histology reveals inflamed trachea, bronchi, bronchioles, and alveoli, and mucous plugging is apparent; alveolar and interstitial exudates contain mostly infiltrating lymphocytes. Radiologically, psittacosis pneumonia is not distinguishable from other atypical pneumonias and X-ray films often show pneumonitis originating from the hilum during the first week and lower lobe consolidation afterwards, with pleural effusions seen in up to 50% of cases. These radiological abnormalities may take up to 5 months to resolve and underscore the severity of lung involvement in psitticosis.[1,18,19]

Although the lung is the organ most frequently involved in psittacosis, the disease can be systemic with damage to multiple organ systems. The mechanism of systemic spread is not known, but as *C. psittaci* can infect and survive within human, murine, and pig alveolar macrophages,[14,20-22] this cell type may contribute to spread of the organism. Neurological and gastrointestinal symptoms such as headache, malaise, vomiting, diarrhea or constipation, and nausea are common, but less common general symptoms such as sore throat, dyspnea, hemoptysis, rash, diaphoresis, and photophobia may complicate the diagnosis. If untreated, psitticosis may result in cardiac, hepatobiliary, neurological, and endocrine involvement with fatal consequences.[1,18,19]

3.3. Diagnosis and Treatment

The differential diagnosis of psittacosis includes other causes of atypical pneumonia including viral, *Mycoplasma, Coxiella, Legionella,* and *C. pneumoniae* pneumonia.[23] Common signs of psittacosis reported in greater than 50% of patients are fever, lung consolidation, and hepatomegaly. Splenomegaly may appear after the first week of onset of symptoms and together with arthralgia or myalgia may help focus the differential diagnosis.[1] An important epidemiological clue is exposure to birds.

The complement fixation assay (CFA), combined with clinical symptoms and a detailed history, currently is the most common diagnostic method for psittacosis,[24] but antigen detection methods such as enzyme immunoassay (EIA) and molecular methods such as the polymerase chain reaction (PCR) soon may provide more sensitive and specific methods of diagnosis. Treatment with tetracycline or doxycycline for up to 3 weeks reduces mortality to below 1%.

Very little is known about host immune responses to *C. psittaci* pneumonia. Immunity to *C. psittaci* infection has not been documented, and reinfections can occur.[24]

4. *C. TRACHOMATIS* PNEUMONIA

Unlike *C. psittaci*, *C. trachomatis* probably is not transmitted via respiratory droplets, although the organism can still cause pneumonia in both infants and adults. In infant pneumonia, *C. trachomatis* is transmitted during childbirth from the mother to the newborn, whereas in adult pneumonia *C. trachomatis* can establish lung infection in the immunocompromised individual, possibly by respiratory tract colonization or systemic dissemination from the genital tract. Cases of *C. trachomatis* pneumonia in immunocompetent adults have been reported in laboratory workers exposed to high titers of the organism,[25] but natural respiratory tract infection is very rare in individuals with intact immunity. *C. trachomatis* is a minor cause of pneumonia even in immunocompromised individuals,[26] but the resulting disease is severe,[26-30] in contrast to the mild pneumonia reported in immunocompetent infants. Thus, although the two syndromes are caused by the same organism, the diseases can manifest in different clinical symptoms, suggesting the contribution of distinct immune mediators in determining the severity of *C. trachomatis* pneumonia. Sections 4.1 to 4.3 discuss *C. trachomatis* infant pneumonia.

4.1. Epidemiology

Pneumonia in infants initially was associated with *C. trachomatis* when Beem and Saxon[31] detected the organism in 90% of infants with a distinct pneumonia syndrome characterized by a chronic, afebrile course, diffuse lung involvement and high serum immunoglobulins (Ig) G and M. Specific antibody titers to *C. trachomatis* also were elevated in these infants and no other respiratory pathogens were consistently associated with the pneumonia. Subsequent prospective studies[32-35] have indicated that 16% to 28% of infants born to *C. trachomatis*–infected mothers develop pneumonia and that the prevalence of disease is 1% to 5% in different communities.

4.2. Pathogenesis and Symptoms

The organism can infect numerous sites in the infant during childbirth including the conjunctiva, nasopharynx, rectum, and vagina.[36] Disease may manifest sequentially, as *C. trachomatis* can be recovered earlier in the conjunctiva compared to the nasopharynx[36] and half of infants with *C. trachomatis* pneumonia also have a history of conjunctivitis.[37] The onset of symptoms usually occurs within 8 weeks of birth when infants present with a staccato cough, tachypnea, and nasal discharge.[37] Importantly, the infants remain afebrile during the course of disease, and respiratory tract obstruction is uncommon.[37–39] Radiological findings may show diffuse interstitial infiltrates and bilateral hyperexpansion whereas pleural effusion and lobar consolidation are not present.[40] Hematological findings include peripheral eosinophilia and elevated serum IgG and IgM levels.[31,37] Although the disease is usually mild, very young infants may have severe symptoms[41,42] and untreated infants may remain ill for months.[31] Complications from acute *C. trachomatis* pneumonia are rare; however, follow-up studies on infants with *C. trachomatis* pneumonia report a significant increase of obstructive airway disease and asthma later in life, suggesting that infection may result in long-term respiratory sequelae.[43,44]

4.3. Diagnosis and Treatment

The recommended diagnostic method is culture of the organism from the pharynx followed by detection of chlamydial inclusions by immunofluorescent antibody staining.[45] The recommended treatment, oral erythromycin 50 mg/kg/day for 10 to 14 days, is only 80% effective and therefore a second antibiotic course may be required.[46,47] In many cases newer macrolides such as azithromycin or clarithromycin may be preferred, especially if the infant is intolerant to erythromycin.[48–51]

4.4. Host Immune Response to *C. trachomatis* Pneumonia

Pneumonia in infants is mild compared to the fulminant pneumonia observed in immunocompromised adults, suggesting that the immune response is important to protection from *C. trachomatis* pneumonia. However, the immune components involved in humans during *C. trachomatis* pneumonia are poorly understood. Instead, the immune mediators in this disease have been described extensively in animal models. These animal model studies are reviewed here, and pertinent correlations to the few human-based reports are provided.

Studies using an immunocompromised mouse model developed by Williams *et al.*[52] have contributed valuable information about the immune response to *C. trachomatis* pneumonia. The authors initially observed that athymic nude mice (*nu/nu*), compared to their immunocompetent littermates (*nu/+*), were more susceptible to pneumonia caused by *C. trachomatis* (strain mouse pneumonitis, MoPn) as determined by increased mortality and decreased pulmonary clearance of the organism.[52] Transplantation of thymuses from *nu/+* mice to *nu/nu* resulted in increased resistance, indicating that T cells were important to protection.[52] The contribution of cell-mediated immunity (CMI) was demonstrated further when adoptive transfer of T cells from immunized *nu/+* mice to *nu/nu* mice conferred protective immunity in these animals.[53] Subsequent studies suggested a role for humoral immunity in protection as adoptive transfer of immune serum from *nu/+* to *nu/nu* mice increased resistance to intranasal MoPn challenge.[54] Indeed, human infants with *C. trachomatis* pneumonia had increased numbers of peripheral blood B cells that secreted large amounts of IgG, IgM, and IgA antibody in the absence of mitogens *in vitro*.[55] However, B-cell-deficient mice were as susceptible to MoPn as control animals, suggesting the importance of a multifactoral response to *C. trachomatis* pneumonia.[56]

    The diversity of immune mediators involved in *C. trachomatis* pneumonia was supported further in histopathological studies with *nu/+*, *nu/nu*, and immunized *nu/nu* animals. These studies revealed that protection correlated with the presence of a variety of cell types including plasma cells, lymphocytes, monocytes, and macrophages.[57] A protective role for the latter also was indicated by the observation that alveolar macrophages were activated in infected *nu/+* (but not *nu/nu*) mice.[53] Importantly, Nakajo *et al.*[58] showed that human adult alveolar macrophages killed *C. trachomatis*, and the authors proposed that differences in bactericidal capacities of adult vs. infant alveolar macrophages[59,60] may explain the susceptibility of infants to *C. trachomatis* pneumonia; however, these studies did not examine the capacity of infant alveolar macrophages to kill *C. trachomatis*.

    The presence of interferon-γ (IFN-γ)[61] tumor necrosis factor-α (TNF-α)[62] interleukin-1 (IL-1),[63] IL-6,[63] and transforming growth factor-β (TGF-β)[64] have been demonstrated in the lungs of immunocompetent mice inoculated with MoPn, and high serum levels of colony stimulating factors have been detected in infected *nu/nu* and *nu/+* mice.[65] Neutralizing antibody to IFN-γ[61] and to TNF-α[62] exacerbated disease in *nu/+* mice, indicating a protective role for these cytokines in *C. trachomatis* pneumonia. A protective role for IFN-γ also was suggested in a recent report by Yang *et al.*[66] using BALB/c mice, which die from *C. trachomatis* infection, and C57BL/6 mice, which are resistant to infection. These authors showed that BALB/c mice secreted higher levels of IL-10 and less IFN-γ compared with C57BL/6 mice that produced high levels of IFN-γ but minimal IL-10. Importantly, injection of neutralizing antibody to IL-10 initiated a delayed-type hypersensitivity (DTH) response in BALB/c mice,[66] indicating that IL-10 may inhibit Th1-like responses in BALB/c mice and that these Th1-like responses may be important in conferring immunity to C57BL/6 animals. Future studies with IFN-γ-knockout animals should elucidate further the role of this cytokine in *C. trachomatis* pneumonia.

Many of the protective components in the MoPn model for *C. trachomatis* pneumonia are similar to the MoPn model for *C. trachomatis* genital tract infections, recently reviewed by Cotter and Byrne.[67] Unlike in MoPn genital tract infections,[68] however, the role of specific T-cell subsets in MoPn pneumonia is not well understood. Recently, a dual role for γδ T cells, which may be induced following infection of *nu/nu* mice,[61] was suggested by Williams *et al.*[69] The authors showed that compared to control mice, γδ T-cell knockout mice and higher levels of pulmonary MoPn at days 3 and 7 but lower levels of MoPn at day 14,[69] suggesting that γδ T cells may be protective earlier but harmful later in *C. trachomatis* pneumonia. Additional studies are needed to elucidate the role of different T-cell subsets in MoPn pneumonia. Nevertheless, the MoPn murine model for *C. trachomatis* pneumonia has yielded valuable insight into immune responses during infection.

In summary, immunity to *C. trachomatis* pneumonia probably involves multiple cellular and cytokine-mediated effects, including induction of a T-cell-dependent CMI response with secretion of IFN-γ, activation of alveolar macrophages with subsequent secretion of TNF-α and other monokines, and recruitment of B lymphocytes followed by antibody production. Few studies have examined mediators of immunity to *C. trachomatis* pneumonia in humans and future work must focus on human cellular and molecular components involved in *C. trachomatis* pneumonias.

5. *C. PNEUMONIAE* PNEUMONIA

Of the three chlamydial species that cause diseases in humans, *C. pneumoniae* is the most common cause of chlamydial pneumonia in humans. *C. pneumoniae*, previously named the TWAR agent, was originally identified as an atypical strain of *C. psittaci*[70] in a mild epidemic of pneumonia in two northern Finnish communities. In 1989, *C. pneumoniae* received its own species designation,[71] partly due to its lack of DNA homology (<10%) with *C. trachomatis* and *C. psittaci*[72] and its unique, pear-shaped EB morphology.[73] Since its speciation 8 years ago, the organism has been recognized as an important cause of acute respiratory infections including community-acquired pneumonia, bronchitis, and sinusitis, and has been associated with a number of chronic pulmonary and extrapulmonary diseases including adult-onset asthma[3] and atherosclerosis.[4] Although clinical and epidemiological studies identify the organism as a major cause of community-acquired pneumonias (Table I), few studies thus far have examined the role of host immune responses to *C. pneumoniae* pneumonia.

TABLE I

Results of Major Clinical and Epidemiological Studies Examining the Role of *C. pneumoniae* in Community-Acquired Pneumonias

Year(s), location	Type of population	No. of cases	Percent of cases with etiologic diagnosis	Most common pathogen (% of cases)	Method(s) to detect *C. pneumoniae*[†]	No. *C. pneumoniae* diagnoses (% of cases)	Percent of *C. pneumoniae* cases with mixed etiology
1980–1 Seattle, USA[111]	Hospitalized patients	198	NR	Influenza A virus (11)[††]	Serology (MIF[a], CF)	20 (10)	NR
1981–4 Halifax, Canada[112]	Hospitalized patients	301	63	*Streptococcus pneumoniae* (9)	Serology (MIF[a])	18 (6)	61
1983–5 Seattle, USA[113]	University students	76	47	*Mycoplasma pneumoniae* (22)[††]	Serology (MIF[a], CF) and culture	9 (12)	NR
1983–7 Seattle, USA[98]	University students	149	32	*Mycoplasma pneumoniae* (11)[††]	Serology (MIF[a], CF) and culture	14 (9)	NR
1985 Little Rock, USA[114]	Hospitalized patients	154	51	*Legionella pneumophila* (8)	Serology (MIF[a])	12 (8)	33
1985–7 Gavle, Sweden[115]	Hospitalized patients	188	66	*Streptococcus pneumoniae* (20)	Serology (MIF[c])	23 (12)	52
1986–7 Oulu, Finland[116]	Hospitalized patients	125	88	*Streptococcus pneumoniae* (55)	Serology (MIF[b], CF)	54 (43)	66
1986–7 Pittsburgh, USA[117]	Hospitalized patients	359	66	*Steptococcus pneumoniae* (15)	Serology (MIF[a], CF)	22 (6)	NR

1987–8 South Africa[118]	Hospitalized patients	92	C. pneumoniae (21)††	Serology (MIF^g)	19 (21)	NR
1988 New Zealand[119]	Hospitalized patients	92	S. pneumoniae (33)	Serology (MIF, CF) and culture	1 (1)	NR
1990–1 Barcelona, Spain[82]	Outpatients, population-based study	105	C. pneumoniae (15)	Serology (MIF^f)	16 (15)	44
1991–2 Beer-Sheva, Israel[120]	Hospitalized patients	346	S. pneumoniae (43)	Serology (MIF^c)	62 (18)	69
1991–2 Berlin, Germany[121]	Hospitalized patients	236	S. pneumoniae (13)	Serology (CF, MIF^a and culture)	27 (11)	NR
1991–2 Milan, Italy[122]	Hospitalized patients	108	M. pneumoniae (14)	Serology (MIF^a)	14 (13)	0
1991–3 Scandinavia[123]	Hospitalized patients and outpatients	303	S. pneumoniae (14)	Serology (MIF)	26 (9)	20
1991–4 Halifax, Canada[84]	Outpatients	149	M. pneumoniae (23)††	Serology (MIF^a)	16 (11)	31
1991–4 San Patrignano, Italy[83]	Injection drug users in residential community, population-based study	210 total 149 HIV$^+$ 61 HIV$^-$	S. pneumoniae (18) S. pneumoniae (22) C. pneumoniae (26)	Serology (MIF^a)	36 (17) 20 (13) 16 (26)	11

(continued)

TABLE I
(Continued)

Year(s), location	Type of population	No. of cases	Percent of cases with etiologic diagnosis	Most common pathogen (% of cases)	Method(s) to detect C. pneumoniae[†]	No. C. pneumoniae diagnoses (% of cases)	Percent of C. pneumoniae cases with mixed etiology
1991–4 Murcia, Spain[124]	Hospitalized patients	342	29	S. pneumoniae (13)	Serology (MIF[f])	21 (6)	NR
1992–3 Multicenter study USA[85]	Ambulatory pediatric patients	260	47	C. pneumoniae (28)[††]	Serology (MIF[a]), culture	74 (28)	30
1992–4 Multicenter study Barcelona, Spain[100]	Hospitalized COPD patients	124	64	S. pneumoniae (26)	Serology (MIF[a])	9 (7)	22
1993–4 Multicenter study Ohio, USA[125]	Hospitalized patients	227	65	C. pneumoniae (18)	Serology (MIF[a]), PCR, culture	40 (18)	28
1995–6 Connecticut, USA[126]	Outpatients	50	54	C. pneumoniae (36)[††]	Serology (MIF[a]), PCR	18 (36)	NR

MIF = microimmunofluorescence; CF = complement fixation; PCR = polymerase chain reaction; NR = not recorded.

[¶]Adapted with permission from Kauppinen and Saikku.[103]

[*]Denotes mixed infections with pyogens.

[†]A four-fold rise in IgM or IgG titers by MIF was one diagnostic criterion used in all studies.
Additional MIF diagnostic criteria included: [a]IgM ≥ 16 or IgG ≥ 512[104]; [b]IgM ≥ 16, or IgG or IgA ≥ 512; [c]IgM ≥ 16 or IgA ≥ 512; [d]IgM ≥ 16, or IgG or IgA ≥ 64 or IgG ≥ 512; [e]IgM ≥ 32; [f]IgM ≥ 16;
[f]presence of IgM[+]; [g]IgG ≥ 512.

[††]Presence of S. pneumoniae not systematically sought.

5.1. Epidemiology

The population prevalence of *C. pneumoniae* in adults, as estimated by the microimmunofluorescence (MIF) test, is high (up to 50%) in all geographical locations examined.[74-77] Aldous *et al.*[78] used sera from a long-term family study to estimate an incidence of infection (70% asymptomatic) as 6% to 9% per year in children ages 5 to 14, and also noted declining incidence over time. Indeed, the prevalence of MIF antibody increases rapidly up to 40% to 50% between ages 5 and 20 but rises only gradually thereafter,[77] indicating that most primary infections occur in children and young adults. Even though a minority of *C. pneumoniae* infections probably result in pneumonia,[79] a role for the organism in severe community-acquired pneumonias requiring hospitalization has been reported in 2% to 43% of cases (Table I), with most estimates ranging between 6% and 18%. Because the pneumonia caused by *C. pneumoniae* also may be mild, many cases could go undetected[79-81] and the proportion of cases in the general population may be underestimated by hospital-based studies.

Since its first association with pneumonia less than 2 decades ago, *C. pneumoniae* has acquired a place among the top causes of community-acquired pneumonia in adults and also is important in children (Table I). Compared to pneumonia caused by *Streptococcus pneumoniae, C. pneumoniae* pneumonia frequently is milder and therefore may not lead as often to hospitalization or even to outpatient medical visits.[70] In adults, *S. pneumoniae* remains the number one cause of pneumonia in hospitalized patients, but two population-based studies in immunocompetent adults show *C. pneumoniae* as the most commonly identified pathogen in ambulatory patients diagnosed with pneumonia.[82,83] Studies targeting adult outpatients have detected *C. pneumoniae* in 11% to 36% of pneumonia cases.[82-84] Furthermore, a multicenter study in the United States[85] that examined in ambulatory pediatric population (ages 3 to 12) found a large number of cases attributable to *C. pneumoniae* (28%) and *M. pneumoniae* (27%), indicating a potential causative role for these atypical pathogens in the majority of pneumonias in this population.

5.2. Pathogenesis and Clinical Symptoms

C. pneumoniae initially is delivered by aerosol droplets into the upper respiratory tract, where it may cause ciliostasis[86] to gain access into the lungs. The organism has been shown to multiply within human alveolar macrophages[87] as well as endothelial cells[12] *in vitro*, which conceivably may serve as host cells during the infection. Growth of *C. pneumoniae* may initiate an inflammatory process, which induces lymphocyte recruitment[88] and subsequent manifestations of the pneumonia syndrome.

Although limited knowledge is available on the pathogenesis of *C. pneumoniae* pneumonia, intranasal infection of mice,[89-93] nonhuman primates,[94,95] and rabbits[96,97] has shown that (1) infected animals develop a prolonged, mild pneumonia with evidence of acute polymorphonuclear cell infiltrates and later, mononuclear cells; and (2) the organism can be isolated from extrapulmonary tissues. Upon reinfection, recovery of *C. pneumoniae* becomes increasingly difficult in both the murine[93] and cynomolgus monkey models,[95] suggesting that partial protective immunity occurs as a result of infection. These observations correlate well with human infections which often take a mild but chronic course, with reinfections resulting in fewer cases of pneumonia.[80,81,98]

Clinically, *C. pneumoniae* pneumonia resembles other atypical pneumonias, and symptoms specific for *C. pneumoniae* pneumonia do not exist. However, a number of characteristic features of *C. pneumoniae* pneumonia have been documented.[88] The incubation period is about 4 weeks,[99] and most cases develop with a gradual onset. Furthermore, often a biphasic illness is noted with initial onset of pharyngitis, hoarseness, and fever that may resolve before the onset of cough and other signs of lower respiratory tract illness.[88] Headache is another common symptom and auscultation often reveals rales, but neither finding is specific for *C. pneumoniae* pneumonia. Radiography may show pneumonitis in mild disease and pleural effusions in severe illness, but these findings also are not helpful in differentiating *C. pneumoniae* from other pneumonias.[88]

Although most *C. pneumoniae* pneumonias are mild, recovery from infection is slow even with antibiotic therapy[81] and severe cases do occur. An underlying disease such as chronic obstructive pulmonary disease (COPD) predisposes to *C. pneumoniae* pneumonia[100] and may aggravate the course of the disease. An important finding in *C. pneumoniae* pneumonias is the high rate of coinfection by *C. pneumoniae* and other organisms (Table I). This high coinfection rate observed in *C. pneumoniae* pneumonias suggests that the organism may predispose to pyogenic infections which may increase disease severity,[101] although additional studies are needed to address this hypothesis.

5.3. Diagnosis and Treatment

Diagnostic methods available to detect *C. pneumoniae* infection have been reviewed recently.[102,103] As Table I indicates, most studies make use of the MIF test to diagnose *C. pneumoniae* infections, and MIF has been useful in showing a high prevalence of *C. pneumoniae* pneumonias. However, because the prevalence of *C. trachomatis* infections also is high in selected populations, a certain portion of pneumonia patients may have cross-reactive antibodies to *C. trachomatis*. Comparison of results between studies (Table I) is further complicated because some groups define arbitrary MIF criteria for acute infection even though standard diagnostic criteria have been proposed.[104] Thus, as with other chlamydial species, *C. pneumoniae* diagnoses based solely on serological criteria are less preferable to diagnoses made by multiple methods.

In the absence of controlled trials, treatment with 2 g of tetracycline or erythromycin daily for a minimum of 14 days has been recommended. The newer macrolides clarithromycin and azithromycin also appear effective.[105] Notably, slow resolution and/or relapse after treatment are observed frequently.

5.4. Host Immune Response to *C. pneumoniae* Pneumonia

Little is known about the immune mechanisms involved in *C. pneumoniae* pneumonia. Yang *et al.*[89,93] infected mice with a high infective dose (10^7 infectious units) and observed an acute, patchy pneumonia with PMN infiltration and alveolar and bronchiolar exudate, followed by monocytic infiltration. Using a 10-fold lower inoculum, Laitinen *et al.*[106] observed a chronic inflammation developing gradually with perivascular and peribronchial lymphocytic infiltrations. Both groups reported histological changes for several weeks after infection and the organism could be isolated from the lungs of infected mice for up to 2 weeks following challenge. A strong antibody response that peaked 3 to 4 weeks after intranasal challenge also was present by EIA, and an inverse relationship existed between recovery of pulmonary infectious units and specific antibody titers. An IgM isotype was common in primary infections whereas IgG and IgA were markedly increased in reinfections.[81]

T-cell-lymphoproliferative responses to *C. pneumoniae* antigen were increased in patients with recent *C. pneumoniae* pneumonia,[107] suggesting a role for CMI in this disease. CMI responses may be modulated by *C. pneumoniae*–alveolar macrophage interactions, as *C. pneumoniae* induced the secretion of IL-1β, IL-6, and TNF-α by human monocytic cells[108] and IL-1β, IL-6, TNF-α, and IFN-α by human peripheral blood mononuclear cells.[109] The contribution of these cytokines to induction of cellular and humoral immune responses and the importance of these immune mediators in *C. pneumoniae* pneumonia currently are not understood. In murine models, corticosteroid administration during secondary infection allows recovery of previously noncultivatable organisms, suggesting that persistent infection may occur in the lung following the acute phase of pneumonia.[110] Thus in some cases the immune response to *C. pneumoniae* may suppress active infection but not totally eliminate the organism.

6. CONCLUSION

As outlined in Table II, this review has delineated similarities and differences in the epidemiology, pathogenesis, clinical symptoms, and immune responses to chlamydial pneumonias. Each organism may induce unique immune responses, as different pneumonia syndromes result from infection with different chlamydiae. Understanding such species differences in the context of one disease may help

TABLE II
Similarities and Differences between Chlamydial Pneumonias

	C. psittaci	C. trachomatis	C. pneumoniae
Epidemiology	Mainly zoonosis from birds, rare human-to-human transmission	Infant pneumonia from infected mothers during childbirth, adult pneumonia in immunocompromised individuals	Most common chlamydial pneumonia. Rare in infants and preschoolers; common in older children, adolescents, and adults
Pathogenesis	Primary infection in lungs, may become systemic. 1–3 week incubation period	Primary infection in infants results in mild pneumonia, may predispose to chronic pulmonary sequelae later in life. < 8 week incubation period	Primary infections and reinfections occur associated with chronic pulmonary and extrapulmonary diseases including adult-onset asthma, atherosclerosis. 3–5 week incubation period
Clinical symptoms	Initially as atypical pneumonia with fever, cough, headache, later with multiple organ-system involvement and fulminant psittacosis	Infant pneumonia—chronic, mild, afebrile disease with staccato cough. Adult pneumonia—acute, fulminant disease	Atypical pneumonia with gradual onset and biphasic illness (URT symptoms may resolve before LRT symptoms). Also severe pneumonia in hospitalized patients
Treatment	Tetracycline 500 mg q.i.d. or doxycycline 100 mg b.i.d. × 14–21 days	Erythromycin 50 mg/kg × 10–14 days	Tetracycline or erythromycin 2 g × 14 days. Newer macrolides (e.g., azithromycin, clarithromycin)
Immune response	Protective immunity not shown. Reinfections may occur.	Murine model exists. CMI, alveolar macrophages, humoral response (?) important. IFN-γ, TNF-α have protective effects. Little known on human immune responses.	Partial immunity as reinfections less severe in younger adults. CMI and alveolar macrophages may be important. Some animal models available.

CMI = cell-mediated immunity; URT = upper respiratory tract; LRT = lower respiratory tract.

establish common principles applicable to understanding the pathogenesis of these chlamydial infections. Clearly, the use of murine models for *C. trachomatis* pneumonia has described important immune mediators, and whether these mediators are equally applicable to recently developed *C. pneumoniae* animal models awaits to be seen. In either case, the immune response to pneumonia may be different in humans, and future studies therefore must define immune mediators in human chlamydial pneumonias.

REFERENCES

1. Crosse, B. A., 1990, Psittacosis: A clinical review, *J. Infect.* **21:**251–259.
2. Weinstock, H., Dean, D., and Bolan, G., 1994, *Chlamydia trachomatis* infections, *Infect. Dis. Clin. North. Am.* **8:**797–819.
3. Hahn, D. L., Dodge, R. W., and Golubjatnikov, R., 1991, Association of *Chlamydia pneumoniae* (strain TWAR) infection with wheezing, asthmatic bronchitis, and adult-onset asthma, *JAMA* **266:**225–230.
4. Kuo, C. C., Jackson, L. A., Campbell, L. A., and Grayston, J. T., 1995, *Chlamydia pneumoniae* (TWAR), *Clin. Microbiol. Rev.* **8:**451–461.
5. Ward, M., 1995, The immunobiology and immunopathology of chlamydial infections, *APMIS* **103:** 769–796.
6. Rockey, D. D., Fischer, E. R., and Hackstadt, T., 1996, Temporal analysis of the developing *Chlamydia psittaci* inclusion by use of fluorescence and electron microscopy, *Infect. Immun.* **64:**4269–4278.
7. Hackstadt, T., Scidmore, M. A., and Rockey, D. D., 1995, Lipid metabolism in *Chlamydia trachomatis*-infected cells: Directed trafficking of Golgi-derived sphingolipids to the chlamydial inclusion, *Proc. Natl. Acad. Sci. USA* **92:**4877–4881.
8. Hackstadt, T., Rockey, D. D., Heinzen, R. A., and Scidmore, M. A., 1996, Chlamydia trachomatis interrupts an exocytic pathway to acquire endogenously synthesized sphingomyelin in transit from the golgi apparatus to the plasma membrane, *EMBO J.* **15:**964–977.
9. Scidmore, M. A., Fischer, E. R., and Hackstadt, T., 1996, Sphingolipids and glycoproteins are differentially trafficked to the *Chlamydia trachomatis* inclusion, *J. Cell Biol.* **134:**363–374.
10. Moulder, J., 1991, Interaction of *chlamydiae* and host cells *in vitro*, *Microbiol. Rev.* **55:**143–190.
11. La Verda, D., and Byrne, G., 1994, Interactions between macrophages and *chlamydiae*, *Immunol. Ser.* **60:**381–399.
12. Gaydos, C. A., Summersgill, J. T., Sahney, N. N., Ramirez, J. A., and Quinn, T. C., 1996, Replication of Chlamydia pneumoniae *in vitro* in human macrophages, endothelial cells, and aortic artery smooth muscle cells, *Infect. Immun.* **64:**1614–1620.
13. Godzik, K. L., O'Brien, E. R., Wang, S. K., and Kuo, C. C., 1995, *In vitro* susceptibility of human vascular wall cells to infection with *Chlamydia pneumoniae*, *J. Clin. Microbiol.* **33:**2411–2414.
14. Manor, E., and Sarov, I., 1986, Fate of *Chlamydia trachomatis* in human monocytes and monocyte-derived macrophages, *Infect. Immun.* **54:**90–95.
15. Suwa, T., Ando, S., Hashimoto, N., and Itakura, C., 1990, Pathology of experimental chlamydiosis in chicks, *J. Vet. Med. Sci.* **52:**275–283.
16. Kuo, C., Shor, A., Campbell, L., Fukushi, H., Patton, D., and Grayston, J., 1993, Demonstration of *Chlamydia pneumoniae* in atherosclerotic lesions of coronary arteries, *J. Infect. Dis.* **167:**841–849.

17. Potter, M., Kaufmann, A., and Plikaytis, B., 1983, Psittacosis in the United States 1979, CDC Surveillance Summaries. *MMWR* **32:**27–31.
18. Yung, A., and Grayston, M., 1988, Psittacosis—a review of 135 cases, *Med. J. Aust.* **148:**228–233.
19. Schaffner, W., Drutz, D., and Duncan, G., 1967, The clinical spectrum of endemic psittacosis, *Arch. Intern. Med.* **119:**433–443.
20. Hood, J. W., McMartin, D. A., and Harris, J. W., 1984, Growth of *Chlamydia* in pig lung alveolar macrophages; preparation of macrophages and demonstration of growth, *Vet. Res. Commun.* **8:**15–23.
21. Brownridge, E., and Wyrick, P. B., 1979, Interaction of *Chlamydia psittaci* reticulate bodies with mouse peritoneal macrophages, *Infect. Immun.* **24:**697–700.
22. Wyrick, P. B., and Brownridge, E. A., 1978, Growth of *Chlamydia psittaci* in macrophages, *Infect. Immun.* **19:**1054–1060.
23. Seibert, R., Jordan, W., and Dingle, J., 1956, Clinical variations in the diagnosis of psittacosis, *N. Eng. J. Med.* **254:**925–930.
24. Bowman, P., Wilt, J., and Sayed, H., 1973, Chronicity and recurrence of psittacosis, *Can. J. Pub. Health* **64:**167–173.
25. Bernstein, D. I., Hubbard, T., Wenman, W. M., Johnson, B. L., Jr., Holmes, K. K., Liebhaber, H., Schachter, J., Barnes, R., and Lovett, M. A., 1984, Mediastinal and supraclavicular lymphadenitis and pneumonitis due to *Chlamydia trachomatis* serovars L1 and L2, *N. Eng. J. Med.* **311:**1543–1546.
26. Moncada, J. V., Schachter, J., and Wofsy, C., 1986, Prevalence of *Chlamydia trachomatis* lung infection in patients with acquired immune deficiency syndrome, *J. Clin. Microbiol.* **23:**986.
27. Tack, K. J., Peterson, P. K., Rasp, F. L., O'Leary, M., Hanto, D., Simmons, R. L., and Sabath, L. D., 1980, Isolation of *Chlamydia trachomatis* from the lower respiratory tract of adults, *Lancet* **i:**116–120.
28. Ito, J. I., Jr., Comess, K. A., Alexander, E. R., Harrison, H. R., Ray, C. G., Kiviat, J., and Sobonya, R. E., 1982, Pneumonia due to *Chlamydia trachomatis* in an immunocompromised adult, *N. Eng. J. Med.* **307:**95–98.
29. Meyers, J. D., Hackman, R. C., and Stamm, W. E., 1983, *Chlamydia trachomatis* infection as a cause of pneumonia after human marrow transplantation, *Transplantation* **36:**130–134.
30. Kroon, F. P., van 't Wout, J. W., Weiland, H. T., and van Furth, R., 1989, *Chlamydia trachomatis* pneumonia in an HIV-seropositive patient, *N. Eng. J. Med.* **320:**806–807.
31. Beem, M. O., and Saxon, E. M., 1977, Respiratory-tract colonization and a distinctive pneumonia syndrome in infants infected with *Chlamydia trachomatis*, *N. Eng. J. Med.* **296:**306–310.
32. Heggie, A. D., Lumicao, G. G., Stuart, L. A., and Gyves, M. T., 1981, *Chlamydia trachomatis* infection in mothers and infants. A prospective study, *Am. J. Dis. Child.* **135:**507–511.
33. Limudomporn, S., Prapphal, N., Nanthapisud, P., and Chomdej, S., 1989, Afebrile pneumonia associated with chlamydial infection in infants less than 6 months of age: Initial results of a three year prospective study, *Southeast Asian J. Trop. Med. Public Health* **20:**285–290.
34. Schachter, J., Grossman, M., Sweet, R. L., Holt, J., Jordan, C., and Bishop, E., 1986, Prospective study of perinatal transmission of *Chlamydia trachomatis*, *JAMA* **255:**3374–3377.
35. Schachter, J., Grossman, M., Holt, J., Sweet, R., Goodner, E., and Mills, J., 1979, Prospective study of chlamydial infection in neonates, *Lancet* **2:**377–380.
36. Schachter, J., Grossman, M., Holt, J., Sweet, R., and Spector, S., 1979, Infection with *Chlamydia trachomatis:* Involvement of multiple anatomic sites in neonates, *J. Infect. Dis.* **139:**232–234.
37. Tipple, M. A., Beem, M. O., and Saxon, E. M., 1979, Clinical characteristics of the afebrile pneumonia associated with *Chlamydia trachomatis* infection in infants less than 6 months of age, *Pediatrics* **63:**192–197.

38. Brewster, D. R., De Silva, L. M., and Henry, R. L., 1981, *Chlamydia trachomatis* and respiratory disease in infants, *Med. J. Aust.* **2:**328–330.
39. Embil, J. A., Ozere, R. L., and MacDonald, S. W., 1978, *Chlamydia trachomatis* and pneumonia in infants: Report of two cases, *Can. Med. Assoc. J.* **119:**1199–1203.
40. Radkowski, M. A., Kranzler, J. K., Beem, M. O., and Tipple, M. A., 1981, *Chlamydia* pneumonia in infants: Radiography in 125 cases, *AJR Am. J. Roentgenol.* **137:**703–706.
41. Wheeler, W. B., Kurachek, S. C., Lobas, J. G., and Einzig, M. J., 1990, Acute hypoxemic respiratory failure caused by *Chlamydia trachomatis* and diagnosed by flexible bronchoscopy, *Am. Rev. Respir. Dis.* **142:**471–473.
42. Broadbent, R., and O'Learly, L., 1988, Chlamydial infections in young infants—a cause for concern, *N. Z. Med. J.* **101:**44–45.
43. Brasfield, D. M., Stagno, S., Whitley, R. J., Cloud, G., Cassell, G., and Tiller, R. E., 1987, Infant pneumonitis associated with cytomegalovirus, *Chlamydia, Pneumocystis,* and *Ureaplasma:* Follow-up, *Pediatrics* **79:**76–83.
44. Weiss, S., Newcomb, R., and Beem, M., 1986, Pulmonary assessment of children after chlamydial pneumonia of infancy, *J. Pediatr.* **108:**659–664.
45. CDC 1993. Sexually transmitted diseases treatment guidelines, *MMWR* **42:**1–102.
46. Pereira, L. H., Embil, J. A., Haase, D. A., and Manley, K. M., 1990, Cytomegalovirus infection among women attending a sexually transmitted disease clinic: Association with clinical symptoms and other sexually transmitted diseases, *Am. J. Epidemiol.* **131:**683–692.
47. Heggie, A. D., Jaffe, A. C., Stuart, L. A., Thombre, P. S., and Sorensen, R. U., 1985, Topical sulfacetamide vs. oral erythromycin for neonatal chlamydial conjunctivitis, *Am. J. Dis. Child.* **139:**564–566.
48. Lode, H., and Schaberg, T., 1992, Azithromycin in lower respiratory tract infections, *Scand. J. Infect. Dis. Suppl.* **83:**26–33.
49. Ridgway, G. L., 1996, Azithromycin in the management of *Chlamydia trachomatis* infections, *Int. J. STD AIDS* **7:**5–8.
50. Guay, D. R., 1996, Macrolide antibiotics in paediatric infectious diseases, *Drugs* **51:**515–536.
51. Lode, H., Borner, K., Koeppe, P., and Schaberg, T., 1996, Azithromycin—review of key chemical, pharmacokinetic and microbiological features, *J. Antimicrob. Chemother.* **37:**1–8.
52. Williams, D. M., Schachter, J., Drutz, D., and Sumaya, C. V., 1981, Pneumonia due to *Chlamydia trachomatis* in the immunocompromised mouse, *J. Infect. Dis.* **143:**238–241.
53. Williams, D. M., Schachter, J., Coalson, J. J., and Grubbs, B., 1984, Cellular immunity to the mouse pneumonitis agent, *J. Infect. Dis.* **149:**630–639.
54. Williams, D. M., Schachter, J., Grubbs, B., and Sumaya, C. V., 1982, The role of antibody in host defense against the agent of mouse pneumonitis, *J. Infect. Dis.* **145:**200–205.
55. Levitt, D., Newcomb, R. W., and Beem, M. O., 1983, Excessive numbers and activity of peripheral blood B cells in infants with *Chlamydia trachomatis* pneumonia, *Clin. Immunol. Immunopathol.* **29:**424–432.
56. Williams, D. M., Grubbs, B., and Schachter, J., 1987, Primary murine *Chlamydia trachomatis* pneumonia in B-cell-deficient mice, *Infect. Immun.* **55:**2387–2390.
57. Coalson, J. J., Winter, V. T., Bass, L. B., Schachter, J., Grubbs, B. G., and Williams, D. M., 1987, *Chlamydia trachomatis* pneumonia in the immune, athymic and normal BALB mouse, *Br. J. Exp. Pathol.* **68:**399–411.
58. Nakajo, M. N., Roblin, P. M., Hammerschlag, M. R., Smith, P., and Nowakowski, M., 1990, Chlamydicidal activity of human alveolar macrophages, *Infect. Immun.* **58:**3640–3644.
59. Kurland, G., Cheung, A., Miller, M., Ayin, S., Cho, M., and Ford, E., 1988, The ontogeny of pulmonary defenses: Alveolar macrophage function in neonatal and juvenile rhesus monkeys, *Ped. Res.* **23:**293–297.
60. Chida, K., Myrvik, Q., Leake, E., Gordon, M., Wood, P., and Ricardo, M., 1987, Chem-

iluminescent responses of alveolar macrophages from normal and *Mycobacterium bovis* BCG-vaccinated rabbits as a function of age, *Infect. Immun.* **55:**1476–1483.

61. Williams, D. M., Grubbs, B. G., Schachter, J., and Magee, D. M., 1993, Gamma interferon levels during *Chlamydia trachomatis* pneumonia in mice, *Infect. Immun.* **61:**3556–3558.

62. Williams, D. M., Magee, D. M., Bonewald, L. F., Smith, J. G., Bleicker, C. A., Byrne, G. I., and Schachter, J., 1990, A role *in vivo* for tumor necrosis factor alpha in host defense against *Chlamydia trachomatis, Infect. Immun.* **58:**1572–1576.

63. Magee, D. M., Smith, J. G., Bleicker, C. A., Carter, C. J., Bonewald, L. F., Schachter, J., and Williams, D. M., 1992, *Chlamydia trachomatis* pneumonia induces *in vivo* production of inter-leukin-1 and -6, *Infect. Immun.* **60:**1217–1220.

64. Williams, D. M., Grubbs, B. G., Park-Snyder, S., Rank, R. G., and Bonewald, L. F., 1996, Activation of latent transforming growth factor beta during *Chlamydia trachomatis*-induced murine pneumonia, *Res. Microbiol.* **147:**251–262.

65. Magee, D. M., Williams, D. M., Wing, E. J., Bleicker, C. A., and Schachter, J., 1991, Production of colony-stimulating factors during pneumonia caused by *Chlamydia trachomatis, Infect. Immun.* **59:**2370–2375.

66. Yang, X., Hayglass, K. T., and Brunham, R. C., 1996, Genetically determined differences in interleukin-10 and interferon-gamma responses correlate with clearance of *Chlamydia trachomatis* mouse pneumonitis infection, *J. Immunol.* **156:**4338–4344.

67. Cotter, T., and Byrne, G., 1997, Immunity to *Chlamydia:* Comparison of human infections and murine models. Submitted.

68. Morrison, R., Feilzer, K., and Tumas, D., 1995, Gene knockout mice establish a primary protective role for major histocompatibility complex class II-restricted responses in *Chlamydia trachomatis* genital tract infection, *Infect. Immun.* **63:**4661–4668.

69. Williams, D. M., Grubbs, B. G., Kelly, K., Pack, E., and Rank, R. G., 1996, Role of gamma-delta T cells in murine *Chlamydia trachomatis* infection, *Infect. Immun.* **64:**3916–3919.

70. Saikku, P., Wang, S. P., Kleemola, M., Brander, E., Rusanen, E., and Grayston, J. T., 1985, An epidemic of mild pneumonia due to an unusual strain of *Chlamydia psittaci, J. Infect. Dis.* **151:**832–839.

71. Grayston, J., Kuo, C.-C., Campbell, L., and Wang, S., 1989, *Chlamydia pneumoniae* sp nov. for *Chlamydia* sp. strain TWAR, *Intern. J. Syst. Bacteriol.* **39:**88–90.

72. Cox, R., Kuo, C.-C., Grayston, J., and Campbell, L., 1988, Deoxyribonucleic acid relatedness of *Chlamydia* sp. strain TWAR to *Chlamydia trachomatis* and *Chlamydia psittaci, Int. J. Syst. Bacteriol.* **38:**265–268.

73. Chi, E., Kuo, C.-C., and Grayston, J., 1990, Unique ultrastructure in the elementary body of *Chlamydia* sp. strain TWAR, *J. Bacteriol.* **169:**3757–3763.

74. Wang, S.-P., and Grayston, J., 1990, Population prevalence antibody to *Chlamydia pneumoniae*, strain TWAR, in: *Chlamydial Infections* (W. R. Bowie, H. D. Caldwell, R. P. Jones, P. A. Mardh, G. L. Ridgway, J. Schachter, W. E. Stamm, and M. E. Ward, eds.), Cambridge University Press, England, pp. 402–405.

75. Kanamoto, Y., Ouchi, K., Mizui, M., Ushio, M., and Usui, T., 1991, Prevalence of antibody to *Chlamydia pneumoniae* TWAR in Japan, *J. Clin. Microbiol.* **29:**816–818.

76. Forsey, T., Darougar, S., and Treharne, J. D., 1986, Prevalence in human beings of antibodies to *Chlamydia* IOL-207, an atypical strain of *chlamydia, J. Infect.* **12:**145–152.

77. Grayston, J. T., 1992, Infections caused by *Chlamydia pneumoniae* strain TWAR, *Clin. Infect. Dis.* **15:**757–761.

78. Aldous, M., Grayston, J., Wang, S.-P., and Foy, H., 1990, Seroepidemiology of *Chlamydia pneumoniae* TWAR infection in Seattle families, 1966–1979, *J. Infect. Dis.* **166:**646–649.

79. Kleemola, M., Saikku, P., Visakorpi, R., Wang, S. P., and Grayston, J. T., 1988, Epidemics of

pneumonia caused by TWAR, a new *Chlamydia organism, in military trainees in Finland, J. Infect. Dis.* **157:**230–236.

80. Berdal, B. P., Scheel, O., Ogaard, A. R., Hoel, T., Gutteberg, T. J., and Anestad, G., 1992, Spread of subclinical *Chlamydia pneumoniae* infection in a closed community, *Scand. J. Infect. Dis.* **24:**431–436.

81. Ekman, M. R., Grayston, J. T., Visakorpi, R., Kleemola, M., Kuo, C. C., and Saikku, P., 1993, An epidemic of infections due to *Chlamydia pneumoniae* in military conscripts, *Clin. Infect. Dis.* **17:**420–425.

82. Almirall, J., Morato, I., Riera, F., Verdaguer, A., Priu, R., Coll, P., Vidal, J., Murgui, L., Valls, F., Catalan, F., Balanz, 1993, Incidence of community-acquired pneumonia and *Chlamydia pneumoniae* infection: A prospective multicentre study, *Eur. Resp. J.* **6:**14–18.

83. Boschini, A., Smacchia, C., Fine, M., Schiesari, A., Ballarini, P., Arlotti, M., Gabrielli, C., Castellani, G., Genova, M., Pantani, P., Lepri, A., and Rezza, G., 1996, Community-acquired pneumonia in a cohort of former injection drug users with and without human immunodeficiency virus infection: Incidence, etiologies, and clinical aspects, *Clin. Infect. Dis.* **23:**107–113.

84. Marrie, T., Peeling, R., Fine, M., Singer, D., Coley, C., and Kapoor, W., 1996, Ambulatory patient swith community-acquired pneumonia: The frequency of atypical agents and clinical course, *Am. J. Med.* **101:**508–515.

85. Block, S., Hedrick, J., Hammerschlag, M. R., Cassell, G. H., and Craft, J. C., 1995, *Mycoplasma pneumoniae* and *Chlamydia pneumoniae* in pediatric community-acquired pneumonia: Comparative efficacy and safety of clarithromycin vs. erythromycin ethylsuccinate, *Ped. Infect. Dis. J.* **14:**471–477.

86. Shemer-Avni, Y., and Lieberman, D., 1995, *Chlamydia pneumoniae*-induced ciliostasis in ciliated bronchial epithelial cells, *J. Infect. Dis.* **171:**1274–1278.

87. Black, C., and Perez, R., 1990, *Chlamydia pneumoniae* multiplies within human pulmonary macrophages, in: *Program and Abstracts of the 90th Annual Meeting of the American Society for Microbiology* (Anaheim), American Society for Microbiology Press, Washington, D. C.

88. Kauppinen, M., Kujala, P., Leinonen, M., Saikku, P., Herva, E., and Syrjala, J., 1994, Clinical features of community-acquired *Chlamydia pneumoniae*-pneumonia, in: *Chlamydial Infections* (J. Orfila, G. I. Byrne, M. A. Chernesky, J. T. Grayston, R. B. Jones, G. L. Ridgway, P. Saikku, J. Schachter, W. E. Stamm, and R. S. Stephens, eds.), Societa Editrice Esculapio, Bologna, pp. 457–60.

89. Yang, Z. P., Kuo, C. C., and Grayston, J. T., 1993, A mouse model of *Chlamydia pneumoniae* strain TWAR pneumonitis, *Infect. Immun.* **61:**2037–2040.

90. Yang, Z. P., Kuo, C. C., and Grayston, J. T., 1995, Systemic dissemination of *Chlamydia pneumoniae* following intranasal inoculation in mice, *J. Infect. Dis.* **171:** 736–738.

91. Malinverni, R., Kuo, C. C., Campbell, L. A., Lee, A., and Grayston, J. T., 1995, Effects of two antibiotic regimens on course and persistence of experimental *Chlamydia pneumoniae* TWAR pneumonitis, *Antimicrob. Agents Chemother.* **39:**45–49.

92. Masson, N. D., Toseland, C. D., and Beale, A. S., 1995, Relevance of *Chlamydia pneumoniae* murine pneumonitis model to evaluation of antimicrobial agents, *Antimicrob. Agents Chemother.* **39:**1959–1964.

93. Yang, Z., Cummings, P., Patton, D., and Kuo, C., 1994, Ultrastructural lung pathology of experimental *Chlamydia pneumoniae* pneumonitis in mice, *J. Infect. Dis.* **170:**464–467.

94. Bell, T. A., Kuo, C. C., Wang, S. P., and Grayston, J. T., 1989, Experimental infection of baboons (*Papio cynocephalus anubis*) with *Chlamydia pneumoniae* strain 'TWAR', *J. Infect.* **19:**47–49.

95. Holland, S. M., Taylor, H. R., Gaydos, C. A., Kappus, E. W., and Quinn, T. C., 1990, Experimental infection with *Chlamydia pneumoniae* in nonhuman primates, *Infect. Immun.* **58:**593–597.

96. Moazed, T. C., Kuo, C. C., Patton, D. L., Grayston, J. T., and Campbell, L. A., 1996, Experimental rabbit models of *Chlamydia pneumoniae* infection, *Am. J. Pathol.* **148:**667–676.

97. Fong, I. W., Chiu, B., Viira, E., Fong, M. W., Jang, D., and Mahony, J., 1997, Rabbit model for *Chlamydia pneumoniae* infection, *J. Clin. Microbiol.* **35:**48–52.

98. Thom, D., Grayston, J., Wang, S., Kuo, C., and Altman, J., 1990, Chlamydia pneumoniae, strain TWAR, *Mycoplasma pneumoniae* and viral infections in acute respiratory disease in a university student health clinic population, *Am. J. Epidemiol.* **132:**248–256.

99. Mordhorst, C. H., Wang, S. P., and Grayston, J. T., 1992, Outbreak of *Chlamydia pneumoniae* infection in four farm families, *Eur. J. Clin. Microbiol. Infect. Dis.* **11:**617–620.

100. Torres, A., Dorca, J., Zalacain, R., Bello, S., Elebiary, M., Molinos, L., Arevalo, M., Blanquer, J., Celis, R., Iriberri, M., Prats, E., Fernandez, R., Irigaray, R., and Serra, J., 1996, Community-acquired pneumonia in chronic obstructive pulmonary disease—a Spanish multicenter study, *Am. J. Respir. Crit. Care. Med.* **154:**1456–1461.

101. Kauppinen, M., Saikku, P., Kujala, P., Herva, E., and Syrjala, H., 1996, Clinical picture of community-acquired *Chlamydia pneumoniae* pneumonia requiring hospital treatment: A comparison between chlamydial and pneumococcal pneumonia, *Thorax* **51:**185–189.

102. Peeling, R., and Brunham, R., 1996, *Chlamydiae* as pathogens: New species and new issues, *Emerg. Infect. Dis.* **2:**307–319.

103. Kauppinen, M., and Saikku, P., 1995, Pneumonia due to *Chlamydia pneumoniae:* Prevalence, clinical features, diagnosis, and treatment, *Clin. Infect. Dis.* **21:**5244–5252.

104. Grayston, J. T., Campbell, L. A., Kuo, C. C., Mordhorst, C. H., Saikku, P., Thom, D. H., and Wang, S. P., 1990, A new respiratory tract pathogen: *Chlamydia pneumoniae* strain TWAR, *J. Infect. Dis.* **161:**618–625.

105. Williams, J. D., and Sefton, A. M., 1993, Comparison of macrolide antibiotics, *J. Antimicrob. Chemother.* **31:**11–26.

106. Laitinen, K., Laurila, A., Leinonen, M., and Saikku, P., 1994, Experimental *Chlamydia pneumoniae* infection in mice: Effect of reinfection and passive protection by immune serum, in: *Proceedings of the 8th International Symposium on Human Chlamydial Infections* (J. Orfila, G. L. Byrne, M. A. Chernesky, J. T. Grayston, R. B. Jones, G. L. Ridgway, P. Saikku, J. Schachter, W. E. Stamm, and R. S. Stephens, eds.), Esculapio, Bologna, pp. 545–548.

107. Surcel, H. M., Syrjala, H., Leinonen, M., Saikku, P., and Herva, E., 1993, Cell-mediated immunity to *Chlamydia pneumoniae* measured as lymphocyte blast transformation *in vitro*, *Infect. Immun.* **61:**2196–2199.

108. Heinemann, M., Susa, M., Simnacher, U., Marre, R., and Essig, A., 1996, Growth of *Chlamydia pneumoniae* induces cytokine production and expression of CD14 In a human monocytic cell line, *Infect. Immun.* **64:**4872–4875.

109. Kaukorantatolvanen, S. S. E., Teppo, A. M., Laitinen, K., Saikku, P., Linnavuori, K., and Leinonen, M., 1996, Growth of *Chlamydia pneumoniae* in cultured human peripheral blood mononuclear cells and induction of a cytokine response, *Microb. Pathog.* **21:**215–221.

110. Malinverni, R., Kuo, C. C., Campbell, L. A., and Grayston, J. T., 1995, Reactivation of *Chlamydia pneumoniae* lung infection in mice by cortisone, *J. Infect. Dis.* **172:**593–594.

111. Grayston, J. T., Diwan, V. K., Cooney, M., and Wang, S. P., 1989, Community- and hospital-acquired pneumonia associated with *Chlamydia* TWAR infection demonstrated serologically, *Arch. Int. Med.* **149:**169–173.

112. Marrie, T. J., Grayston, J. T., Wang, S. P., and Kuo, C. C., 1987, Pneumonia associated with the TWAR strain of *Chlamydia*, *Ann. Int. Med.* **106:**507–511.

113. Grayston, J. T., Kuo, C. C., Wang, S. P., and Altman, J., 1986, A new *Chlamydia psittaci* strain, TWAR, isolated in acute respiratory tract infections, *N. Eng. J. Med.* **315:**161–168.

114. Bates, J., Campbell, G., Barron, A., McCracken, G., Morgan, P., Moses, E., and Davis, C., 1992, Microbial etiology of acute pneumonia in hospitalized patients, *Chest* **101:**1005–1012.

115. Sundelof, B., Gnarpe, J., Gnarpe, H., Grillner, L., and Darougar, S., 1993, *Chlamydia pneumoniae* in Swedish patients, *Scand. J. Infect. Dis.* **25:**429–433.

116. Kauppinen, M. T., Herva, E., Kujala, P., Leinonen, M., Saikku, P., and Syrjala, H., 1995, The etiology of community-acquired pneumonia among hospitalized patients during a *Chlamydia pneumoniae* epidemic in Finland, *J. Infect. Dis.* **172:**1330–1335.

117. Fang, G. D., Fine, M., Orloff, J., Arisumi, D., Yu, V. L., Kapoor, W., Grayston, J. T., Wang, S. P., Kohler, R., Muder, R. R., Yee, Y., Rins, J. D., and Vickers, R. M., 1990, New and emerging etiologies for community-acquired pneumonia with implications for therapy. A prospective multicenter study of 359 cases, *Medicine* **69:**307–316.

118. Maartens, G., Lewis, S., Goveia, C., Bartie, C., Roditi, D., and Klugman, K., 1994, Atypical bacteria are a common cause of community-acquired pneumonia in hospitalized adults, *S. Afr. Med. J.* **84:**678–682.

119. Karalus, N. C., Cursons, R. T., Leng, R. A., Mahood, C. B., Rothwell, R. P., Hancock, B., Cepulis, S., Wawatai, M., and Coleman, L., 1991, Community acquired pneumonia: Aetiology and prognostic index evaluation, *Thorax* **46:**413–418.

120. Lieberman, D., Ben-Yaakov, M., Lazarovich, Z., Porath, A., Schlaeffer, F., Lieberman, D., Leinonen, M., Saikku, P., Horovitz, O., and Boldur, I., 1996, *Chlamydia pneumoniae* community-acquired pneumonia: A review of 62 hospitalized adult patients, *Infection* **24:**109–114.

121. Steinhoff, D., Lode, H., Ruckdeschel, G., Heidrich, B., Rolfs, A., Fehrenbach, F. J., Mauch, H., Hoffken, G., and Wagner, J., 1996, *Chlamydia pneumoniae* as a cause of community-acquired pneumonia in hospitalized patients in Berlin, *Clin. Infect. Dis.* **22:**958–964.

122. Blasi, F., Cosentini, R., Legnani, D., Denti, F., and Allegra, L., 1993, Incidence of community-acquired pneumonia caused by *Chlamydia pneumoniae* in Italian patients, *Eur. J. Clin. Microbiol. Infect. Dis.* **12:**696–699.

123. Ortqvist, A., and Jean, C., 1994, Sparflloxacin (SPX) compared to roxithromycin (R) for the treatment of community-acquired pneumonia [abstract M53], in: *Program and Abstracts of the 34th Interscience Conference on Antimicrobial Agents and Chemotherapy* (Orlando), American Society for Microbiology Press, Washington, D. C.

124. Gomez, J., Banos, V., Gomez, J. R., Soto, M. C., Munoz, L., Nunez, M. L., Canteras, M., and Valdes, M., 1996, Prospective study of epidemiology and prognostic factors in community-acquired pneumonia, *Eur. J. Clin. Microbiol. Infect. Dis.* **15:**556–560.

125. Plouffe, J., Herbert, M., File, T., Baird, I., Parsons, J., Kahn, J., Rielly-Gauvin, K., and Group, P. S., 1996, Ofoxacin versus standard therapy in treatment of community-acquired pneumonia requiring hospitalization, *Antimicrob. Agents Chemother.* **40:**1175–1179.

126. Virata, M., Tirrellpeck, S., Meek, J., Ryder, R., Delbene, J., Messmer, T., Skelton, S., Talkington, D., Thacker, L., Fields, B., and Butler, J., 1996, Comparison of serology and throat swab PCR for diagnosis of *Chlamydia pneumoniae* and *Mycoplasma pneumoniae* among out-patients with pneumonia, *Clin. Infect. Dis.* **23:**895.

15

Brucella Infections and Immunity

CYNTHIA L. BALDWIN and R. MARTIN ROOP II

1. INTRODUCTION

Brucellosis, caused by several species of Gram-negative intracellular bacteria in the genus *Brucella*, is a zoonotic disease that has a significant impact on both human and animal health worldwide.[1] Animal species infected include companion (dogs) and agricultural species (sheep, cattle, swine, camels, and water buffalo) as well as wildlife (bison, elk, caribou, and African buffalo).[2,3] *Brucella* spp. infective for humans in order of virulence are *B. melitensis*, whose primary hosts are sheep and goats; *B. suis*, whose primary host is swine; *B. abortus*, whose primary host is cattle; and *B. canis*, whose primary host is dogs. The first three species are classified as "smooth" organisms based upon the length of their lipopolysaccharide *O*-side chains, while *B. canis* is a naturally occurring "rough" strain. Although the severity of disease is variable, ranging from lethal to subclinical in humans, in most cases the brucellae establish long-term parasitic relationships with their hosts whether human or animal. Survival and replication of brucellae in macrophages is critical to the maintenance of these chronic infections[4,5] and our current understanding of this process is the primary focus of this chapter.

CYNTHIA L. BALDWIN • Department of Veterinary and Animal Sciences, Paige Laboratory, University of Massachusetts, Amherst, Massachusetts 01003.   R. MARTIN ROOP II • Department of Microbiology and Immunology, Louisiana State University Medical Center, Shreveport, Louisiana 71130-3932.

Opportunistic Intracellular Bacteria and Immunity, edited by Lois J. Paradise *et al*. Plenum Press, New York, 1999.

2. ZOONOTIC NATURE OF THE INFECTION
AND CLINICAL SYMPTOMS

Humans most often acquire brucellosis through direct contact with infected animals or animal products; therefore the incidence of human disease is closely linked to the occurrence of infection in food animals.[6] Pregnant animals are the most susceptible to infection due to the propensity of the brucellae to replicate in the gravid uterus.[3] As a consequence, enormous numbers of brucellae are expelled from infected animals during abortion or parturition and thus these animals pose a significant risk for spreading the disease to humans and other animals.[6] Infected animals also shed the organisms in milk and uterine discharges.[1] Infection of people and other animals occurs through aerosol inhalation, entry via the conjunctiva and wounds, and following ingestion of the bacteria. Humans are known to become infected while engaged in animal husbandry, butchering, and from consumption of unpasteurized milk or dairy products. In addition to the threat of zoonotic infection posed to veterinarians ministering to field-strain-infected animals, these individuals also face the potential for infection as the result of accidental injection with the attenuated live *B. abortus* strain 19 or *B. melitensis* Rev-1 vaccines, which are virulent in humans.[7] *Brucella* spp. are also highly infectious in a laboratory setting and have the dubious distinction of being the most frequently acquired laboratory infection, infecting workers involved in diagnostic testing of farm animals, preparation of veterinary vaccines, or performing research.[8]

At present there is no safe, effective brucellosis vaccine available for use in humans and thus control of human disease relies on preventing exposure. In areas of the world where successful brucellosis eradication programs are in effect, and thus the incidence of the disease in food animals is low, and where routine pasteurization of milk occurs, human brucellosis is primarily an occupational hazard for slaughterhouse workers, veterinarians, and laboratory personnel.[6] Because infections may be latent in young animals, introduction of inapparent infected carriers into uninfected herds can result in rapid transmission of the disease through the herd.[1] This, as well as exposure of domestic animals to infected wildlife, can be an important mechanism by which brucellosis is maintained in food animals even in geographical regions where strict surveillance and quarantine measures are practiced. Thus, human brucellosis remains a serious public health problem, with *B. melitensis* being responsible for the greatest number of reported cases, occurring in regions where the disease is endemic in food animals such as Middle Eastern countries. As evidence of the importance of brucellosis to the world agricultural and public health communities, some experts have regarded this disease as the most economically devastating zoonotic disease due to the fact that it causes abortion, infertility, and decreased milk production in food animals.

Following infection, the onset of clinical symptoms in humans may be insidious or abrupt, taking days to months to appear, and is characterized by malaise, anorexia, fever, and muscle weaknesses.[9] Unlike the situation in animals, abortion does not appear to be a clinical presentation associated with human *Brucella* infections. However, serious complications such as endocarditis, arthritis, spondylitis, and neurological disorders may occur. The symptoms of human brucellosis are generally the same regardless of the infecting organism, with the severity of disease varying according to the infecting species. Treatment of human brucellosis is difficult owing to the intracellular nature of the infection, and prolonged antibiotic therapy is necessary.[10] Relapses are not uncommon, and in some cases, chemotherapy may be unsuccessful, leaving the individual with a lifelong, often debilitating disease.

3. SURVIVAL OF BRUCELLAE IN MACROPHAGES

Brucellae are resistant to killing by phagocytes from a number of species, including cattle,[11] goats,[12] guinea pigs,[13] mice,[14] and humans.[15] Moreover, *Brucella* has been shown by *in vitro* experiments to multiply both in mononuclear phagocytes as well as in other cells such as fibroblasts and trophoblasts. Inside host cells bacteria are inaccessible to humoral immune responses. Such immune responses include direct activation of complement, which brucellae are known to induce, and acquired immunity such as brucella-specific antibodies, which are readily induced by lipopolysaccharide (LPS) and shown by adoptive transfer to provide some degree of protection against infection. In addition to providing a safe haven for the brucellae, it is postulated that infected macrophages provide a vehicle for systemic spread.[5] Thus, intracellular survival and multiplication are believed to contribute to the ability of brucellae to infect hosts chronically.

Support for the contention that intracellular survival of *Brucella* spp. is essential to establishing and maintaining a chronic infection comes from the observations that in cattle and goats brucellae are sequestered or harbored in the reproductive organs, udder, and supramammary lymph nodes,[3] where they have been observed by histological examination to be inside macrophages and trophoblasts.[16–18] In experimentally infected mice, *Brucella* spp. are found associated with tissues rich in mononuclear phagocytes, such as the spleen and liver.[19] A correlation also exists between the virulence of *B. abortus* strains *in vivo* and their ability to survive in macrophages *in vitro*. For instance, LPS *O*-chain-deficient rough variants of *B. abortus* do not resist killing by cultured neutrophils and macrophages as well as their smooth counterparts[13] and are correspondingly less virulent in experimentally infected mice,[20] goats,[21] and cattle.[22] The limited survival of the *B. abortus* vaccine strain 19 in cultured macrophages also reflects its attenuation in both the mouse model and in ruminants.[5] Moreover, recent evidence suggests that resistance to *B. abortus* is linked to expression of a homolog of the *BCG / Ity / Lsh*^{resistance} gene[23]—a gene known to have its effect by influencing the ability of macrophages to prevent intracellular survival of microbes. Finally, it is well documented that the induction of specific cell-mediated immunity and subsequent activation of macrophages is required for host clearance of *Brucella* infections.[4,5,24,25]

4. *BRUCELLA* COMPONENTS THAT CONTRIBUTE TO SURVIVAL IN MACROPHAGES

Brucellae do not escape from the phagosome into the cytoplasm of host macrophages (see Fig. 1). Moreover, although there are considerable experimental data suggesting that the brucellae can inhibit phagosome–lysosome fusion in neutrophils,[26–28] evidence for interference with this process in macrophages is limited.[29] Likewise, there is no evidence that intracellular brucellae actively inhibit the oxidative burst of host macrophages following uptake.[26] However, there is evidence that *B. abortus* enters cultured macrophages in the absence of opsonization[30–32] and that entry in this fashion leads to a diminished or nonexistent oxidative burst. In this scenario entry would be mediated by direct binding of bacteria to surface receptors on these phagocytes and induced endocytosis, an important mechanism by which other intracellular pathogens such as *Legionella pneumophila*[33] and *Mycobacterium tuberculosis*[34] avoid intracellular killing.

Nevertheless, regardless of the mechanism by which they enter host macrophages, the environmental conditions within the phagosomal compartment are likely to be adverse. Thus the intracellular microbial parasites must either be able to prevent or alter the normal processes of endosomal acidification and maturation or withstand this harsh environment. Cellular components that help brucellae appropriately adapt to the harsh conditions in the macrophage phagosomal compartment are likely to make substantial contributions to the pathogenicity and chronicity of the infection. A number of genes encoding proteins predicted to assist *Brucella* spp. in this task have been identified and are described here (summarized in Table I). In many instances genetic approaches have been used to evaluate their contributions to the ability of brucellae to resist killing by host macrophages *in vitro* and to produce chronic infections and / or patent disease in natural or experimental hosts. Such studies not only provide us with important information concerning the roles played by various gene products in the pathogenesis of *Brucella* infections but they also provide insight into the environmental conditions encountered by the brucellae within the host macrophages. This is particularly relevant for *Brucella* spp., as presently a comprehensive understanding of the nature of the phagosomal compartment in which these successful intra

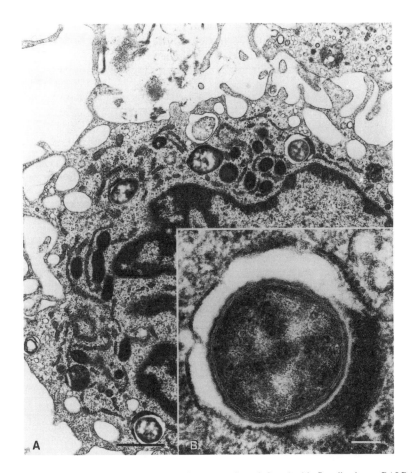

FIGURE 1. Electron micrograph of a murine macrophage infected with *Brucella abortus*. BALB/c mice were inoculated intraperitoneally with *B. abortus* 2308 and peritoneal cells harvested 3 h postinfection. Intracellular breucellae are contained within phagosomes and are surrounded by an electron-dense material. (Courtesy of Allen Jensen, National Animal Disease Center, Ames, IA)

cellular pathogens maintain their long-term residence is lacking (and thus is not discussed further here).

4.1. Defenses against Reactive Oxygen Intermediate (ROI)-Mediated Killing

Oxidative killing is a primary mechanism by which murine macrophages eliminate intracellular brucella.[14] Therefore, bacterial components that contribute to the resistance of these pathogens to ROI-mediated killing represent impor-

TABLE I
Genes of *Brucella* spp. Predicted to Contribute to Survival in Macrophages and Bacterial Virulence *in Vivo*

Gene	Identity of gene product	Function of gene product	Effect of deletion or disruption of the gene
katE	Catalase	Detoxify reactive oxygen intermediates (ROI)	(Not known)
sodC	CuZn superoxide dismutase	Detoxify ROI	Effect on growth *in vivo* ambivalent; no effect on growth in macrophages
unnamed	Mn superoxide dismutase	Detoxify ROI	(Not known)
htrA	Stress response protease of high temperature requirement A (HtrA) family	Degrades oxidatively damaged proteins	Increased sensitivity to ROI; increased sensitivity to macrophage killing; attenuated *in vivo*
htrA-like	Putative protease, HtrA-like	Unknown	Attenuated *in vivo;* no increased sensitivity to ROI
lon	Stress response protease Lon	Generalized degradation of damaged proteins and regulator of SOS response	Increased sensitivity to DNA damage; attenuated *in vivo;* no increase in ROI sensitivity
recA	Rec A (Recombinase A)	Homologous recombination, DNA repair	Attenuated *in vivo;* increased sensitivity to ROI
uvrA	UvrA (Ultraviolet repair A)	DNA repair	Attenuated *in vivo;* no increase in sensitivity to ROI
dnaKJ	Heat-shock protein DnaK and DnaJ	Molecular chaperone, protein folding	Needed for intracellular replication; increased sensitivity to acidic conditions
groELS	Heat-shock proteins GroEL and GroES	Molecular chaperone, protein folding	Essential in other prokaryotes
asp24	Acid-shock protein	Unknown	(Not known)
fur	Ferric uptake regulator	Transcriptional repressor of siderophore biosynthesis for iron acquisition and regulator of acid tolerance response genes	(Not known)

TABLE I
(Continued)

Gene	Identity of gene product	Function of gene product	Effect of deletion or disruption of the gene
ent	Dihydroxybenzoic acid biosynthesis operon (iron acquisition)	Siderophore bio-synthesis	(Not known)
bfn	Bacterioferritin	Iron storage protein	(Not known)
purE	5'-phosphorribosyl-*N*-carboxyaminoamida-zole isomerase	Purine biosynthesis	Attenuated *in vivo;* needed for intracellu-lar replication
unnamed	?	LPS *O*-side chain bio-synthesis	Attenuated *in vivo;* re-duced survival intra-cellularly; increased sensitivity to anti-microbial peptides

tant virulence determinants. Such components identified for intracellular bacteria include antioxidants that detoxify the reactive oxygen intermediates, stress response proteases[35] that degrade proteins that are denatured or otherwise damaged before they can accumulate to toxic levels,[36] and DNA repair enzymes.[37]

Two types of primary antioxidants have been identified and characterized in *Brucella. B. abortus* produces a single periplasmic catalase that appears to be a homolog of the RpoS-regulated *katE* gene product of *E. coli.*[38] Unlike the *katE* of *E. coli,* however, the *B. abortus katE* is inducible in response to exposure of H_2O_2 (J. Mayfield, personal communication). The inducible nature and high-level specific activity of the *Brucella* KatE suggest that this protein represents an important primary defense mechanism against ROI-mediated killing. Earlier studies suggest that there is a direct correlation between catalase activity and virulence in *Brucella* strains,[39] but a genetic evaluation of this relationship is clearly needed. *B. abortus* also produces both the Mn and CuZn forms of superoxide disumtase (SOD), and the combined specific activities of these enzymes is 10- to 100-fold higher than what has previously been reported for other intracellular pathogens.[40] Contrasting results have been obtained by investigators examining the virulence of *B. abortus* CuZn SOD deficient (*sodC*) mutants in BALB/c mice.[41,42] One of these groups reported that *sodC* mutants showed no significant difference from the parental strain with respect to their capacity to survive and replicate in the murine macrophage cell line J774 but showed a reduction in colony-forming units (CFUs) recovered from infected mice.[41] The other group found no difference *in vivo* with an *sodC* deletion mutant of *B. abortus* strain 2308.[42] It seems likely that the identification and characterization of the gene encoding the *Brucella* Mn SOD will be necessary before a definitive evaluation of the contributions of these primary antioxidants to the successful intracellular replication of brucellae can be performed.

Bacterial stress response proteases of the high-temperature requirement A (HtrA) family are able to degrade oxidatively damaged proteins before they accumulate to toxic levels within cells.[35] Genetic studies in *Salmonella typhimurium* and *Yersinia enterocolitica* have confirmed the participation of the HtrA proteases in cellular defense against oxidative damage and further suggest that these proteases contribute to the survival and replication of these facultative intracellular pathogens in host macrophages[43,44] and to their virulence in mice.[44,45] The *Brucella htrA* has been cloned,[46–50] and *B. abortus* and *B. melitensis htrA* mutants show increased sensitivity to oxidative killing *in vitro*, a reduced capacity to resist killing by murine neutrophils and macrophages, and significant attenuation in the mouse model in the early stages of infection. These mutants are also cleared more rapidly and fail to induce abortion in their natural hosts, cattle[51] and goats,[52] respectively, and *B. abortus htrA* mutants are more susceptible to killing by bovine macrophages in culture than the parental strain.[51] These results indicate that the *Brucella* HtrA plays a critical role in the resistance to ROI-mediated killing by host macrophages.

Another gene encoding a putative protease showing considerable amino acid identity with the *Brucella* HtrA has recently been cloned and given the designation *htrA*-like.[53] The initial description of *B. abortus htrA*-like mutants indicated that these strains showed a spleen colonization profile in BALB/c mice similar to that reported for *B. abortus htrA* mutants, that is, significant attenuation limited to the early stages of infection. These results suggested that the HtrA and HtrA-like proteases might perform similar biological functions, for example, the degradation of oxidatively damaged proteins. Recently completed experiments indicate that this is probably not the case, however, as *B. abortus htrA*-like mutants do not demonstrate increased susceptibility to ROI *in vitro*, and introduction of an *htrA*-like mutation into the *B. abortus htrA* mutant PHE1 did not increase the sensitivity of this strain to oxidative killing *in vitro* nor enhance its attenuation in BALB/c mice.[54] The biological function of the *B. abortus* HtrA-like protease is unknown at present, but this protein does not appear to be involved in resistance to oxidative killing.

DNA repair mechanisms represent an important secondary line of defense against oxidative damage, and studies with *S. typhimurium recA* mutants suggest that functional DNA repair pathways are critical for resisting ROI-mediated killing in host macrophages. In fact, *S. typhimurium recA* mutants[55] appear to be more susceptible to killing by murine macrophages in culture than catalase-deficient *S. typhimurium katE katG* double mutants.[55] Two major DNA repair proteins have been identified in *Brucella*, RecA and UvrA. *B. abortus recA* mutants showed increased sensitivity to oxidative killing *in vitro*[56] and attenuation in BALB/c mice.[56,57] *B. abortus uvrA* mutants, on the other hand, are also attenuated in mice, but do not show increased ROI sensitivity *in vitro*.[58] The capacity of *B. abortus recA* and *uvrA* mutants to resist intracellular killing by murine macrophages is under investigation at present.

4.2. Resistance to Killing by Low pH

Acidification of the phagosome is an important component in the destruction of microbes by phagocytes. Indeed, the capacity to interfere with this process has been proposed to be important in the pathogenesis of several bacterial pathogens that persist for prolonged periods within host macrophages, including *Mycobacterium tuberculosis*[59] and *Legionella pneumophila*.[60] Other organisms adapt to this stressful environment, including *B. abortus*, which undergoes a global regulation of gene expression reminiscent of the acid tolerance response described in *S. typhimurium* and *E. coli*.[61] It seems likely that this physiological adaptation to low pH plays an important role in facilitating prolonged survival of the brucellae in host macrophages. In this regard one of the prominent phenotypic characteristics of *B. suis dnaK* mutants (see below) is their increased susceptibility to acidic conditions *in vitro*,[62] suggesting that inappropriate adaptation to the low pH encountered in the phagosome may account for the inability of these mutants to survive and replicate in cultured macrophages. Two other genes that have been cloned and likely contribute to the ability of *Brucella* to mount an effective acid tolerance responses are *fur*,[63] which is discussed below with regard to its role in preventing nutrient deprivation, and a newly identified locus designated *asp*.[64]

4.3. Resistance to Nutrient Deprivation

Iron restriction appears to be a key mechanism by which activated macrophages control the intracellular replication of facultative intracellular pathogens.[65,66] Because the brucellae survive and may even replicate within interferon-γ (IFN-γ)-activated macrophages,[67] it is likely that iron acquisition systems play an important role in allowing these intracellular pathogens to survive the prolonged periods of iron starvation that may be encountered within the phagosomal compartment of activated macrophages.[68] Similarly, iron storage proteins such as bacterioferritin also may play a role. *B. abortus* has been reported to produce a single siderophore, 2,3-dihydroxybenzoic acid (DHBA), under conditions of iron limitation,[69] and experimental evidence suggests that DHBA promotes intracellular survival and replication of this organism in host macrophages.[70] The addition of exogenous DHBA to *B. abortus*-infected murine macrophages resulted in increased numbers (or, alternatively, enhanced survival) of intracellular brucellae when evaluated at both 12 and 48 h after infection. This included recovery from macrophages activated with IFN-γ and supplemented with Fe^{3+}. This latter finding is particularly interesting, as Fe^{3+} supplementation has been shown to increase the brucellacidal activity of IFN-γ-activated murine macrophages in culture through production of hydroxyl radicals.[71] The genetic locus responsible for DHBA biosynthesis in *B. abortus* (*ent*) has been cloned,[72] as well as the bacterioferritin gene (*bfn*) from *B. melitensis*.[73] The *ent* and *bfn* mutants constructed from virulent *Brucella* strains will be useful for evaluating the contribution of iron acquisition and storage pathways to the pathogenesis of *Brucella* spp. in animal models and in cultured macrophages.

In addition to iron, there is also considerable evidence that intracellular pathogens that are restricted to the phagosome are starved of a variety of other nutrients. Purine and aromatic amino acid auxotrophs of *S. typhimurium*, for example, *purA* and *aroA* mutants, show a dramatic defect in their capacity to replicate in cultured macrophages.[74] An operon involved in purine biosynthesis (*purEK*) has recently been characterized in *B. melitensis*.[75] A *purE* deletion mutant constructed from *B. melitensis* 16M was unable to replicate in cultured human monocyte-derived macrophages and showed significant and stable attenuation in the BALB/c mouse model.[75,76] These results support the contention that the brucellae, like salmonellae, remain enclosed within the phagosome of host macrophages.

4.4. Resistance to Antimicrobial Peptides

A direct correlation between the presence of intact *O*-chain and virulence in a variety of experimental and natural hosts has been established for *B. abortus*. Studies employing spontaneously arising LPS *O*-chain-deficient rough variants of *B. abortus* have also shown that these strains do not resist killing by cultured macrophages as well as their smooth counterparts.[13] Genes involved in the biosynthesis of smooth LPS by *B. abortus* have recently been identified by Tn5 mutagenesis.[77] *O*-chain-deficient mutants constructed in this fashion are attenuated in BALB/c mice and show reduced intracellular survival in the J774 murine macrophage cell line and in bovine monocytes cultured *in vitro* (T. A. Ficht, personal communication). These mutants show an increased sensitivity to killing by defensins *in vitro*, suggesting that the *O*-chain of the smooth *Brucella* spp. protects these organisms from the antimicrobial peptides of host macrophages.

4.5. Generalized Resistance to a Variety of Environmental Stresses

Stress response or "heat-shock" proteins assist bacterial cells in adapting to a variety of adverse environmental conditions, including exposure to oxidative stress and acidic conditions. In general these proteins fall into two classes. Molecular chaperones such as DnaK, DnaJ, GroEL, and GroES maintain the proper folding of cellular proteins, while proteases such as Lon and HtrA (also known as DegP) degrade proteins that become denatured or otherwise damaged before they accumulate to toxic levels.[78]

The *Brucella gro ESL*[79–81] and *dnaKJ*[82] operons have been cloned, and studies with *B. suis dnaK* mutants indicate that a functional DnaK proteins is required for wild-type intracellular replication in the human U937 macrophage cell line.[62] In addition to their defective stress response phenotype, the *B. suis dnaK* mutants are sensitive to acidic conditions (see earlier). There is experimental evidence that *groELS* expression is increased during intracellular growth.[61,83] Based on the importance of the corresponding gene products for both normal cell physiology as well as the bacterium's capacity to deal with environmental stresses, it seems quite likely that these proteins play a critical role in allowing brucellae to adapt to their intracellular environment. Moreover, the *groES* and *groEL* genes appear to be essential in all prokaryotes that have been examined.[84] However, direct evidence is unavailable at this point, specifically for brucellae.

Another stress response protein that apparently contributes to the adaptation of *Brucella* spp. to survival in the host is the Lon protease.[85] In *E. coli*, this particular protein not only makes a major contribution to the elimination of damaged or abnormal proteins from the cell, but it also helps regulate the SOS response, an important cellular DNA repair pathway.[86] *B. abortus lon* mutants show increased susceptibility to DNA damaging agents *in vitro*, as well as significant attenuation during the early stages of infection in BALB/c mice.[85] These mutants do not, however, show increased sensitivity to ROI-mediated killing *in vitro*. The physiological basis for their attenuation in the mouse model is presently under investigation, as is their interaction with murine macrophages.

As described previously, iron represents a vital micronutrient but accumulation of excess iron can be toxic to bacterial cells.[87] For example, it is well established that the accumulation of excess intracellular iron can lead to ROI-mediated damage. This is particularly relevant for *B. abortus* based on the fact that oxidative killing is thought to be a primary mechanism by which host macrophages kill intracellular brucellae,[14] and the recent observation that excess intracellular iron apparently enhances the ROI-mediated killing of brucellae by these host phagocytes.[71] The expression of bacterial genes encoding the components of iron acquisition pathways are usually tightly regulated in response to environmental iron levels, with siderophores being maximally produced only under conditions of iron limitation.[83] In many bacteria, a highly conserved transcriptional repressor known as Fur (*f*erric *u*ptake *r*egulator) becomes active when it binds intracellular Fe^{2+} and, in doing so, represses genes encoding both siderophore biosynthesis and iron transport functions.[88] Interestingly, Fur also regulates the expression of other genes in *E. coli* and *Salmonella typhimurium* which are apparently unrelated to iron acquisition, including those encoding the Mn superoxide dismutase (*sodA*)[89] and those involved in the acid tolerance response. These results suggest that Fur is an important global regulatory protein that likely plays a critical role in facilitating the physiological adaptation of bacteria to a variety of ever-changing environmental conditions. The *B. abortus fur* has been cloned,[63] and studies employing *B. abortus fur* mutants will provide us with important information regarding the mechanisms by which these organisms adapt to a variety of adverse conditions encountered in the host phagosome including iron deprivation and exposure to ROI and acidic pH.

5. IMMUNE RESPONSES CONTROLLING INFECTION

As discussed previously, the susceptibility of strains of *Brucella* to killing by macrophages often correlates with virulence of the strains *in vivo*. However, factors in addition to the intrinsic capacity of macrophages to inhibit intracellular growth of *B. abortus* also contribute to resistance. This is demonstrated by the observation that some *Brucella*-resistant cattle actually have macrophages that are permissive for *B. abortus* growth rather than resistant.[23] Also there is no apparent difference in the abilities of macrophages from resistant (C57BL/10) and susceptible (BALB/c) mice to kill or control replication of the virulent *B. abortus* strain 2308 (unpublished data). Differences in acquired cellular immune responses to *Brucella* spp. and production of inflammatory cytokines that promote development of protective acquired responses among hosts are likely to contribute to the differences among individuals to control the infection. With regard to this, T cells and a number of cytokines involved in cellular immune responses have been shown to enhance control of brucellosis and are discussed here. Although antibodies also play a significant role in protection during the initial period of the infection by acting as opsonins, cellular immunity is more important once the infection is intracellular[24] and is the focus of the discussion here.

5.1. Role of IFN-γ

There is much evidence indicating that IFN-γ,[90–92] a cytokine produced by T cells and natural killer (NK) cells, is an important factor in the control of brucellosis. For instance, neutralization of endogenous IFN-γ *in vivo* results in a decreased ability of mice to control infection with the attenuated *B. abortus* strain 19 or the virulent strain 2308 during the first week of infection.[90,91] Furthermore, Stevens *et al.* showed that supplementing BALB/c mice with recombinant IFN-γ results in enhanced control of infection with *B. abortus* strain 2308 at 1 week postinfection.[92] *In vitro* studies have shown that IFN-γ functions by increasing the antibrucellae activities of macrophages.[67,90,93,94] Whereas production of IFN-γ by NK cells has been shown to be principally responsible for early control of other intracellular bacteria such as listeriae, NK cells apparently do not play a role in protection against *B. abortus* during the initial infection phase,[95] a time when

IFN-γ is crucial.[90-92] Thus, the IFN-γ important for the early control of brucellosis is likely to be a product of T cells.

Both CD4 and CD8 T cells have been shown to contribute to immunity by adoptive transfer studies as well as by *in vivo* depletion studies in mice.[96-99] CD4 T cells from *B. abortus*-infected mice have been shown to produce IFN-γ at 1 week postinfection in response to stimulation with *Brucella* antigens.[100] These data support the suggestion that they are the primary source of IFN-γ. IFN-γ has also been shown to be a product of CD8 T cells from infected C57BL/10 mice.[99] In several experimental systems CD8 T cells have been shown to be more potent mediators of protective immunity to murine brucellosis than CD4 T cells.[96,97,99] Nevertheless, CD8 T cells generally produce less IFN-γ than CD4 T cells,[101] and thus their principle role in protection may be cytolysis of *Brucella*-infected macrophages as it is with *Listeria monocytogenes*.[102,103] As *in vitro* studies have shown that macrophages have to be activated with IFN-γ before or coincident with infection to have an anti-*Brucella* effect,[67] lysis of *Brucella*-infected macrophages to expose *Brucella* to extracellular mechanisms of immunity and to IFN-γ-activated macrophages is likely to be an important component of immunity to brucellosis (at least to mediate clearance if not to control the initial infection level). The role of cytotoxic cells in control of *B. abortus* are alluded to by studies of Splitter and coworkers[99] since they showed that class I major histocompatibility complex (MHC)-restricted CD8 T cells were important in control of brucellosis in mice and that CD8 T cells from infected mice are cytolytic for *Brucella*-infected macrophages *in vitro*.

5.2. Th1 vs. Th2 Responses

Following infection with a virulent strain of *B. abortus* there is apparently a simultaneous production of Th1 and Th2 cytokines in susceptible BALB/c mice. This is based upon the observation that when splenocytes from BALB/c mice infected with *B. abortus* 2308 are stimulated *in vitro* with *Brucella* antigens, CD4 T cells produced both IFN-γ and IL-10.[100] Thus a concomitant production of IL-10 and IFN-γ is most likely occurring *in vivo* following infection. A similar conclusion was reached by investigators measuring cytokine mRNA and exploring the response of human and mouse cells to heat-killed *B. abortus* strain 19[104,105] and the response of CD1 mice to *B. abortus* strain 2308 infections.[106]

In contrast with the effects of IFN-γ described previously, IL-10 negatively affects the ability of the susceptible BALB/c mice to control infections with *B. abortus* strain 2308. This effect is revealed when mice are infected with a low dose of *B. abortus* (5 × 10³ CFUs) and occurs even in the presence of the known beneficial cytokine, IFN-γ.[90] The negative effect of interleukin-10 (IL-10) is exerted at two levels: the cytokine decreases production of IFN-γ by spleen cells stimulated with *B. abortus* and decreases the anti-*Brucella* response of macrophages stimulated with IFN-γ *in vitro*.

These results with *Brucella* contrast with the polarity of the cytokine response induced by the intracellular protozoan *Leishmania tropica*. In that model, resistant mice have Th1 CD4 T cells that produce IFN-γ and IL-2 in response to stimulation with antigen and these cytokines are responsible for "healing," while susceptible mice have Th2 CD4 T cells that produce IL-4 and IL-10 resulting in chronic disease or "nonhealing." Cytokine responses following infection of the resistant C57BL/10 mice with *B. abortus* are more in accordance with the Th1/Th2 paradigm. That is, while unfractionated populations of splenocytes from *Brucella*-infected C57BL/10 mice produced both IFN-γ and IL-10, the IL-10 was produced by cells other than CD4 T cells, indicating that there was not a concurrent CD4 Th2 response. Moreover, *in vivo* studies indicated that when IL-10 and IL-4 were neutralized there was not a statistically significant decrease in the number of *B. abortus* recovered from C57BL/10 mice.[100] Thus, Th2 cytokines seem to contribute to susceptibility to *Brucella* infections more prominently in the susceptible BALB/c mice.

However, even when Th2 cytokines are neutralized, BALB/c mice are less able than C57BL/10 mice to control infections. This may be due to the lower levels of IFN-γ produced in these mice. This contention was supported by experiments in mice infected with a high challenge dose of *B. abortus* (i.e., 5×10^6 CFUs). The *in vivo* injection of anti-IL-10 and anti-IL-4 mAb did not affect the outcome of infection of the BALB/c mice when infected with a high dose of *B. abortus*, suggesting that neither IL-10 nor IL-4 influenced control. Rather, resistance and susceptibility correlated with the amount of IFN-γ produced by splenocytes in response to antigenic stimulation with splenocytes and purified CD4 T-cell populations. Those cells from BALB/c mice produced less IFN-γ and the development of IFN-γ-producing cells was delayed compared to C57BL/10 splenocytes.[100] Thus we hypothesize that under conditions of high levels of IFN-γ production, such as occurs in mice infected with a high dose of brucellae, the effects of Th2 cytokines are less evident and the level of IFN-γ produced has a more profound effect on determining resistance and susceptibility. A similar situation occurs in mice infected with *L. donovani* in that Th2 cytokines, although present, do not influence resistance but rather resistance is determined by the strength of the Th1 response.[107]

5.3. Role of IL-12

Recent studies have indicated that administration of antigens with the cytokine IL-12 results in a clonal expansion of IFN-γ-producing Th1 cells that is sufficient to protect against challenge with *Leishmania*.[108] Other studies have indicated an adjuvant role for recombinant IL-12. It promoted development of a protective immune response in mice infected with many other intracellular microbes, including *Listeria monocytogenes*, *Toxoplasma gondii*, *Mycobacterium tuberculosis*, *Plasmodium yoelii*, *Histoplasma capsulatum*,[109] and *M. avium*.[110] Conversely, treatment of mice with anti-IL-12 antibodies has been shown to exacerbate infections with intracellular pathogens known to rely on Th1 type responses for protection including mice infected with *B. abortus* strain 19.[111] The protective effect of IL-12 has been shown generally to be mediated by enhancing IFN-γ production by NK cells and T cells. It is known that both IL-12 and IFN-γ must act together on T cells to promote Th1 cell development.[112]

B. abortus has a potent ability to induce IL-12 production by mononuclear phagocytes through its interaction with the macrophage LPS-receptor, CD14.[113,114] Yet, *in vitro* analyses of CD4 T cells suggest that the production of IFN-γ is reduced after the first week of infection in *B. abortus*-infected BALB/c mice[100] and more recently we have shown by *in vivo* neutralization studies that IFN-γ does not contribute to control of infection when evaluated 3 weeks postinfection (unpublished data). The decrease in IFN-γ may result from a cessation of IL-12 production once the brucellae have been phagocytosed, and thus are no longer available to induce signal transduction through the LPS receptor. Alternatively, cytokines such as TNF-α or IL-1 that promote IL-12 production may be suboptimally expressed during later stages of the infection.

The importance of TNF-γ in controlling *Brucella* infections has been shown by Zhan and Cheers,[111] as when TNF-γ was neutralized during the first 2 weeks of infection there was about a 10-fold increase in the total number of brucellae in the spleens of mice. Moreover, the role of TNF-α was overlapping with that of IL-12 as simultaneous neutralization of both did not have a synergistic or additive effect on control of the number of brucellae in the spleen. *B. abortus*, *B. suis* and *B. canis* reportedly produce an extracellular protein that has been shown to inhibit TNF-α by the human U937 macrophage cell line.[115] Such a protein could affect production of TNF-α, and thereby IL-12, once the infection is established. Similarly, Cheers *et al.* showed that addition of recombinant IL-1 increased clearance of *B. abortus* strain 19 from mice[116] (perhaps through promoting IL-12 production) yet infection of bovine macrophages with *B. abortus* in combination with IFN-γ activation results in decreased expression of IL-1 and thus an inability of antigen presenting cells to signal antigen-specific T cell responses[117]. Although lack of optimal TNF-α and IL-1 levels could affect IL-12 and thereby IFN-γ levels, more direct effects are also possible. For instance, TNF-α is necessary for full activation of macrophage brucellacidal activity in response to IFN-γ.[14] Thus the ability of *Brucella* infections to inhibit TNF-α production may ultimately result in ineffective macrophage activation even when IFN-γ is present.

Other cytokines have an inhibitory effect on IL-12 production. Granulocyte/macrophage-colony-stimulating factor (GM-CSF) has been shown to turn off IL-12 production and IL-10 inhibits IL-12 activity. It is known that in brucellosis a large influx of macrophages accounts for the splenomegaly that accompanies infection and that these macrophages do not contribute to control of the infection.[97] Using mice specifically depleted of splenic macrophages, inoculation of *Brucella* organisms and extracts of it have been shown to result in rapid repopulation of liver and spleen by macrophages, suggesting that brucellae stimulate high concentrations of colony-stimulating factors.[118] More specifically, large amounts of GM-CSF have been shown to be produced by spleen cells from infected mice when stimulated *in vitro*.[119] We speculate that the GM-CSF may be responsible for turning off IL-12 production. With regard to Th2 cytokines, a recent study by Scott *et al.*[120] has shown that the impaired ability of BALB/c mice to control infections with *L. major* was not due to a lack of IL-12 production but to the simultaneous production of IL-4 and IL-10 that inhibited the function of IL-12. We have already discussed the negative impact that these cytokines have on control of brucellosis at 1 week postinfection although we have not shown a direct effect on IL-12 production.

The decreased proportion of T cells that occurs in *Brucella*-infected mice at 3 weeks postinfection[121] may also mean that even if IL-12 is produced there are too few T cells to produce adequate levels of IFN-γ in response to it. The decrease in T cells accompanying brucellosis may be caused by programmed cell death of CD4 T cells due to inappropriate TcR signaling or inappropriate cytokine signaling. Moreover, although TNF-α is needed for optimal production of IL-12, it may also contribute to subsequent death of T cells. Conversely, IL-12 has been shown to prevent apoptosis of CD4 T cells.[122] We hypothesize that sustaining a higher level of IL-12 might also sustain the T-cell population and thus IFN-γ production. However, lack of CD4 T cells is not the only explanation for decreased IFN-γ production because even when purified CD4 T cells from *Brucella*-infected BALB/c mice were evaluated on a per cell basis there was less IFN-γ produced by them during the first several weeks of infection than occurred when clearance began. Increased production of IFN-γ by CD4 T cells[100] correlated with the ability to adoptively transfer resistance after 8 weeks postinfection.[24] This does not seem to be due to a skewing toward the Th1 axis, as the CD4 T cells also produced more IL-10 in response to *Brucella* antigens at this time.

Thus using the mouse model it has become clear that IL-12, IFN-γ, IL-1, and TNF-α are necessary for effective control of brucellosis whereas IL-10 may be detrimental to control. However, the event that alters the status quo and thus triggers clearance around 6 to 8 weeks after infection in mice is still unknown. There is evidence that it may be caused by a change in cytokine production, but not by cytolytic CD8 T cell activity (E. Murphy, J. Satniyaseelan, and C. L. Baldwin, unpublished data).

6. FUTURE VACCINES: ANTIGENS AND INDUCTION OF CELLULAR IMMUNE RESPONSES

Although it is clear that antibodies are largely generated to the LPS in the outer membrane of smooth strains of *Brucella* and to other outer membrane components such as the porins in rough strains,[123] to design vaccines against brucellosis it is necessary to precisely define the *Brucella* antigens that can most effectively stimulate protective T-cell responses. Using nitrocellulose blotting of *Brucella* extracts and recombinant antigens produced from cloned *Brucella* genes, the proliferative responses of T cells obtained from *Brucella* vaccinated or infected cattle or mice have been evaluated. Results of cellular immunoblotting suggest that 38 proteins induce lymphocytes from vaccinated cattle to proliferate, with a protein of 12 kDa inducing the strongest response. In other studies using recombinant proteins, lymph node cells from *B. abortus* strain 19-vaccinated cattle proliferated to the recombinant SOD protein.[124] Proteins coded for by the *uvrA*, *groES*, and *groEL* genes stimulated T cells from *Brucella*-vaccinated mice to produce Th1-type cytokines *in vitro* including IFN-γ and also induced DTH responses in guinea pigs.[125]

Killed vaccines circumvent many hazards associated with live vaccines and also allow incorporation of antigens that might necessarily be deleted from live vaccines to achieve attenuation. It has been suspected for many years that the inability of killed vaccines to evoke protection against intracellular pathogens was due to the lack of processing and presentation of antigens by the endogenous pathway, thereby resulting in an inability to engage CD8 T cells. (A vaccine against *Brucella* spp. may need to be able to activate CD8 T cells to produce IFN-γ and lyse infected host cells, as virulent strains apparently have the capacity to rapidly hide in cells.) However, recent studies provide evidence that "killed antigen" is not necessarily excluded from the endogenous pathway if it is in a particulate form.[126] With regard to this, heat-killed *B. abortus* has been shown to act as a carrier for human immunodeficiency virus (HIV) proteins for induction of CD8 T-cell responses.[127]

The inefficiency of killed vaccines might be attributable at least in part to suboptimal stimulation of IL-12 due either to the rapid phagocytosis of whole killed brucellae or to the lack of appropriate IL-12 stimulatory molecules in subcellular vaccines. Killed bacteria also stimulate IL-10 production, which inhibits the bioactivity of any IL-12 produced.[128] In support of this, Smith *et al.* have shown that purified proteins from the outer wall of *B. abortus* are less efficient at inducing cellular immune responses in cattle, even when given in adjuvant, compared to more complex outer membrane subcellular preparations.[129] Cheers and coworkers also have shown that soluble *Brucella* proteins stimulate Th2 CD4 T cell responses in mice and that these T cells do not adoptively transfer resistance to naive mice.[130] Finally, *B. abortus* CuZn SOD does not stimulate T-cell responses when mice are immunized with the recombinant proteins[131] even in adjuvant whereas mice undergoing a *Brucella* infection have T cells responsive to SOD. These observations suggest that the antigenic complexity of the vaccine and the milieu of cytokines it evokes influence both the ability to respond to particular proteins and the type of immune response that ensues. Therefore determining the role of particular *Brucella* proteins in induction of protective immune responses will not be as simple as immunizing animals with the recombinant protein and challenging with field strains.

REFERENCES

1. Acha, P. N., and Szyfres, B., 1980, *Zoonoses and Communicable Diseases Common to Man and Animals*, Pan American Health Organization, Washington, D.C., pp. 28–45.
2. Young, E. J., 1983, Human brucellosis. *Rev. Infect. Dis.* **5:**821–842.
3. Nicoletti, P., 1980, The epidemiology of bovine brucellosis. *Adv. Vet. Sci. Comp. Med.* **24:**69–98.
4. Enright, F. M., 1990, The pathogenesis and pathobiology of *Brucella* infection in domestic animals, in: *Animal Brucellosis* (K. H. Nielsen and J. R. Duncan, eds.), CRC Press, Boca Raton, FL, pp. 301–320.
5. Baldwin, C. L., and Winter, A. J., 1994, Macrophages and *Brucella*, in: *Macrophage–Pathogen Interactions* (B. S., Zwilling and T. K. Eisenstein, eds.), Marcel Dekker, New York, pp. 363–380.
6. Nicoletti, P., 1989, Relationship between animal and human disease, in: *Brucellosis: Clinical and Laboratory Aspects* (J. Young and M. J. Corbel, eds.), CRC Press, Boca Raton, FL, pp. 41–51.
7. Spink, W. W., Hall, J. W., Finstad, J., and Malle, E., 1962, Immunization with viable *Brucella* organisms. Results of a safety test in humans. *Bull. WHO* **26:**409.
8. United States Department of Health and Human Services, 1988, *Biosafety in Microbiological and Biomedical Laboratories*, H.H.S. Publication No. (NIH) 88-8395, U.S. Government Printing Office, Washington, D. C.
9. Young, E. J., 1989, Clinical manifestations of human brucellosis, in: *Brucellosis: Clinical and Laboratory Aspects* (E. J. Young and M. J. Corbel, eds.), CRC Press, Boca Raton, FL, pp. 97–126.
10. Young, E. J., 1989, Treatment of brucellosis in humans, in: *Brucellosis: Clinical and Laboratory Aspects* (E. J. Young and M. J. Corbel, eds.), CRC Press, Boca Raton, FL, pp. 127–141.
11. Campbell, G. A., and Adams, L. G., 1992, The long-term culture of bovine-derived macrophages and their use in the study of intracellular proliferation of *Brucella abortus*. *Vet. Immunol. Immunopathol.* **34:**291–305.
12. Gallego, M. C., Cuello, F., and Garrido, A., 1989, *In vitro* determination of phagocytosis and intracellular killing of *Brucella melitensis* by goat polymorphonuclear phagocytes. *Comp. Immun. Microbiol. Infect. Dis.* **12:**9–15.
13. Kreutzer, D. L., Dreyfus, L. A., and Robertson, D. C., 1979, Interaction of polymorphonuclear leukocytes with smooth and rough strains of *Brucella abortus*. *Infect. Immun.* **23:**737–742.
14. Jiang, X., Leonard, B., Benson, R., and Baldwin, C. L., 1993, Macrophage control of *Brucella abortus:* Role of reactive oxygen intermediates and nitric oxide. *Cell. Immunol.* **151:**309–319.
15. Young, E. J., Borchert, M., Kreutzer, F. L., and Musher, D. M., 1985, Phagocytosis and killing of *Brucella* by human polymorphonuclear leukocytes. *J. Infect. Dis.* **151:**682–690.
16. Meador, V. P., and Deyoe, B. L., 1989, Intracellular localization of *Brucella abortus* in bovine placenta. *Vet. Pathol.* **26:**513–515.
17. Ackermann, M. R., Cheville, N. F., and Deyoe, B. L., 1988, Bovine ileal dome lymphoepithelial cells: Endocytosis and transport or *Brucella abortus* strain 19. *Vet. Pathol.* **25:**28–35.
18. Meador, V. P., Deyoe, B. L., and Cheville, N. F., 1989, Pathogenesis of *Brucella abortus* infection of the mammary gland and supramammary lymph node of the goat. *Vet. Pathol.* **26:**357–368.
19. Cheers, C., and Pagram, F., 1979, Macrophage activation during experimental murine brucellosis: A basis for chronic infection. *Infect. Immun.* **23:**197–205.
20. Schurig, G. G., Roop, R. M. II, Bagchi, T., Boyle, S., Buhrman, D., and Sriranganathan, N., 1991, Biological properties of RB51, a stable rough strain of *Brucella abortus*. *Vet. Microbiol.* **28:**171–188.
21. Roop, R. M. II, Jeffers, G., Bagchi, T., Walker, J., Enright, F. M., and Schurig, G. G., 1991, Experimental infection of goat fetuses *in utero* with a stable, rough mutant of *Brucella abortus*. *Res. Vet. Sci.* **51:**123–127.
22. Cheville, N. F., Jensen, A. E., Halling, S. M., Tatum, F. M., Morfitt, D. C., Hennager, S. G., Frerichs, W. M., and Schurig, G., 1992, Bacterial survival, lymph node changes, and immu-

nologic responses of cattle vaccinated with standard and mutant strains of *Brucella abortus. Am. J. Vet. Res.* **53:**1881–1888.

23. Price, R. E., Templeton, J. W., Smith, R. III, and Adams, L. G., 1990, Ability of mononuclear phagocytes from cattle naturally resistant or susceptible to brucellosis to control *in vivo* intracellular survival of *Brucella abortus. Infect. Immun.* **58:**879–886.

24. Araya, L. N., Elzer, P. H., Rowe, G. E., Enright, F. M., and Winter, A. J., 1989, Temporal development of protective cell-mediated and humoral immunity in BALB/c mice infected with *Brucella abortus. J. Immunol.* **143:**3330–3337.

25. Nicoletti, P. L., and Winter, A. J., 1990, The immune response to *Brucella abortus*—the cell-mediated response to infections, in: *Animal Brucellosis* (K. H. Nielsen and J. R. Duncan, eds.), CRC Press, Boca Raton, FL, pp. 83–96.

26. Canning, P. C., 1990, Phagocyte function in resistance to brucellosis, in: *Advances in Brucellosis Research* (L. G. Adams, ed.), Texas A & M University Press, College Station, TX, pp. 151–163.

27. Orduña, A., Orduña, C., Eiros, J. M., Bratos, M. A., Gutiérrez, P., Alonso, P., and Torres, A. R., 1991, Inhibition of degranulation and myeloperoxidase activity of human polymorphonuclear neutrophils by *Brucella melitensis. Microbiol. Semin.* **7:**113–119.

28. Riley, L. K., and Robertson, D. C., 1984, Brucellacidal activity of human and bovine polymorphonuclear leukocyte granule extracts against smooth and rough strains of *Brucella abortus. Infect. Immun.* **46:**231–236.

29. Frenchick, P. J., Markham, R. J., and Cochrane, A. H., 1985, Inhibition of phagosome–lysosome fusion in macrophages by soluble extracts of virulent *Brucella abortus. Am. J. Vet. Res.* **46:**332–335.

30. Elzer, P. H., Robertson, G. T., Phillips, R. W., and Roop, R. M. II, 1995, Evaluation of a *Brucella abortus* high-temperature-requirement A (*htrA*) deletion mutant in cultured murine macrophages. *Abstr. 95th Annu. Meet. Am. Soc. Microbiol.*, Abstr. B-336, p. 224.

31. Canning, P. C., Deyoe, B. L., and Roth, J. A., 1988, Opsonin-dependent stimulation of bovine neutrophil oxidative metabolism by *Brucella abortus. Am. J. Vet. Res.* **49:**160–163.

32. Harmon, B. G., Adams, L. G., and Frey, M., 1988, Survival of rough and smooth strains of *Brucella abortus* in bovine mammary gland macrophages. *Am. J. Vet. Res.* **49:**1092–1097.

33. Payne, N. R., and Horwitz, M. A., 1987, Phagocytosis of *Legionella pneumophila* is mediated by human monocyte complement receptors. *J. Exp. Med.* **166:**1377–1389.

34. Schlesinger, L. S., Bellinger-Kawahara, C. G., Payne, N. R., and Horwitz, M. A., 1990, Phagocytosis of *Mycobacterium tuberculosis* is mediated by human monocyte complement receptors and complement component C3. *J. Immunol.* **133:**2771–2780.

35. Davies, K. J. A., and Lin, S. W., 1988, Oxidatively damaged proteins are degraded by an ATP-independent proteolytic pathway in *Escherichia coli. Free Rad. Biol. Med.* **5:**225–236.

36. Gross, C., 1996, Function and regulation of the heat shock proteins, in: Escherichia coli *and* Salmonella: *Cellular and Molecular Biology*, 2nd Ed. (F. C. Neidhardt, ed.), American Society for Microbiology Press, Washington, D. C., pp. 1382–1399.

37. Farr, S. B., and Kogoma, T., 1991, Oxidative stress responses in *Escherichia coli* and *Salmonella typhimurium. Microbiol. Rev.* **55:**561–585.

38. Sha, Z., Stabel, T. J., and Mayfield, J. E., 1994, *Brucella abortus* catalase is a periplasmic protein lacking a standard signal sequence. *J. Bacteriol.* **176:**7375–7377.

39. Fitzgeorge, R. B., Keppie, J., and Smith, H., 1965, The relation between resistance to hydrogen peroxide and virulence in brucellae. *J. Pathol.* **89:**745–747.

40. Sriranganathan, N., Boyle, S. M., Schurig, G. G., and Misra, H., 1990, Superoxide dismutases of virulent and avirulent strains of *Brucella abortus. Vet. Microbiol.* **26:**359–366.

41. Tatum, F. M., Detilleux, P. G., Sacks, J. M., and Halling, S. M., 1992, Construction of Cu-Zn superoxide dismutase deletion mutants of *Brucella abortus:* Analysis of survival *in vitro* in epithelial and phagocytic cells and *in vivo* in mice. *Infect. Immun.* **60:**2863–2869.

42. Latimer, E., Simmers, J., Sriranganathan, N., Roop, R. M. II, Schurig, G. G., and Boyle, S. M., 1992, *Brucella abortus* deficient in copper / zinc superoxide dismutase is virulent in BALB / c mice. *Microb. Pathogen.* **12:**105–113.

43. Bäumler, A. J., Kusters, J. G., Stojiljkovic, I., and Heffron, F., 1994, *Salmonella typhimurium* loci involved in survival within macrophages. *Infect. Immun.* **62:**1623–1630.

44. Li, S.-R., Dorrell, N., Everest, P. H., Dougan, G., and Wren, B. W., 1996, Construction and characterization of a *Yersinia enterocolitica* O:8 high-temperature requirement (*htrA*) isogenic mutant. *Infect. Immun.* **64:**2088–2094.

45. Johnson, K., Charles, I., Dougan, G., Pickard, D., O'Gaora, P., Costa, G., Ali, T., Miller, I., and Hormaeche, C., 1991, The role of a stress-response protein in *Salmonella typhimurium* virulence. *Mol. Microbiol.* **5:**401–407.

46. Tatum, F., Cheville, N. F., and Morfitt, D., 1994, Cloning, characterization and construction of *htrA* and *htrA*-like mutants of *Brucella abortus* and their survival in BALB / c mice. *Microb. Pathog.* **17:**23–26.

47. Elzer, P. H., Phillips, R. W., Kovach, M. E., Peterson, K. M., and Roop, R. M. II, 1994, Characterization and genetic complementation of a *Brucella abortus* high-temperature-requirement A (*htrA*) deletion mutant. *Infect. Immun.* **62:**4135–4139.

48. Elzer, P. H., Phillips, R. W., Robertson, G. T., and Roop, R. M. II, 1996, The HtrA stress response protease contributes to resistance of *Brucella abortus* to killing by murine phagocytes. *Infect. Immun.* **64:**4838–4841.

49. Phillips, R. W., Elzer, P. H., and Roop, R. M. II, 1995, A *Brucella melitensis* high-temperature-requirement-A (*htrA*) deletion mutant demonstrates a stress response defective phenotype *in vitro* and transient attenuation in the BALB / c mouse model. *Microb. Pathogen.* **19:**277–284.

50. Robertson, G. T., Elzer, P. H., and Roop, R. M. II, 1996, *In vitro* and *in vivo* phenotypes resulting from the deletion of the high-temperature-requirement A (*htrA*) gene from the bovine vaccine strain *B. abortus* S19. *Vet. Microbiol.* **49:**197–207.

51. Edmonds, M. D., O'Reilly, K. L., Hagius, S. D., Walker, J. V., Enright, F. M., Roop, R. M. II, and Elzer, P. H., 1997, The evaluation of the decreased pathogenicity of a *Brucella abortus htrA* mutant in cattle. *Proc. 50th Annu. Meet. Anim. Dis. Res. Work. So. States*, Abstr. 3.

52. Phillips, R. W., Elzer, P. H., Robertson, G. T., Hagius, S. D., Walker, J. V., Fatemi, M. B., Enright, F. M., and Roop, R. M. II, 1997, A *Brucella melitensis* high-temperature-requirement A (*htrA*) deletion mutant is attenuated in goats and protects against abortion. *Res. Vet. Sci.* **63:**165–167.

53. Tatum, F. M., Cheville, N. F., and Morfitt, D., 1994, Cloning, characterization and construction of *htrA* and *htrA*-like mutants of *Brucella abortus* and their survival in BALB / c mice. *Microb. Pathogen.* **17:**23–26.

54. Phillips, R. W., and Roop, R. M. II, 1996, What's in a name? The HtrA and HtrA-like proteins of *Brucella abortus*. *Proc. 77th Annu. Conf. Res. Work. Anim. Dis.*, Abstr. 2, p. 6.

55. Buchmeier, N. A., Libby, S. J., Xu, Y., Loewen, P. C., Switala, J., Guiney, D. G., and Fang, F. C., 1995, DNA repair is more important than catalase for *Salmonella* virulence in mice. *J. Clin. Invest.* **5:**1047–1053.

56. Kovach, M. E., and Roop, R. M. II, 1996, First proteins and now DNA: The effect of DNA repair mutations on the reactive oxygen intermediate (ROI)-sensitive phenotype of a *Brucella abortus htrA* mutant. *Proc. 77th Annu. Conf. Res. Work. Anim. Dis.*, Abstr. 8, p. 7.

57. Tatum, F. M., Morfitt, D. C., and Halling, S. M., 1993, Construction of a *Brucella abortus* RecA mutant and its survival in mice. *Microb. Pathogen.* **14:**177–185.

58. Xhu, Y., Oliveira, S. C., and Splitter, G. A., 1993, Isolation of *Brucella abortus ssb* and *uvrA* genes from a genomic library by use of lymphocytes as probes. *Infect. Immun.* **61:**5339–5344.

59. Xu, S., Cooper, A., Sturgill-Koszycki, S., van Heyningen, T., Chatterfee, D., Orme, I., Allen, P., and Russell, D. G., 1994, Intracellular trafficking in *Mycobacterium tuberculosis* and *Mycobacterium avium*-infected macrophages. *J. Immunol.* **153:**2568–2578.

60. Horwitz, M. A., and Maxfield, F. R., 1984, *Legionella pneumophila* inhibits acidification of its phagosome in human monocytes. *J. Cell Biol.* **99:**1936–1943.

61. Lin, J., and Ficht, T. A., 1995, Protein synthesis in *Brucella abortus* induced during macrophage infection. *Infect. Immun.* **63:**1409–1414.

62. Köhler, S., Teyssier, J., Cloeckaert, A., Rouot, B., and Liautard, J.-P., 1996, Participation of the molecular chaperone DnaK in intracellular growth of *Brucella suis* within U937-derived phagocytes. *Mol. Microbiol.* **20:**701–712.

63. Phillips, R. W., Seastone, D. J., Norton, D. D., Farris, M. A., Kovach, M. E., Elzer, P. H., Baldwin, C. L., and Roop, R. M. II, 1996, Molecular cloning of the *Brucella abortus* iron uptake regulation (*fur*) gene. *Abstr. 96th Annu. Meet. Am. Soc. Microbiol.*, Abstr. D-24, p. 245.

64. Song, G., and Ficht, T. A., 1996, A putative calcium-binding protein is expressed by *Brucella abortus* in response to acid shock and phagocytosis. *Abstr. 96th Annu. Meet. Am. Soc. Microbiol.*, Abstr. B-136, p. 178.

65. Fortier, A. H., Green, S. J., Polsinelli, T., Jones, T. R., Crawford, R. M., Leiby, D. A., Elkins, K. L., Meltzer, M. S., and Nacy, C. A., 1994, Life and death of an intracellular pathogen: *Francisella tularensis* and the macrophage, in: *Macrophage–pathogen interactions* (B. S. Zwilling and T. K. Eisenstein, eds.), Marcel Dekker, New York, pp. 349–361.

66. Byrd, T. F., and Horwitz, M. A., 1989, Interferon gamma-activated human monocytes downregulate transferrin receptors and inhibit the intracellular multiplication of *Legionella pneumophila* by limiting the availability of iron. *J. Clin. Invest.* **83:**1457–1465.

67. Jiang, X., and Baldwin, C. L., 1993, Effects of cytokines on the intracellular growth of *Brucella abortus*. *Infect. Immun.* **61:**124–134.

68. Morrison, N. E., 1995, *Mycobacterium leprae* iron nutrition: Bacterioferritin, mycobactin, exochelin and intracellular growth. *Int. J. Leprosy* **63:**86–91.

69. Lopez-Goni, I., Moriyon, I., and Neilands, J. B., 1992, Identification of 2,3-dihydroxybenzoic acid as a *Brucella abortus* siderophore. *Infect. Immun.* **60:**4496–4503.

70. Leonard, B. A., Benson, R., Lopez-Goni, I., and Baldwin, C. L., 1997, *Brucella abortus* siderophore, 2,3-dihydroxybenzoic acid (DHBA) protects brucellae from killing by macrophages. *Vet. Res.* **28:**87–92.

71. Jiang, X., and Baldwin, C. L., 1993, Iron augments macrophage-mediated killing of *Brucella abortus* alone and in conjunction with interferon-γ. *Cell. Immun.* **148:**397–407.

72. Bellaire, B. H., Schuetze, P. L., Roop, R. M. II, Baldwin, C. L., and Elzer, P. H., 1996, Identification and characterization of a siderophore biosynthesis gene from *Brucella abortus*. *Proc. 77th Annu. Conf. Res. Work. Anim. Dis.*, Abstr. 3, p. 6.

73. Denoel, P. A., Zygmunt, M. S., Weynants, V., Tibor, A., Lichtfouse, B., Briffeuil, P., Limet, J. N., and Letesson, J.-J., 1995, Cloning and sequencing of the bacterioferritin gene of *Brucella melitensis* 16M strain. *FEBS Lett.* **361:**238–242.

74. Fields, P. I., Swanson, R. V., Haidaris, C. G., and Heffron, F., 1986, Mutants of *Salmonella typhimurium* that cannot survive within the macrophage are avirulent. *Proc. Natl. Acad. Sci. USA* **83:**5189–5193.

75. Drazek, E. S., Houng, H. S., Crawford, R. M., Hadfield, T. L., Hoover, D. L., and Warren, R. L., 1995, Deletion of *purE* attenuates *Brucella melitensis* 16M for growth in human monocytederived macrophages. *Infect. Immun.* **63:**3297–3301.

76. Crawford, R. M., van de Berg, L., Yuan, L., Hadfield, T. L., Warren, R. L., Drazek, E. S., Houng, H. H., Hammack, C., Sasala, K., Polsinelli, T., Thompson, J., and Hoover, D. L., 1996, Deletion of *purE* attenuates *Brucella melitensis* infection in mice. *Infect. Immun.* **64:**2188–2192.

77. Allen, C. A., Bearden, S. W., and Ficht, T. A., 1994, Complement and macrophage mediated killing of transposon derived rough mutants of *Brucella abortus*. *Abstr. 94th Annu. Meet. Am. Soc. Microbiol.*, Abstr. B-371, p. 95.

78. Gross, C., 1996, Function and regulation of the heat shock proteins, in: Escherichia coli *and* Salmonella: *Cellular and Molecular Biology*, 2nd Ed. (F. C. Neidhardt, ed.), American Society for Microbiology Press, Washington, D. C., pp. 1382–1399.

79. Lin, J., Adams, L. G., and Ficht, T. A., 1992, Characterization of the heat shock response in *Brucella abortus* and isolation of the genes encoding the GroE heat shock proteins. *Infect. Immun.* **60:**2425–2431.

80. Gor, D., and Mayfield, J. E., 1992, Cloning and nucleotide sequence of the *Brucella abortus groE* operon. *Biochim. Biophys. Acta* **1130:**120–122.

81. Roop, R. M. II, Price, M. L., Dunn, B. E., Boyle, S. M., Sriranganathan, N., and Schurig, G. G., 1992, Molecular cloning and nucleotide sequence analysis of the gene encoding the immunoreactive *Brucella abortus* Hsp60 protein, BA60K. *Microb. Pathogen.* **12:**47–62.

82. Cellier, M. F., Teyssier, J., Nicolas, M., Liautard, J. P., Marti, J., and Sri Widada, 1992, Cloning and characterization of the *Brucella ovis* heat shock protein DnaK functionally expressed in *Escherichia coli. J. Bacteriol.* **174:**8036–8042.

83. Rafie-Kolpin, M., Essenberg, R. C., and Wyckoff, J. H., III, 1996, Identification and comparison of macrophage-induced proteins and proteins induced under various stress conditions in *Brucella abortus. Infect. Immun.* **64:**5274–5283.

84. Fayet, O., Ziegelhoffer, T., and Georgopoulos, C., 1989, The *groES* and *groEL* heat shock genes of *Escherichia coli* are essential for bacterial growth at all temperatures. *J. Bacteriol.* **171:**1379–1385.

85. Robertson, G. T., Kovach, M. E., and Roop, R. M. II, 1996, Genetic evidence that the *Brucella abortus* Lon functions as a stress response protease. *Proc. 77th Annu. Conf. Res. Work. Anim. Dis.*, Abstr. 1, p. 6.

86. Gottesman, S., and Maurizi, M. R., 1992, Regulation by proteolysis: Energy-dependent proteases and their targets. *Microbiol. Rev.* **56:**59–6212.

87. Touati, D., Jacques, M., Tardat, B., Bouchard, L., and Despied, S., 1995, Lethal oxidative damage and mutagenesis are generated by iron in D*fur* mutants of *Escherichia coli:* Protective role of superoxide dismutase. *J. Bacteriol.* **177:**2305–2314.

88. Earhardt, C. F., 1996, Uptake and metabolism of iron and molybdenum, in: Escherichia coli *and* Salmonella: *Cellular and Molecular Biology*, 2nd Ed. (F. C. Neidhardt, ed.), American Society for Microbiology, Press, Washington, D. C., pp. 1075–1090.

89. Neiderhoffer, E. C., Naranjo, C. M., Bradley, K. L., and Fee, J. A., 1990, Control of *Escherichia coli* superoxide dismutase (*sodA* and *sodB*) genes by the ferric uptake regulation (*fur*) locus. *J. Bacteriol.* **172:**1930–1938.

90. Fernandes, D. M., and Baldwin, C. L., 1995, IL-10 downregulates protective immunity to *Brucella abortus. Infect. Immun.* **63:**1130–1133.

91. Khan, Y., and Cheers, C., 1993, Endogenous gamma interferon mediates resistance to *Brucella abortus* infection. *Infect. Immun.* **61:**4899–4901.

92. Stevens, M. G., Pugh, G. W., Jr., and Tabatabai, L. B., 1992, Effects of gamma interferon and indomethacin in preventing *Brucella abortus* infections in mice. *Infect. Immun.* **60:**4407–4409.

93. Jones, S. M., and Winter, A. J., 1992, Survival of virulent and attenuated strains of *B. abortus* in normal and gamma-interferon-activated murine peritoneal macrophages. *Infect. Immun.* **60:**3011–3014.

94. Jiang, X., and Baldwin, C. L., 1993, Iron augments macrophage-mediated killing of *Brucella abortus* alone and in conjunction with IFN-γ. *Cell. Immunol.* **148:**397–407.

95. Fernandes, D. M., Benson, R., and Baldwin, C. L., 1995, Lack of a role for natural killer cells in early control of *Brucella abortus. Infect. Immun.* **63:**4029–4033.

96. Pavlov, H., Hogarth, M., McKenzie, I. F. C., and Cheers, C., 1992, *In vivo* and *in vitro* effects of monoclonal antibody to Ly antigens on immunity to infection. *Cell. Immunol.* **7:**127–138.

97. Mielke, M. E. A., 1991, T cell subsets in granulomatous inflammation and immunity to *L. monocytogenes* and *B. abortus*. *Behring Inst. Mitt.* **88:**99–111.

98. Araya, L. N., Elzer, P. H., Rowe, G. E., Enright, F. M., and Winter, A. J., 1989, Temporal development of protective cell-mediated and humoral immunity in BALB/c mice infected with *Brucella abortus*. *J. Immunol.* **143:**3330–3337.

99. Oliveira, S. C., and Splitter, G. A., 1995, CD8 type 1 CD44^hi CD45RB^lo T lymphocytes control intracellular *Brucella abortus* infection as demonstrated in major histocompatibility complex class I and class II deficient mice. *Eur. J. Immunol.* **25:**2551–2557.

100. Fernandes, D. M., Jiang, X., Jung, J. H., and Baldwin, C. L., 1996, Comparison of T cell cytokines in resistant and susceptible mice infected with virulent *Brucella abortus* strain 2308. *FEMS Immunol. Med. Microbiol.* **16:**193–203.

101. Coffman, R. L., Varkila, K., Scott, P., and Chatelain, R., 1991, Role of cytokines in the differentiation of CD4+ T-cell subset *in vivo*. *Immunol. Rev.* **123:**189–207.

102. Harty, J. T., and Bevan, M. J., 1995, Specific immunity to *Listeria monocytogenes* in the absence of IFN-γ. *Immunity* **3:**109–117.

103. Kagi, D., Ledermann, B., Burki, K., Hengartner, H., and Zinkernagel, R. M., 1994, CD8 T cell-mediated protection against an intracellular bacterium by perforin-dependent cytotoxicity. *Eur. J. Immunol.* **24:**3068–3072.

104. Svetic, A., Jian, Y. C., Finkleman, F. D., and Gause, W. C., 1993, *Brucella abortus* induces a novel cytokine gene expression pattern characterized by elevated IL-10 and IFN-γ in CD4+ T cells. *Int. Immunol.* **5:**877–883.

105. Zaitseva, M. B., Golding, H., Betts, M., Yamauchi, A., Bloom, E. T., Butler, L. E., Stevan, L., and Golding, B., 1995, Human peripheral blood CD4+ and CD8+ T cells express Th1-like cytokine mRNA and proteins following *in vitro* stimulation with heat-inactivated *Brucella abortus*. *Infect. Immun.* **63:**2720–2728.

106. Fernandez-Lago, L., Monte, M., and Chordi, A., 1996, Endogenous gamma interferon and interleukin-10 in *Brucella abortus* 2308 infection in mice. *FEMS Immunol. Med. Microbiol.* **15:**109–115.

107. Satoskar, A., Bleuthmann, H., and Alexander, J., 1995, Disruption of the murine IL-4 gene inhibits disease progression during *Leishmania mexicana* infection but does not increase control of *Leishmania donovani* infection. *Infect. Immun.* **63:**4894–4899.

108. Wang, Z. E., Zheng, S., Corry, D. B., and Dalton, D. K., 1994, Interferon gamma-independent effects of interleukin 12 administered during acute or established infection due to *Leishmania major*. *PNAS* **91:**12932–12936.

109. Wynn, T. A., Reynolds, A., James, S., Cheever, A. W., Caspar, P., Hieny, S., Jankovic, D., Strand, M., and Sher, A., 1996, IL-12 enhances vaccine-induced immunity to schistosomes by augmenting both humoral and cell-mediated immune responses against the parasite. *J. Immunol.* **157:**4068–4078.

110. Castro, A. G., Silva, R. A., and Appelberg, R., 1995, Endogenously produced IL-12 is required for the induction of protective T cells during *Mycobacterium avium* infections in mice. *J. Immunol.* **155:**2013–2019.

111. Zhan, Y., Liu, Z., and Cheers, C., 1996, Tumor necrosis factor alpha and interleukin-12 contribute to resistance to the intracellular bacterium *Brucella abortus* by different mechanisms. *Infect. Immun.* **64:**2782–2786.

112. Wenner, C. A., Guler, M. L., Macaonia, S. E., O'Garra, A., and Murphy, K. M., 1996, Roles of IFN-gamma and IFN-α in IL-2-induced T helper cell-1 development. *J. Immunol.* **156:**1442–1447.

113. Zaitseva, M., Golding, H., Manischewitz, J., Webb, D., and Golding, B., 1996, *Brucella abortus* as a potential vaccine candidate: Induction of interleukin-12 secretion and enhanced B7.1 and B7.2 and intercellular adhesion molecule 1 surface expression in elutriated human monocytes stimulated by heat-inactivated *B. abortus*. *Infect. Immun.* **46:**3109–3117.

114. Baldwin, C. L., Benson, R. M., and Sathiyaseelan, J., 1996, Role of IL-12 in control of brucellosis. *Abstr. 49th Annu. Meet. Brucellosis Res. Workers,* Chicago, IL.
115. Caron, E., Gross, A., Liautard, J.-P., and Dornand, J., 1996, *Brucella* species release a specific, protease-sensitive, inhibitor of TNF-α expression, active on human macrophage-like cells. *J. Immunol.* **156:**2885–2893.
116. Zhan, Y. F., Stanley, E. R., and Cheers, C., 1991, Prophylaxis or treatment of experimental brucellosis with interleukin-1. *Infect. Immun.* **59:**1790–1794.
117. Splitter, G. A., and Everlith, K. A., 1989, *Brucella abortus* regulates bovine macrophages-T-cell interaction by major histocompatibility complex class II and interleukin-1 expression. *Infect. Immun.* **57:**1151–1157.
118. Buiting, A. M. J., de Rover, Z., and van Rooijen, N., 1995, *Brucella abortus* causes an accelerated repopulation of the spleen and liver of mice by macrophages after their liposome-mediated depletion. *J. Med. Microbiol.* **42:**133–140.
119. Zhan, Y., Kelso, A., and Cheers, C., 1993, Cytokine production in the murine response to brucella infection or immunization with antigenic extracts. *Immunology* **80:**458–464.
120. Scharton-Kersten, T., Afonso, L. C., Wysocka, M., Trinchieri, G., and Scott, P., 1995, IL-12 is required for natural killer cell activation and subsequent T helper 1 cell development in experimental leishmaniasis. *J. Immunol.* **154:**5320–5330.
121. Araya, L. N., and Winter, A. J., 1990, Comparative protection of mice against virulent and attenuated strains of *Brucella abortus* by passive transfer of immune T cells or serum. *Infect. Immun.* **58:**254–256.
122. Estaquier, J., Idziorek, T., Zou, W., Emilie, D., Farber, C. M., Bourez, J. M., and Ameisen, J. C., 1995, T helper type 1/T helper type 2 cytokines and T cell death: Preventive effect of interleukin 12 on activation-induced and CD95 (FAS/APO-1)-mediated apoptosis of CD4+ T cells from human immunodeficiency virus-infected persons. *J. Exp. Med.* **182:**1759–1767.
123. Winter, A. J., Rowe, G. E., Duncan, J. R., Eis, M. J., Widom, J., Ganem, B., and Morein, B., 1988, Effectiveness of natural and synthetic complexes of porin and O-polysaccharide as vaccines against *Brucella abortus* in mice. *Infect. Immun.* **56:**2808–2817.
124. Stevens, M. G., Tabatabai, L. B., Olsen, S. C., and Cheville, N. F., 1994, Immune responses to superoxide dismutase and synthetic peptides of superoxide dismutase in cattle vaccinated with *Brucella abortus* strain 19 or RB51. *Vet. Microbiol.* **41:**383–389.
125. Oliveira, S. C., Harms, J. S., Banai, M., and Splitter, G. A., 1996, Recombinant *Brucella abortus* proteins that induce proliferation and gamma-interferon secretion by CD4 T cells from *Brucella*-vaccinated mice and delayed-type hypersensitivity in sensitized guinea pigs. *Cell. Immunol.* **172:**262–268.
126. Shen, Z., Reznikoff, G., Dranoff, G., and Rock, K. L., 1997, Cloned dendritic cells can present exogenous antigens on both MHC class I and class II molecules. *J. Immunol.* **158:**2723–2730.
127. Laphan, C., Golding, B., Inman, J., Balckburn, R., Manischewitz, J., Highet, P., and Golding, H., 1996, *Brucella abortus* comjugated with a peptide derived from the V3 loop of human immunodeficiency virus (HIV) type 1 induces HIV-specific cytotoxic T-cell responses in normal and in CD4 cell-depleted BABL/c mice. *J. Virol.* **70:**3084–3092.
128. Murray, P. J., Wang, L., Onufryk, C., Tepper, R. I., and Young, R. A., 1997, T cell-derived IL-10 antagonizes macrophage function in mycobacterial infection. *J. Immunol.* **158:**315–321.
129. Smith, R. III, Adams, L. G., Ficht, T. A., Sowa, B. A., and Wu, A. M., 1990, Immunogenicity of subcellular fractions of *Brucella abortus:* Measurement by *in vitro* lymphocyte proliferative responses. *Vet. Immunol. Immunopathol.* **25:**83–97.

130. Zhan, Y., Kelso, A., and Cheers, C., 1995, Differential activation of *Brucella*-reactive CD4$^+$ T cells by *Brucella* infection or immunization with antigenic extracts. *Infect. Immun.* **63:**969–975.
131. Tabatabai, L. B., and Pugh, G. W., 1994, Modulation of immune responses in BABL/c mice vaccinated with *Brucella abortus* Cu-Zn superoxide dismutase synthetic peptide vaccine. *Vaccine* **12:**919–924.

16

Antibiotic Treatment of Infections with Intracellular Bacteria

HERBERT HOF

1. THE IMPLICATIONS OF INTRACELLULAR HABITAT OF MICROORGANISMS FOR ANTIBIOTIC EFFECTIVENESS

The choice of an antibiotic is dependent first on its direct antimicrobial activity. Generally, this property is detected *in vitro* by determination of the minimum inhibitory concentration (MIC) or eventually of the minimum bactericidal concentration (MBC) with standardized techniques. In *in vitro* situations the antibiotic has free access to a small number of bacteria, which find abundant nutrients and ideal growth conditions for rapid multiplication. Under such optimized growth conditions, they are particularly vulnerable to antibiotics. Furthermore, interaction between bacteria and antimicrobial agents takes place in a milieu providing fairly good conditions as to pH, ionic strength, O_2 pressure, etc., optimal prerequisites for the action of antibiotics. In addition, the concentration of antibiotics is held constant over quite a long period of up to 24 h.

Obviously the artificial and highly favorable situation during the elaboration of an antibiogram does not mimic the *in vivo* situation. During an infec-

HERBERT HOF • Institute of Medical Microbiology and Hygiene, Faculty of Clinical Medicine Mannheim, University of Heidelberg, Mannheim D-68165, Germany.

Opportunistic Intracellular Bacteria and Immunity, edited by Lois J. Paradise *et al.* Plenum Press, New York, 1999.

tious process in a host, a bacterial cell may undergo a refractory stage induced by the surrounding milieu, when, for example, the porins of the outer membrane of Gram-negative bacteria are closed by certain ion constellations and concentrations, or when a coat of host-derived proteins inhibits the access of antibiotics, or when adverse growth conditions within a host impede multiplication.

Hence, it is indeed astonishing that there is any correlation between MIC and therapeutic efficacy.[1]

Therapeutic success is also dependent on serum levels and half-time properties of the antibiotic, which determine the final antibiotic concentrations within an infected tissue. But distribution to the various regions of a body is highly variable, in part because diffusion to the site of infection depends on architectural peculiarities of the tissue. As two examples, the brain is concealed by a functional blood–brain barrier[2] and the prostate is also barely accessible to most agents. Thus the location of infectious foci and the ability of a drug to penetrate the proper site of infected tissues definitely influence the outcome of therapy. The permeability of both the vessel walls and the underlying tissue layers is definitely perturbed by inflammatory processes.

In abscesses, granulomas, or necrotic areas and other pathological alterations of normal tissue architecture, the access as well as the activity of antibiotics may be altered. In most instances this means reduced. In consequence, the concentration of efficacious drugs at the very site of microbial residence in many instances may be insufficient to kill or even to inhibit multiplication of bacteria, in spite of apparently rational choice with correct amounts applied.

A particular situation occurs in infections with intracellular microorganisms. Intracellular parasites have developed different strategies to survive and may reside in various compartments of a host cell (Table I), that is, in a membrane-bound vesicle, in the cytosol, or even within the nucleus, like *Listeria monocytogenes*.[3] In many instances this behavior is not a rigid and fixed property but may change during a life cycle. Although host cell membranes represent insuperable obstacles for many antibiotics, some drugs cross these barriers readily, either by passive diffusion or by active transport (Fig. 1). Indeed, in some instances intracellular concentrations of agents may reach even higher levels than exist in the extracellular fluid. This does not, however, necessarily mean that this is useful, as for example, when the antibiotic accumulates in a compartment that is not invaded by the pathogen or when the conditions there are unfavorable for optimal antibiotic activity, such as a low pH, which may inactivate certain compounds. Therefore, several particular prerequisites have to be fullfilled to achieve satisfactory therapeutic efficacy in infections with intracellular microorganisms (Table II) in spite of good direct antimicrobial activity predicted by *in vitro* susceptibility testing.

TABLE I
Compartments of Intracellular Residence

Subcellular setting	Pathogen
I. Membrane-bound vacuoles (a) Complete inhibition of fusion with lysosomes, neutral pH, etc.	*Toxoplasma, Mycobacteria, Chlamydia, Legionella*
(b) Partial inhibition of fusion of lysosomes and delayed acidification	*Salmonella*
(c) Fusion of lysosomes, but only weak acidification	*Mycobacteria*
(d) Fusion of lysosomes with phagosome, low pH	*Rickettsia, Francisella, Listeria, Leishmania*
II. Cytosol (a) Surrounded by host-derived proteins, for example, actin	*Listeria, Shigella*
(b) Naked in the cytosol	*Staphylococcus aureus* (small-colony variants)
III. Nucleus	*Listeria*

2. TRANSPORT OF ANTIBIOTICS ACROSS THE HOST CELL MEMBRANE

2.1. Import

The basic structure of the host cell membrane is a lipid bilayer that acts as a definite barrier for free, passive diffusion of most but not all antibiotics from the extracellular fluid to the intracellular space. Nitroimidazoles, for instance, are said to diffuse easily through membranes.[4] Lipid-soluble antibiotics, such as rifampicin,[5] chloramphenicol, trimethoprim, or brodimoprim,[6] also cross this membrane, of living as well as dead host cells. Most penicillin derivatives diffuse at least in their ionized species, reacting like weak organic acids. The absolute amounts of transported agents by this mechanism are, however, rather low.

Polar molecules, on the other hand, such as some other β-lactams, do not penetrate efficiently into host cells.

If it is impossible for passive diffusion to occur, several other pathways for engulfment of chemical compounds (Fig. 1) exist that can be used by antibiotics as well. For example, active uptake of some cephalosporins, such as ceftibuten, starts immediately, within minutes after exposure, and is mediated by a carrier originally designated for dipeptides,[7] that is, via a transport system that is usually

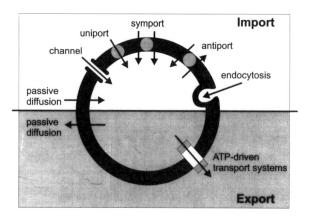

FIGURE 1. Schematic view of transport systems of chemical compounds across biomembranes. In principal import as well as export systems may exist. Most of these examples represent mechanisms, which are not reserved exclusively for antibiotics but are used also for other physiological compounds.

reserved for nutrients. These natural substrates, as well as some chemically related cephalosporins, are able to interfere and to compete with these transport capacities. This transport system is obviously rather discriminatory toward a few particular antimicrobials, as it is not suitable for other cephalosporins closely related to ceftibuten.[7]

Clindamycin uses exactly the same transport vehicles as nucleosides.[8] Nucleoside channels are equally used by macrolides, azalides, and ketolides to enter neutrophils. Obviously, this uptake mechanism is fairly fast, as the maximum level of intracellular macrolides is achieved within a few minutes.[4,9,10] On the other hand, azalides are continuously internalized over a period of several hours.[10] The efficiency of uptake is highly variable from one cell type to another, even within one cell type there may be substantial differences depending on the cell's state of activation. Uptake of macrolides by alveolar macrophages from smokers, for example, was substantially greater than from nonsmokers.[10] It is known that certain chemical agents, for example, pentoxifylline, are able to upregulate this host cell mechanism, which also functions in physiological processes such as phagocytosis.[8] The transport capacity is fairly dependent on Ca^{2+} in the external milieu. Inorganic Ca^{2+}-channel blockers, such as Ni^{2+} and La^{2+}, interfere with macrolide uptake by neutrophils.[11]

Aminoglycosides also are imported actively but via quite a different mechanism, namely fluid-phase pinocytosis. At the plasma membrane of host cells, tiny pits, which invaginate into the cell and pinch off to form intracellular vesicles, develop steadily. Thereby, substances dissolved in the extracellular fluid, including antibiotics, are internalized. The rate at which vesicles are internalized in this

TABLE II
Prerequisites for Good Therapeutic Activities of
Antimicrobials against Intracellular Pathogens

I. *A priori* susceptibility of the microorganism to the given agent
II. Penetration and hopefully high accumulation within the host cell
III. Distribution to the right compartment where the pathogen resides
IV. Favorable conditions to full activity of the antimicrobial agent (pH composition and concentration of ions)
V. Vulnerability of the microbe to a certain drug under the given physiological stage (quiescence, rapid multiplication)

process of pinocytosis varies from one cell type to the other, but is surprisingly high. The amount of drugs transported in this manner is, however, rather low. Nevertheless, if the exposure of host cells continues for several days—for example, during long-term treatment of patients with multiple doses per day—the absolute amount of intracellular aminoglycosides can be remarkable.[4]

In most animal cells yet another pathway provides an efficient manner for taking up macromolecules from the extracellular fluid, that is, receptor-mediated endocytosis.[12] The macromolecules attach to complementary cell-surface receptors, accumulate in clathrin-coated pits, and enter the cell as receptor–macromolecule complexes. Such a mechanism permits a selective concentration of even minor components of the extracellular fluid with high efficiency. The antimycotic drug amphotericin B is said to use the low-density lipoprotein (LDL) receptor of host cells to enter.[13] Intracellular drug delivery can be carefully directed to host cells by using an appropriate vehicle. For example, *p*-aminosalicyclic acid (PAS), an antimycobacterial agent, has been coupled to maleylated bovine serum albumin. This complex was taken up efficiently into macrophages through high-affinity binding sites for the carrier. Within the host cell, the pharmacologically active form of the antimicrobial is released by hydrolysis.[14] An antileishmanial drug, allopurinol riboside, targeted through glycosylated synthetic carriers to a mannose–fucose receptor on the membrane of macrophages was 50 times more effective against intracellular *Leishmania* than the free drug.[15]

Colloidal carriers such as liposomes and nanoparticles are internalized, at least in professional phagocytes, by the usual phagocytotic process. Thus, they may serve as vehicles carrying antibiotics directly to intracellular targets in neutrophils and macrophages.[16,17]

In conclusion, one should keep in mind that there is not one single pathway for all antibiotics to enter every cell. Even within a group of related drugs there may exist quite remarkable differences; the uptake rate is not a stable, regular event; rather it depends definitely on the type of host cells and their physiological state. During infection with an intracellular pathogen the mode and extent of uptake may be quite distinct from those in cells cultured *in vitro* under artificial conditions.

2.2. Export

Some agents that are able to diffuse from the outside of cells to the inside also move in the opposite direction so that the intracellular content remains low, when the extracellular concentration vanishes. This holds true for nitroimidazoles and for most β-lactams.[4]

A bidirectional traffic is maintained also by active carrier systems. Macrolides are eliminated from intracellular sites by an active, carrier-mediated export mechanism, which is almost as rapid and efficient as the import.[9] The export rate of antibiotics also depends, however, on the rate of dissociation from intracellular binding sites.[9] Whereas erythromycin, roxithromycin, and josamycin are only loosely attached to intracellular targets, azithromycin (as well as ketolides) are tightly bound so that excretion is prolonged for several hours.[18] This property contributes to the extended serum half-time of azithromycin, which is measured in days.

Aminoglycosides also are stored in long-lasting reservoirs from which they are continuously released. Once in a host, the internal compartments are loaded with aminoglycosides, which are released over a period of several days, leading to low but consistent levels in the blood plasma.[19]

Certain cells exclude some antibiotics efficiently. This property, called multidrug resistance (MDR), is genetically coded in all cells, but expressed only in certain tissue cells, for example, in the endothelial cells of the brain capillaries and some tumor cells. The gene product is a large membrane protein that belongs to the so-called ABC (ATP binding cassette) transporters, which consist of several extracellular, transmembrane, and intracellular domains. A highly conserved motif for the binding of ATP, a characteristic for this type of transporter, is located at the cytosolic loops.[20] This carrier system functions like a highly efficient vacuum cleaner, because an appropriate substrate is pumped out immediately after its penetration. At least some antibiotics, for example, the macrolides, are transported via this carrier system.[21] Specific blockers of the export pump can restore the import.

Besides MDR, there are still other export pumps acting in certain host cells. Among these the multidrug resistance-related (MRP) is engaged in the export of antibiotics, at least of some quinolones such as difloxacin.[22]

3. INTRACELLULAR ACCUMULATION

In general, quite a number of antibiotics are able to penetrate into animal cells, although to different degrees (Table III). Whereas some are present intra-

TABLE III
Antibiotic Uptake by Eukaryotic Host Cells and Intracellular
Distribution of Antibiotics

	Intracellular distribution in[b]:	
Drug(s)[a]	Cytoplasm	Lysosomes
Group I (ratio, >10)		
Macrolides (erythromycin, roxithromycin, azithromycin, spiramycin)	+	+
Ketolides	NA	NA
Clindamycin	+	+
Rifapentine	+	−
Coumermycin	NA	NA
Streptogramin (RP 59500)	NA	NA
Group II (ratio, 1–10)		
Quinolones (ofloxacin, ciprofloxacin, CI 934)	+	(+)
Rifampicin	+	+
Tetracycline	NA	NA
Chloramphenicol	NA	NA
Vancomycin	NA	NA
Teicoplanin	[c]	−
Fosfomycin	NA	NA
Group III (ratio, < 1)		
Penicillin	+	−
Ampicillin	+	−
Cephalosporins	+	−
Imipenem	+	−
Aminoglycosides (gentamicin, netilmicin, amikacin)	−	+

[a]Intracellular/extracellular ratio.
[b]+, Strong accumulation; (+), minor accumulation; −, no accumulation; NA, no data available.
[c]Sticks to the plasma membrane.

cellularly only in low concentrations, that is, lower than in the extracellular fluid, others have a cellular tropism and accumulate intracellularly. A few of them, for example, azithromycin, may even achieve extremely high concentrations, namely up to 200- to 300-fold the extracellular values, at least in certain host cells and under optimal conditions. The highest concentration of this drug was achieved in polymorphonuclear granulocytes; in monocytes the intracellular yield was six times lower; and in erythrocytes there was no accumulation at all.[18] But even within a single group of cells, heterogeneous levels of activity may be expressed, depending on various stimuli.

The actual intracellular content of a given antibiotic is the result of various processes of import and export that act synergistically in part and antagonistically in part. As stated earlier, the transport capacity of various import mechanisms is quite different for the different antibiotics. The duration of exposure is also important. This topic has been neglected in some publications. For example, the reports about the intracellular concentration of aminoglycosides disagree, because after a short run of only minutes or even few hours the results may still be negative. The intracellular storing sites for macrolides are already saturated after a few minutes.[9,10] Further exposure does not result in a further increase of intracellular contents. On the other hand, azalides, which are weak bases, are trapped in acidic lysosomes, where they are stored and detained. Efflux from the lysosomes into the cytosol can continue over many hours,[10] so that in the end the overall content in host cells may be considerable.

In vivo, the intracellular load is regulated by the pharmacodynamic and pharmacokinetic properties of a drug. Besides the dose, the tissue tropism of a drug and its varying serum levels, in addition to its ensuing tissue fluid concentrations, influence the intracellular yield.

In conclusion, it seems rather arbitrary to give an absolute number or even a relative intracellular concentration of an antibiotic, as is often done (Table III). This rating is, in reality, subjected to many variables.

4. INTRACELLULAR DISTRIBUTION

After penetration, the subcellular distribution of various antibiotics differs widely. An even spread of substances to all compartments is rare and most drugs are, rather, focused in certain organelles. This has an important impact on the therapy.

The intracellular fate of a compound largely depends on the mode of uptake. Materials engulfed either by fluid-phase or receptor-mediated endocytosis, as well as phagocytosed particles, often end up in lysosomes. Aminoglycosides, for example, are therefore located predominantly with these organelles.[4] In addition hydrophobicity, polarity, electrical charge, and other chemical and physiochemical properties of the agent control the allotment to a proper compartment within a host cell. Initially, macrolides are within the cytosol and are transported to some extent from there to lysosomes, so that they can be found and act in both the cytosol and the lysosomes. The relative partition may differ between the various derivatives. Azalides, such as azithromycin, accumulate within acidified vacuoles through an ion-trapping mechanism.[10] β-Lactams are exclusively present in the cytosol. Quinolones stay primarily and predominantly within the cytosol but may spread to other compartments. Teicoplanin, on the other hand, remains adherent to the membrane of the host cell after penetration.[23]

Until now, the exact intracellular location has been determined only for a few antimicrobials.[4,21] (Table III). Therefore, only a rough subdivision has been established; one has to keep in mind that even within the so-called cytosol there are quite dissimilar regions. The various stages of intracellular vesicles, that is, endosome, lysosome, and phagosome, have quite variable milieus. Thus, it remains difficult to predict the precise intracellular path for a definite antibiotic only by its structure.

The impact of uneven intracellular distribution of antibiotics is that, in certain instances at least, the antibiotic and the microorganism may reach quite different sites, so that a therapeutic failure is bound to happen in spite of good susceptibility test results *in vitro*. In consequence, a high intracellular concentration alone is not a guarantee of good therapeutic activity against intracellular pathogens.

5. INTRACELLULAR ACTIVITY

5.1. "Exogenous" Antibiotics

The conditions within the subcellular structures definitely influence the activities of internalized antibiotics. In the endocytic pathway, incoming materials encounter progressively decreasing pH as they move from the early endosome to the late endosome and finally to the lysosome. This is due to the action of ATP-driven proton pumps.[12] When they are entrapped within lysosomes, aminoglycosides adopt a new configuration, especially because of the low pH. In their protonic isoform they are completely inactive.[4]

Macrolides and quinolones also gradually lose their full activity at low, acidic pH. Thus, within acidified phagolysosomal vacuoles, most antibiotics are less active than under the artificial laboratory conditions used for the determination of MIC, although some drugs, for example, rifampicin, actually show enforced antimicrobial properties in acidic conditions.

The altered circumstances within the subcellular structures of a host cell during infection may be specific for the different professional intracellular microorganisms. Thus, the pH in a phagocytic vacuole may be quite low during infection with *Rickettsia,* or only moderately acidic during *Salmonella* infection or even neutral during infection with *Legionella* or others[23] (Table I).

Furthermore, it should be kept in mind that during the transport of one compound across membranes, other quite nonrelated agents may be carried either in the same direction (symport) or in the opposite direction (antiport) (Fig. 1). In particular H^+, Na^+, K^+, and Ca^{2+} or Cl^- and HCO_3^- are shifted concomitantly, thus changing the conditions of the microenvironment in which antimicrobial action must occur.[23]

Another possibility is the influence of conditions by unrelated drugs that may be eventually given to an infected patient. For example, ouabain and amiloride inhibit membrane-associated proton pumps. Lipophilic, weak bases are membrane permeant when uncharged at neutral pH and able to permeate only poorly once protonated. Thus, these agents are trapped and accumulate within acidified vesicles, such as lysosomes. These "lysosomotropic" agents, such as chloroquine, amantadine, etc., elevate the pH within acidic vesicles of living cells by neutralizing protons.[24] Carboxylic ionophores, such as monensin, intercalate into membranes and facilitate exchange of monovalent cations through the membrane. Given the high concentration of K+ in the cytosol, these cations are exchanged for protons, thereby effecting a rise in vacuolar pH. Such alterations may influence the intracellular activity of antibiotics. This was particularly evident in experiments with *Rickettsia*, which normally reside in highly acidic vacuoles. The antibacterial activity of doxycycline was definitely increased when the vacuolar pH was elevated by chloroquine and amantadine.[24]

In conclusion, some antimicrobials may not exhibit equal activity within host cells and *in vitro*. For example, much higher intracellular concentrations of macrolides *in vivo* than *in vitro* are required to inhibit bacterial multiplication.[10]

On the other hand, one should keep in mind that antibiotics exert effects on bacteria even at subinhibitory concentrations, for example, on the architecture of their cell wall.[25] This might not be relevant *in vitro* but will render the pathogen more prone to antimicrobial processes of the host cell, such as intracellular digestion. On the other hand, antibiotics may suppress the production of virulence factors[26] so that intracellular proliferation may be hampered.

The vulnerability of a pathogenic microorganism may be altered during its intracellular life cycle. For example, the multiplication rate of *Listeria monocytogenes* within a permissive host cell is less than half of that seen *in vitro* in Mueller–Hinton broth.[27] Therefore, these bacteria are presumably less susceptible to antimicrobial agents, in particular to β-lactams. Those bacteria that can multiply within the cytosol, such as listeria and shigella, are wrapped by a thick sheet of host-derived actin polymer fibrils,[27] presumably either impermeable for antibiotics or difficult to penetrate. Other microorganisms, such as small-colony variants of *Staphylococcus aureus*[28] sequestered within protected sites of certain host cells, rest in a dormant stage and hence are refractory to antibiotic therapy.

5.2. "Endogenous" Antibiotics

In this context one should also mention the role of "endogenous" antibiotics. In the various compartments of host cells, a microorganism encounters specific innate antimicrobial oligopeptides and proteins including defensins, protegrines, BPI-protein, and others in the lysosomes,[29] or histones,[30] calprotectin,[31] and still others[29] in the cytoplasm.[29] Only those pathogens with inherited peptide-resistance genes are able to successfully colonize host tissues that are rich in antimicrobial peptides.[32] These endogenous antibiotics, together with other oxidative and nonoxidative defense mechanisms,[28] contribute to the final therapeutic efficacy of external antibiotics.

6. CONSEQUENCES OF INTRACELLULAR ACCUMULATION FOR THE HOST CELLS

An ideal antibiotic exhibits exclusively antimicrobial activity without affecting the host. Unfortunately, such a perfect drug does not yet exist. Indeed, several functions of host cells have been found to be influenced by antibiotics, in particular by those drugs that are accumulated intracellularly. Heavy storage of aminoglycosides in the lysosomes of host cells, in particular in the tubular cells of the renal cortex or the hair cells of the inner ear, will inevitably damage these organelles, leading to nephrotoxicity and ototoxicity.[4] Other effects, as on leukocytes, that is, locomotion, phagocytosis, intracellular digestion, cytokine production, etc. are more discrete.[33]

Whereas some of these effects may help to overcome an infection, others damage the host's defenses. Thus, it is difficult to give a final answer as to whether these pleiotropic effects of an antibiotic are deleterious or beneficial. At present, the available data do not yet allow any recommendations for improved use of antibiotics in clinical practice. Obviously, the impact of these consequences on antimicrobial defense is still under debate.

7. ROLE OF ANTIBIOTICS FOR TREATMENT OF INFECTIONS WITH INTRACELLULAR MICROORGANISMS

Some intracellular microorganisms are pathogenic only in immunocompromised hosts, which implies that external support by antibiotic treatment is essential because the body's own defense mechanisms are insufficient. But intracellular pathogens are in protected niches; only a small number of the large list of antibiotics available for clinical use are able to reach the intracellular sites (Table III), so primarily those drugs should be used for therapy.

It should be kept in mind, however, that in many infections with faculatively intracellular bacteria, as in tuberculosis and in listeriosis patients,[21] a considerable number of the bacteria are extracellular during particular stages of their life cycles and are thus freely accessible to antibiotics! Consequently, in practice, many antibiotics are efficient in the therapy of infections with so-called intracellular microorganisms, even those that do not penetrate into host cells.

Intracellularly stored antibiotics contribute still in another way to the killing of extracellular bacteria, insofar that a granulocyte packed with antibiotics will serve as a vehicle and discharge its contents only when it has gained access to its target, that is, a focus of inflammation[18] so elevated drug concentrations are achieved at the right point. On the other hand, for complete eradication of pathogens, one has to eliminate in any case those microorganisms that have retreated into intracellular niches, because otherwise a relapse may occur after cessation of antibiotic therapy. This goal can be achieved only by using intra-cellularly active antibiotics.

REFERENCES

1. Schentag, J. J., 1991, Correlation of pharmacokinetic parameters to efficacy of antibiotics: Rela-tionships between serum concentrations, MIC values, and bacterial eradication in patients with gram-negative pneumonia, *Scand. J. Infect. Dis.* (Suppl) **74:**218–234.
2. Hof, H., 1996, Management of listeriosis, in: *Intracellular Bacterial Infections* (J.-C. Pechére, ed.), Cambridge Medical Publications, Worthing, England, pp. 137–144.
3. Schlüter, D., Chahoud, S., Lassmann, H., Schumann, A., Hof, H., and Deckert-Schlüter, M., 1996, Intracerebral targets and immunomodulation of murine *Listeria monocytogenes* meningoen-cephalitis, *J. Neuropathol. Exp. Neurol.* **55:**14–24.
4. Tulkens, P. M., 1990, The intracellular pharmacokinetics and activity of antibiotics, in: *Frontiers of Infectious Diseases: New Antibacterial Strategies* (H. C. Neu, ed.), Churchill Livingstone, Edinburgh, pp. 243–261.
5. Acocella, G., Carlone, N. A., Cuffini, A. M., and Cavallo, G., 1985, The penetration of rifam-picin, pyrazinamide, and pyrazinoic acid into mouse macrophages, *Am. Rev. Respir. Dis.* **132:**1268–1273.
6. Braga, P. C., Dal Sasso, M., Maci, S., Bondiolotti, G., Fonti, E., and Reggio, S., 1996, Penetra-tion of brodimoprim into human neutrophils and intracellular activity, *Antimicrob. Agents Chemother.* **40:**2392–2398.
7. Muranushi, N., Horie, K., Masuda, K., and Hirano, K., 1994, Characteristics of ceftibuten uptake into Caco-2 cells, *Pharmaceut. Res.* **11:**1761–1765.
8. Hand, W. L., and Hand, D. L., 1995, Influence of pentoxifylline and its derivative on antibiotic uptake and superoxide generation by human phagocytic cells, *Antimicrob. Agents Chemother.* **39:**1574–1579.
9. Laufen, H., and Wildfeuer, A., 1989, Kinetics of uptake of antimicrobial agents by human polymorphonuclear leucocytes, *Drug Res.* **39:**233–235.
10. McDonald, P. J., and Pruul, H., 1991, Phagocyte uptake and transport of azithromycin, *Eur. J. Clin. Microbiol. Infect. Dis.* **10:**828–833.
11. Mtairag, E. M., Abdelghaffar, H., Douhet, C., and Labro, M. T., 1995, Role of extracellular calcium in *in vitro* uptake and intraphagocytic location of macrolides, *Antimicrob. Agents Chemother.* **39:**1676–1682.
12. Mellman, I., Fuchs, R., and Helenius, A., 1986, Acidification of the endocytic and exocytic pathways, *Annu. Rev. Biochem.* **55:**663–700.
13. Brajtburg, J., and Bolard, J., 1996, Carrier effects on biological activity of amphotericin B, *Clin. Microbiol. Rev.* **9:**512–531.
14. Majumdar, S., and Basu, S. K., 1991, Killing of intracellular *Mycobacterium tuberculosis* by receptor-mediated drug delivery, *Antimicrob. Agents Chemother.* **35:**135–140.
15. Nègre, E., Chance, M. L., Hanboula, S. Y., Monsigny, M., Roche, A.-C., Mayer, R. M., and Hommel, M., 1992, Antileishmanial drug targeting through glycosylated polymers specifically internalized by macrophage membrane lectins, *Antimicrob. Agents Chemother.* **36:**2228–2232.

16. Bakker-Woudenberg, I. A. J. M, Lokerse, A. F., ten Kate, M. T., Melissen, P. M. B., van Vianen, W., and van Etten, E. W. M., 1993, Liposomes as carriers of antimicrobial agents or immunomodulatory agents in the treatment of infections, *Eur. J. Clin. Microbiol. Infect. Dis.* **12** (Suppl. 1):61–67.

17. Kreuter, J., 1991, Liposomes and nanoparticles as vehicles for antibiotics, *Infection* **19** (Suppl. 4):224–228.

18. Wildfeuer, A., Laufen, H., and Zimmermann, T., 1996, Uptake of azithromycin by various cells and its intracellular activity under *in vivo* conditions, *Antimicrob. Agents Chemother.* **40:**75–79.

19. Schentag, J. J., Jusko, W. J., Plaut, M. E., Cumbo, T. J., Vance, J. W., and Abrutyn, E., 1977, Tissue persistence of gentamicin in man, *JAMA* **238:**327–329.

20. Gottesman, M. M., and Pastan, I., 1993, Biochemistry of multidrug resistance mediated by the multidrug transporter, *Annu. Rev. Biochem.* **62:**385–427.

21. Hof, H., Nichterlein, T., and Kretschmar, M., 1997, Management of listeriosis, *Clin. Microbiol. Rev.* **10:**345–357.

22. Gollapudi, S., Thadepalli, F., Kim, C. H., and Gupta, S., 1995, Difloxacin reverses multidrug resistance in HL-60/AR cells that overexpress the multidrug resistance-related protein (MRP) gene, *Oncol. Res.* **7:**213–225.

23. Hof, H., 1991, Intracellular microorganisms: A particular problem for chemotherapy, *Infection* **19** (Suppl. 4):193–194.

24. Raoult, D., Drancourt, M., and Vestris G., 1990, Bactericidal effect of doxycycline associated with lysosomotropic agents on *Coxiella burnetii* in P 388D₁ cells, *Antimicrob. Agents Chemother.* **34:**1512–1514.

25. Lorian, V., and Gemmel, C. G., 1991, Effect of low antibiotic concentrations on bacteria: Effects on ultrastructure, virulence, and susceptibility to immunodefenses, in: *Antibiotics in Laboratory Medicine* (V. Lorian, ed.) Williams & Wilkins, London, pp. 493–555.

26. Nichterlein, T., Domann, E., Kretschmar, M., Bauer, M., Hlawatsch, A., Hof, H., and Chakraborty, T., 1996, Subinhibitory concentrations of β-lactams and other cell-wall antibiotics inhibit listeriolysin production by *Listeria monocytogenes*, *Int. J. Antimicrob. Agents* **7:**75–81.

27. Sheehan, B., Kocks, C., Dramsi, S., Gouin, E., Klarsfeld, A. D., Mengaud, J., and Cossart, P., 1994, Molecular and genetic determinants of the *Listeria monocytogenes* infectious process, *Curr. Top. Microbiol. Immunol.* **192:**187–216.

28. Balwit, J. M., van Langevelde, P., Vann, J. M., and Proctor, R. A., 1994, Gentamicin-resistant menadione and hemin auxotrophic *Staphylococcus aureus* persist within cultured endothelial cells, *J. Infect. Dis.* **170:**1033–1037.

29. Hirsch, J. G., 1958, Bactericidal action of histone, *J. Exp. Med.* **108:**925–944.

30. Sohnle, P. G., Collins-Lech, C., and Wiesner, J. H., 1990, Antimicrobial activity of an abundant calcium-binding protein in the cytoplasm of human neutrophils, *J. Infect. Dis.* **163:**187–192.

31. Elsbach, P., and Weiss, J., 1988, Phagocytic cells: oxygen-independent antimicrobial systems, in: *Inflammation: Basic Principles and Clinical Correlates* (J. I. Gallin, I. M. Goldstein, and R. Snyderman, eds.) Raven Press, New York, pp. 445–470.

32. Groisman, E. A., 1994, How bacteria resist killing by host-defense peptides, *Trends Microbiol.* **2:**444–449.

33. Labro, M. T., and El Benna, J., 1992, Effects of anti-infectious agents on polymorphonuclear neutrophils, *Eur. J. Clin. Microbiol. Infect. Dis.* **10:**124–131.

Index

Acanthamoeba, 132
Acid fast bacilli, 120–121
Acid tolerance response, 265
Acinetobacter calcoaceticus, 215
Acta protein, 170
Adhesins, 2
Adrenal steroids, 55–56
Adrenocorticotropic hormone, 64
Adressin, 8
Adult-onset asthma, 233, 239
Aerogenic shedding, 124
AIDS, 20, 39–40, 76, 86–87, 93, 108, 185,
    201, 203–204, 207, 217
Alcoholism, 208–209
Allopurinol riboside, 285
Amantadine, 290
Amikacin, 287
Amiloride, 289
Amino acid sequence identity, 23
Aminoglycosides, 284, 286–288, 291
Amphotericin B, 285
Ampicillin, 287
Anaerobic baccilus, 37
Angiomatosis, 202–205, 209
Antibiotic treatment
    consequences to host cells, 291
    duration of exposure, 288
    effect on virulence factors, 290
    efficiency of, 286–291
    infections with intracellular microorgan-
        isms, 291–292
    intracellular accumulation, 286–288
    intracellular activity, 289–291
        endogenous antibiotics, 290
        exogenous antibiotics, 289

Antibiotic treatment (cont.)
    intracellular distribution, 288–289
    overview of, 281–282
    prerequisites, 285
    subcellular settings, 283
    transport across host cell membrane,
        283–286
        export, 286
        import, 283–286
    uptake in, 287–289
Antiglucocorticoid, 60–63, 66
Antioxidants, 261
Apoptosis, 2, 58, 64
Apoptotic death, 179
Artificial immunization, 224–225
Atherosclerosis, 233, 239
ATP-binding casette transporters, 286
Atrophy, 67–68
Autoimmunity, 56
Azalides, 284, 288
Azithromycin, 217, 237, 286–288

B lymphocytes, 176–177, 222
Baccilus Calmette Guerin susceptible phe-
    notype, 22, 39, 121
Backcross progeny, 22, 25, 31
Bacteremia, 19, 207–208
Bacterial infection
    antigens, 13
    genetic factors, 6–7, 13–14, 94
    host interactions, 1–3, 7
    immune response to, 7–15
        role of cytokines, 3–4, 10, 13
        role of T cells, 7–13
    immunopathological reactions, 95–99